a t l a s   o f

gynecologic Pathology

2 n d   e d i t i o n

a t l a s   o f

Gynecologic Pathology

2 n d   e d i t i o n

J. Donald Woodruff, M.D.

Richard W. TeLinde Professor Emeritus of Gynecologic Pathology
Professor Emeritus of Gynecology & Obstetrics
Johns Hopkins University School of Medicine
Baltimore, Maryland

Teresita L. Angtuaco, M.D.

Associate Professor of Radiology
Assistant Professor of Obstetrics & Gynecology
University of Arkansas for Medical Sciences
Little Rock, Arkansas

Tim H. Parmley, M.D.

Professor of Obstetrics & Gynecology
Professor of Pathology
University of Arkansas for Medical Sciences
Little Rock, Arkansas

Foreword by Robert J. Kurman, M.D.

Richard W. TeLinde Professor of Gynecologic Pathology
Director, Gynecologic Pathology
Johns Hopkins University School of Medicine
Baltimore, Maryland

Raven Press

New York

Distributed in the **USA** and **CANADA** by:

Raven Press
1185 Avenue of the Americas
New York, NY 10036
USA

Library of Congress Cataloging-in-Publication Data

Woodruff, J. Donald (James Donald), 1912–
    Atlas of gynecologic pathology / J. Donald Woodruff, Teresita L.
Angtuaco, Tim H. Parmley ; foreword by Robert J. Kurman. — 2nd ed.
       p.   cm.
    Includes bibliographical references and index.
    ISBN 0-7817-0056-6 (hard cover) :
    1. Pathology, Gynecological—Atlases.   2. Generative organs,
Female—Histopathology—Atlases.   I. Angtuaco, Teresita L., 1949–
.   II. Parmley, Tim H., 1940–   .   III. Title.
    [DNLM: 1. Genital Diseases, Female—pathology—atlases.
2. Pregnancy Complications—pathology—atlases.   WP 17 W893a]
RG79.W66   1993
618.1'07—dc20
DNLM/DLC
for Library of Congress   92-49463
                                                                  CIP

British Library Cataloguing-in-Publication Data

A catalogue record for this book is available from the British Library.

Editors: Susan Suna, Demetrius McDowell, Tim Condon

Illustration supervisor: Carol Kalafatic

Illustrators: Patricia Gast, Kimberly Connors

Designer: Surachara Wirojratana

Printed in Hong Kong by Imago

10   9   8   7   6   5   4   3   2   1

dedication

The second edition of this book
is dedicated not only to those
who look through microscopes
because they like the colors, but
also to those who appreciate
black and white.

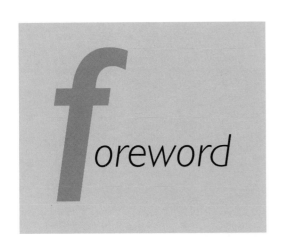

foreword

The second edition of *Atlas of Gynecologic Pathology* has been expanded with the addition of a significant amount of new illustrative material. Many of the new illustrations are radiologic, further enhancing this already superb book.

A knowledge of gynecologic pathology is fundamental to the discipline of obstetrics and gynecology. This is as true today as it was at the turn of the century, when the subspecialty of gynecologic pathology was born. Accordingly, gynecologic pathology has been and continues to be an integral part of the training program in gynecology and obstetrics at the Johns Hopkins University School of Medicine. Recent scientific advances in obstetrics and gynecology have come primarily from the field of molecular biology. In order to direct research meaningfully in this area and apply it to clinical situations, a firm understanding of the pathologic basis of gynecologic disease is essential.

This book admirably fulfills this goal through carefully correlating the clinical and operative findings with the gross and microscopic features of the disease process. The annotated drawings which accompany the photomicrographs facilitate the interpretation of this material to students with limited experience in microscopic examination. Advances in molecular biology have drawn attention to the correlation between embryologic development and the role of oncogenes and suppressor genes in normal proliferation, differentiation, and neoplasia. Accordingly, the focus on embryologic development at the beginning of each chapter is not only timely and appropriate, but also forms an integral part of the discussion of the various disease processes.

Atlas of Gynecologic Pathology is in the tradition of the giants in our specialty who fostered the clinical and pathologic approach to the study of gynecologic disease: Kelly, Cullen, TeLinde, and Novak. Drs. Woodruff, Parmley, and Angtuaco are their scientific heirs and disciples. It is a tribute to their vast breadth of knowledge and their special gifts as teachers that they have been able to present such a large amount of complex material in such a clear and concise fashion.

Robert **J. K**urman, M.D.

Preface to the first edition

The idea for this Atlas of Gynecologic Pathology came from Gower Medical Publishing. And, as any grown child knows, the quality of a book is in direct proportion to the picture–word ratio, so the idea seemed a good one. The attempt has been to present gynecologic pathology in broad terms, giving the novice a general introduction. Obviously, selection is necessary. The process of selecting is educational; it teaches that each case is unique and that typical cases are mostly typical of the initial reports of a given disease. Consequently, there are intrinsic gaps in the presented material that result from the fact that each selected photograph is unique. For this reason, a general visual scanning of the entire volume is a useful preliminary to any detailed study.

The Johns Hopkins medical community is particularly fortunate to have on its premises the photography laboratory run by Raymond Lund. Mr. Lund took the majority of photographs in this volume, and a major portion of the gratification associated with producing it came from the time spent in his facility. In his absence, this pleasant task was shared with Norman Barker. Photographs from other sources are attributed in the legends.

From the original idea to the finished product, Gower has been more than helpful. Particular gratitude is due to Mr. Abe Krieger and Ms. Joy Travalino. They have instructed, guided, and pushed. The fact that the project reached completion is a testimony to their efforts. The large amount of typing required to prepare the manuscript and associated correspondence was handled by Mrs. Susan Skierkowski and Mrs. Ethel Stern, both of whom also tolerated Tim Parmley and James Donald Woodruff.

Tim Parmley, M.D.

J. Donald Woodruff, M.D.

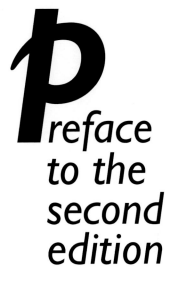

Preface to the second edition

Apparently, we are not alone in liking pictures, so the second edition of this book includes more of them. Not only have more color photographs of gross and microscopic views been included but also black and white radiologic images. We are indebted to Dr. David Bard who kindly supplied many photographs of gross specimens from his extensive collection.

For the radiologic additions we have been happily joined by Dr. T.L. Angtuaco as a co-author. Dr. Angtuaco is actively involved in all phases of the application of imaging techniques to gynecology and obstetrics. Both her professional expertise and personal enthusiasm have contributed to this effort.

Equally important to the second edition have been the people involved in its production. Mr. Abe Kreiger suggested it. Ms. Susan Suna and Mr. Demetrius McDowell edited it, and Ms. Patricia Gast did the artwork required to enhance the labelling of the radiologic images. We are most grateful.

Tim Parmley, M.D.

Contents

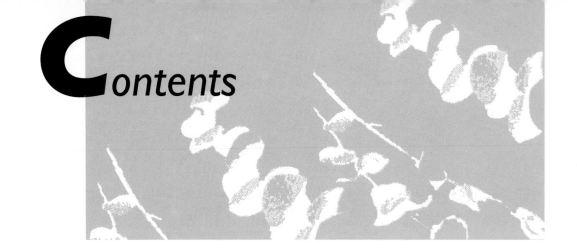

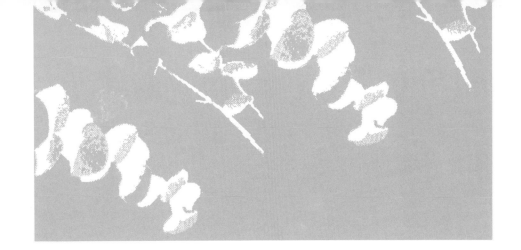

Vulva

c h a p t e r

developmental and Microscopic anatomy

The external form of the vulva is produced by condensations of subepithelial mesoderm that appear during the third and fourth weeks of embryonic life. Figure 1.1 schematically demonstrates the early development of the vulva from 3 weeks of embryonic life, when the primordia of the vulvar structures first appear alongside the anterior cloacal membrane, to 12 weeks, when the external genitalia are formed and differentiated. In the midline, anterior to the cloacal membrane, the first of these condensations results in the genital tubercle. This structure contains the primordia of the corpora cavernosa of the clitoris. Two more condensations occur as paired ridges immediately lateral to the cloacal membrane. These condensations, termed *urogenital folds*, will result in the labia minora. An additional pair of ridges, the *labioscrotal folds*, occur lateral to the urogenital folds and will become the labia majora. An additional condensation, which is more generalized than the rest, develops where the labioscrotal folds join anteriorly to the genital tubercle. This condensation will become the mons pubis. Many of these structures may be viewed histologically in Figure 1.2.

Prior to birth, additional substance and form is given to these folds by sex-steroid-induced growth. The folds develop responsiveness by birth and are enlarged in the newborn due to high levels of maternal hormone, but they regress in size as these levels drop.

The stratified squamous epithelium covering most of this structure is ectodermal in origin, and, consistent with this origin, it is keratinized and has well-developed rete ridges (Fig. 1.3). It also has the expected appendages including hair follicles (Fig. 1.4), sebaceous glands (Fig. 1.5), and sweat glands (Fig. 1.6). The underlying soft tissue of the mons and labia majora is mostly fat (Fig. 1.7). The hair follicles of the labia majora, of the mons pubis, and, in varying amounts, of adjacent abdominal, thigh, and perineal areas respond to the presence of androgens by producing thick pubic-type hair. Sebaceous glands open into these hair follicles and onto the surface of the inner labia minora, external to the vestibule (Fig. 1.8). Apocrine sweat glands are found in the labia majora along its longitudinal axis, as this is the course of the embryonic milk line (Fig. 1.9).

In contrast to the rest of the vulva, the stratified squamous epithelium that forms the mucous membrane lining the vaginal vestibule is of endodermal or urogenital sinus origin, and thus its appendages are more consistent with these types of tissues (Fig. 1.10). Embryologically and histologically similar to salivary glands, the glands of the vestibule consist of acini lined by mucinous epithelium and ducts lined by transitional cell epithelium (Fig. 1.11). Minor vestibular glands

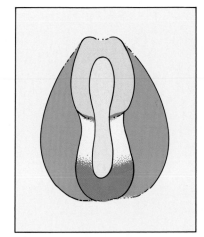

(a) 3 weeks

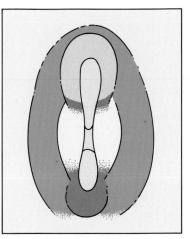

(b) 4 weeks

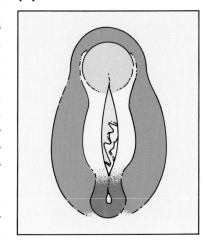

(c) 7 weeks

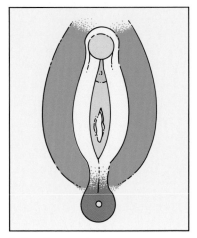

(d) 9 weeks

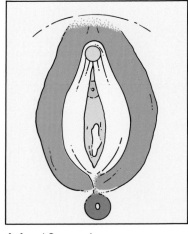

(e) 12 weeks

Genital tubercle	Glans clitoris
Urethral fold	Labia minora
Genital swelling	Labia majora
Anal tubercle	Anus
Cloacal membrane	Hymen
	Urethral meatus

figure 1.1

*Primordia of genital tubercle form on either side of anterior cloacal membrane **(a)**. Primordial tissue migrates and joins anteriorly to form the genital tubercle and develops along sides of cloacal opening to form the cloacal folds **(b)**. Urorectal septum grows to the cloacal membrane to separate urogenital membrane from anal membrane **(c)**. Cloacal membrane disappears totally and urogenital sinus opens at the exterior **(d)**. Clitoris, labia, and urethral and vaginal openings become differentiated **(e)**.*

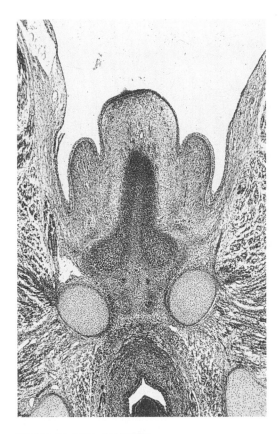

figure 1.2

In this photograph, the genital tubercle is seen protruding between the thighs. Paired labioscrotal folds occupy the angle between the tubercle and the thighs, and condensations of mesoderm destined to become the corpora cavernosa of the clitoris lie in the base and midline of the tubercle. Deep to these are the primary ossification centers of the mons pubis and behind the future pubic symphysis lies the urogenital sinus.

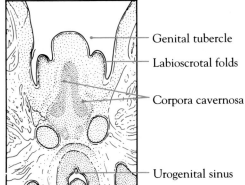

— Genital tubercle

— Labioscrotal folds

— Corpora cavernosa

— Urogenital sinus

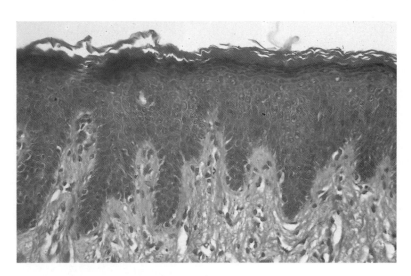

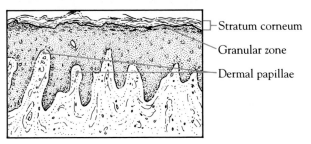

☐ Stratum corneum

— Granular zone

— Dermal papillae

figure 1.3

In this photomicrograph of normal mature vulvar epithelium, a fully developed stratum corneum lies above a granular zone. The rete ridges are well developed and interdigitate with dermal papillae.

1.3

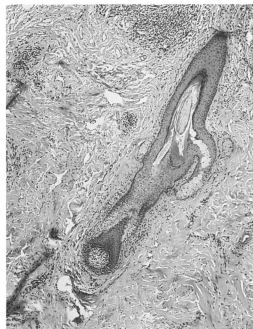

figure 1.4

This longitudinal section of a vulvar hair follicle is characteristic. There is a dermal papilla in the base of the follicle and a sebaceous gland opens into the hair shaft cavity.

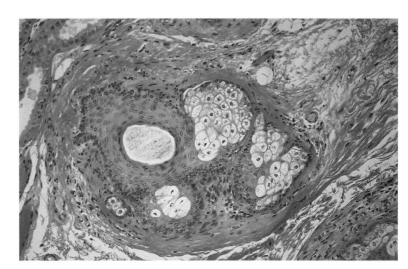

figure 1.5

Cross section multiple sebaceous glands are seen to lie embedded within the epithelium around this vulvar hair shaft. Well illustrated is the fact that both the sebaceous cells and the squamous cells are part of the same epithelium.

vulva

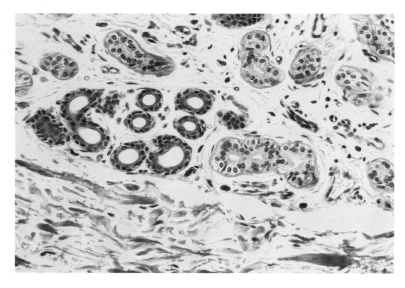

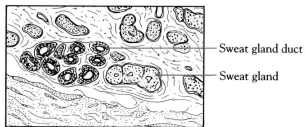

— Sweat gland duct

— Sweat gland

figure 1.6

The eccrine sweat glands seen here are lined by a layer of epithelial cells containing lightly eosinophilic cytoplasm. In contrast, the tightly coiled ducts of these glands are lined by a more eosinophilic cuboidal or flattened epithelium. Note that the surrounding dermis is denser than the island of supportive tissue that immediately invests the glands and ducts.

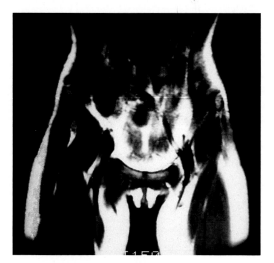

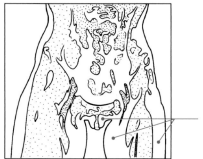

— Subcutaneous fat

figure 1.7

An MRI T1-weighted coronal view of the pelvis. An image of the anterior pelvis at the plane of the symphisis pubis shows the normal vulva. Fat within the labia and beneath the skin of the thigh gives rise to areas of high signal intensity.

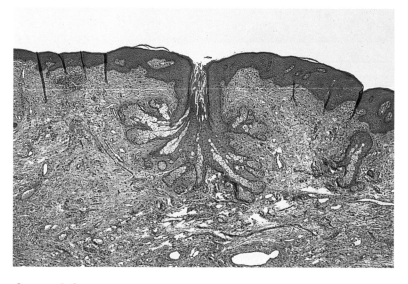

figure 1.8

A complex of sebaceous glands opens onto the skin surface of the inner labia minora. No hair follicle is present, although there is surface keratinization.

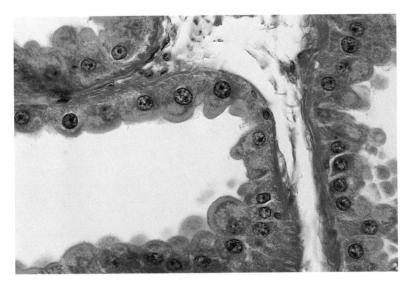

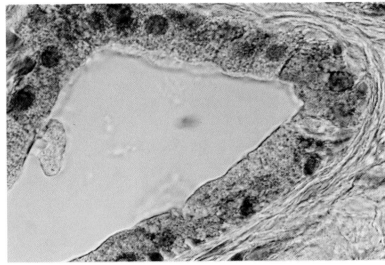

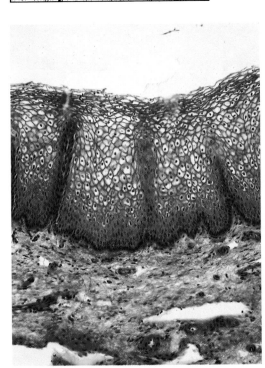

Myoepithelial cell

Secretory vacuoles

figure 1.9

These apocrine glands (left) found in the labia majora show an occasional myoepithelial cell along the basement membrane of the gland. Several of the cells show a prominent secretory vacuole developing in the cytoplasm, prior to its loss. The prominent eosinophilic cytoplasm is characteristic. This apocrine sweat gland (right) is positively stained by the immunoperoxidase technique with antibody to the antigen, CA125. (Courtesy of Dr. H. Hardardottir and Dr. T. O'Brien.)

Vestibular gland duct

Vestibular gland

figure 1.10

The stratified squamous epithelium shown here is a mucous membrane from the vestibule. Consistent with its origin note that there is no keratinization or granular zone.

figure 1.11

The acini of these vestibular glands are lined by a clear mucin-producing-type epithelium. The cells possess small dark basal nuclei that do not fill even the base of the cell. The acini open into ducts lined by darker, more cuboidal cells that comprise a transitional cell epithelium.

vulva

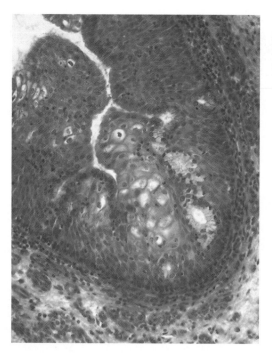

figure 1.12

These minor vestibular glands are embedded directly in the vestibular epithelium. They open directly onto its surface.

1.6

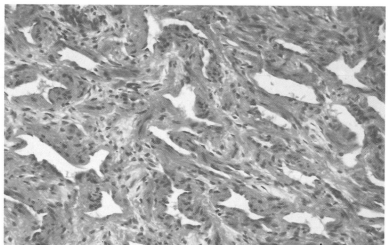

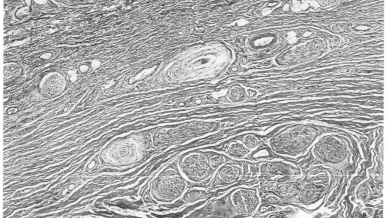

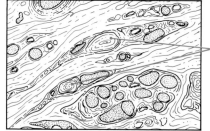

Pacinian corpuscles

figure 1.13

Multiple collapsed vascular channels (top) are seen within the muscle-containing corpora of the clitoris. When these vascular channels become engorged, the corpora expand and produce sensation in the pacinian corpuscles as seen in the bottom illustration. The edge of one corpus (bottom) is seen below and to the right. It is surrounded by a linear layer of connective tissue and nerves. Two well-developed pacinian corpuscles are present.

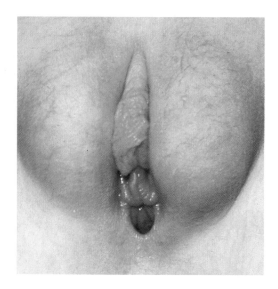

figure 1.14

This photograph of a vulvar developmental anomaly shows the genitalia of a female, but the labia contain testes.

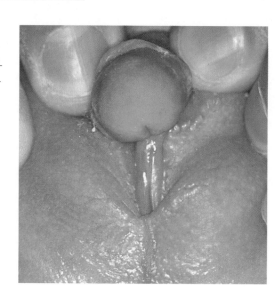

figure 1.15

In this patient with masculinized external genitalia, not only is the clitoris enlarged, but labioscrotal fusion has partially developed as well.

atlas of gynecologic pathology

open directly onto the surface, and those that do not open directly possess short ducts (Fig. 1.12). The major vestibular glands, or *Bartholin's* glands, open onto the surface of the vestibule through a long duct.

The underlying dermis of the vulva is arranged in papillary ridges that lie between the rete of the epidermis. Below this is a looser more reticular layer that contains epidermal appendages, lymphatics, and vasculature. Even lower is a denser layer containing much fat. Specific erectile tissue is found occasionally in the labia minora and routinely in the corpora cavernosa of the clitoris. The corpora are surrounded by a sheath of connective tissue containing many nerves and pressure-sensitive nerve endings, or pacinian corpuscles (Fig. 1.13).

developmental anomalies

Vulvar developmental anomalies occur in several patterns. One such pattern is the presence of normal female external genitalia in a genetic male, with testes found in the labia majora (Fig. 1.14). Similarly, varying degrees of masculinization of the external genitalia may occur, consisting of enlargement of the clitoris and/or varying degrees of posterior to anterior fusion of the labia (Fig. 1.15). Labial fusion may be simulated in small children in whom chronic irritation and denudation of the epithelium has resulted in secondary adherence of normal labia. Such cases respond readily to local estrogen therapy. Rarely, a similar process may occur in adults (Fig. 1.16). Labial fusion should be distinguished from an imperforate hymen (Fig. 1.17).

Prolapse of the urethral mucosa also responds well to local estrogen therapy. Such prolapse can result in an apparent tumor, pain, and bleeding. As for other developmental anomalies, double vulvas have been reported, though rarely, and absence of the vulva is a part of the syndrome of sirenomelia.

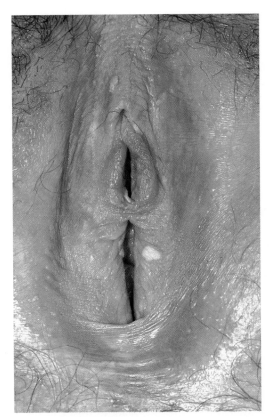

figure 1.16

Fusion of the labia minora in this adult resulted from trauma. (Courtesy of Dr. D. Bard.)

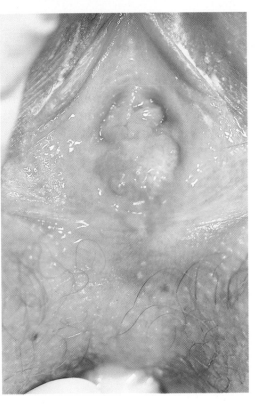

figure 1.17

The labia are widely separated in this example of an imperforate hymen. (Courtesy of Dr. D. Bard.)

Anomalous enlargement of otherwise normal labia majora may occur during pregnancy or immediately following, due to the presence of aberrant breast tissue (Fig. 1.18). This condition resembles that of vulvar edema, which may occur as the result of a pelvic malignancy (Fig. 1.19) or during pregnancy, and may be confused with the anomaly shown in Figure 1.18.

Cystic Masses and Vascular lesions

Cystic masses in the vulva may be developmental in origin or they may occur following obstruction or trauma. Developmental cysts include cysts of the canal of Nuck, which present in the labia majora. Their successful operative removal requires thorough dissection up to the external inguinal ring as well as the excision of all peritoneal remnants. Cysts arising from wolffian or müllerian duct remnants usually are paravaginal in origin, but they too may extend into the vulva (Fig. 1.20).

Nondevelopmental cysts, such as inclusion cysts, may develop in the vulva when hair follicles become obstructed, resulting in the accumulation of large quantities of sebum (Fig. 1.21). They also may develop secondary to trauma, occurring most commonly at the site of a previous episiotomy incision (Fig. 1.22). Moreover, the implantation of decidua into an episiotomy site will result in vulvar endometriosis. The presence of functioning endometrial tissue in an episiotomy incision site also may be the cause of cyclic or persistent pain in that area and of dyspareunia. In such cases, the classic blue appearance of subepithelial blood may be present or the cyst simply may look necrotic (Fig. 1.23). Vulvar endometriosis also may occur in the inguinal canal. In most of the above cases, surgical excision is usually therapeutic.

1.8

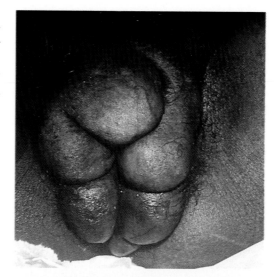

figure 1.18

Associated with postpartum breast engorgement, the labia have become nodular masses consisting of lactating breast tissue.

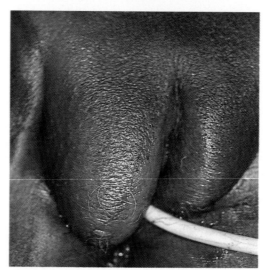

figure 1.19

In this example of vulvar edema, generalized enlargement of the labia has occurred as a result of pelvic malignancy.

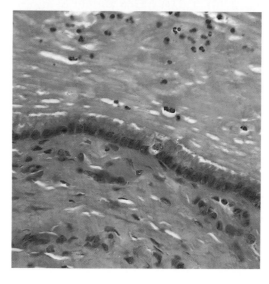

figure 1.20

This vulvar cyst is lined by a mucus-secreting-type epithelium. A single ciliated cell is seen in the center. These epithelial types suggest the müllerian duct origin of this cyst.

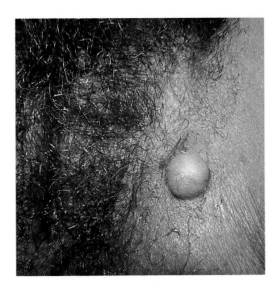

figure 1.21

A skin appendage, most likely a hair follicle, has become obstructed, resulting in the collection of a large quantity of desquamated keratinized cells and lipid.

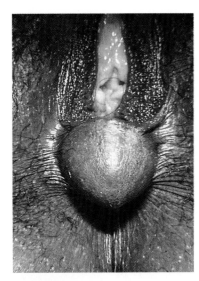

figure 1.22

The location of this inclusion cyst in the fourchette (top) suggests that it occurred secondary to a previous episiotomy repair. Normal stratified squamous epithelium (bottom) covers the surface above the cyst, but the stratified squamous epithelium that lines it is flattened due to the pressure from within.

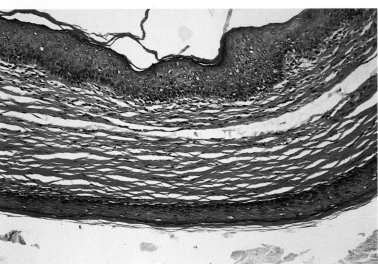

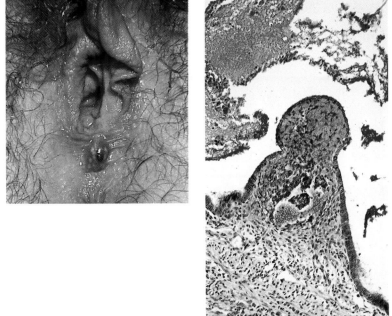

figure 1.23

This example of perineal endometriosis (left) has a yellowish edge suggesting necrosis, but the center is blue, consistent with subepithelial blood. The site is characteristic. (Courtesy of Dr. Jennifer Niebyl.) This perineal cyst (right) is lined by endometrium that is functioning. Tissue breakdown characteristic of endometrial bleeding is seen in the center, and blood fills the cyst.

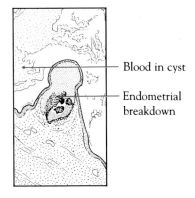

— Blood in cyst

— Endometrial breakdown

Finally, vascular lesions of the vulva will simulate cysts. Congenital hemangiomas of the vulva may resolve and should be treated expectantly (Fig. 1.24). Varicosities nearly always are found in older parous women (Fig. 1.25), and hematomas, which are sometimes confused with melanomas and vice versa, are secondary to trauma, which can be determined historically (Fig. 1.26). Unless they continue to extend, they should be managed expectantly.

Vulvar Inflammation

DERMATITIS AND FUNGAL INFECTION

The more common vulvar inflammations are those associated with some type of reactive dermatitis, either acute or chronic. In the case of an acute reaction, the presence of an inflammatory infiltrate may be the only histologic abnormality. The gross appearance is one of erythema and secondary excoriation (Fig. 1.27). The histologic picture produced by chronic dermatitis is one of blunting and hyperplasia of the rete ridges and hyperkeratosis with varying amounts of inflammation and scarring. The clinical appearance is that of thickened excoriated skin with white areas corresponding to areas of hyperkeratosis (Fig. 1.28). If this process is found in the body creases between the labia and thighs, then intertrigo secondary to maceration resulting from chronic heat and moisture may occur.

Moreover, fungal infections are commonly found in moist, warm environments, and tinea, which produces sharp bordered erythematous patches, is often seen in this area (Fig. 1.29). If the vagina and vestibule are involved, then the vulvar inflammation probably is secondary to vaginitis.

VESTIBULAR GLAND INFLAMMATION

Erythema that usually is associated with dyspareunia, pain on contact, and burning in an area confined to the vestibule often represents an inflammation of the minor vestibular glands (Fig. 1.30). This condition may be associated with punctate elevations in the vestibule that consist of the glandular orifices. Minor vestibular gland adenomas also are seen in this clinical setting.

Inflammation of Bartholin's gland usually is bacterial and is frequently associated with abscess formation in the lower wall of the vestibule (Fig. 1.31). These abscesses may become so large as to involve the entire vulva on the affected side, and a frequent sequela of these abscesses is a cyst of

1.10

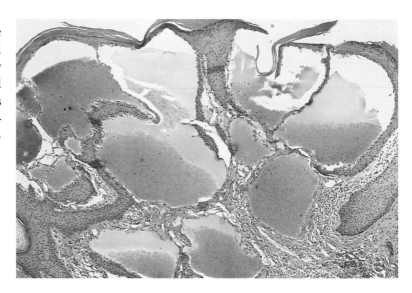

figure 1.24

This photomicrograph of a congenital vulvar hemangioma shows multiple dilated vascular channels covered by an elevated and thinned squamous epithelium. There is associated hyperkeratosis.

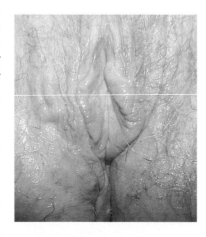

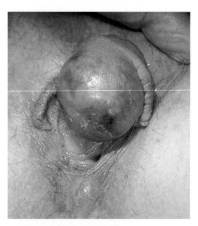

figure 1.25

As seen in this photograph, dilated varices produce tortuous patterns beneath the skin of the labia majora.

figure 1.26

This large blue mass is firm and tender. It contains blood secondary to the traumatic rupture of vessels in the soft tissue of the labia. This hematoma should be managed expectantly.

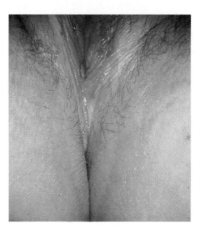

figure 1.27

Diffuse erythema with some linear markings suggestive of scratching is seen in this case of acute dermatitis. The distribution of the rash suggests the contribution of heat and moisture produced by contact when the thighs are together.

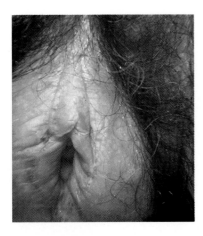

figure 1.28

In this example of chronic dermatitis, the alternating white and red patches are characteristic of varying amounts of hyperkeratosis. The apparent thickening suggests long-term changes.

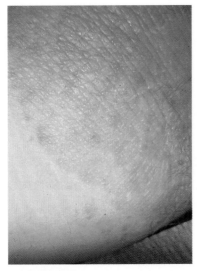

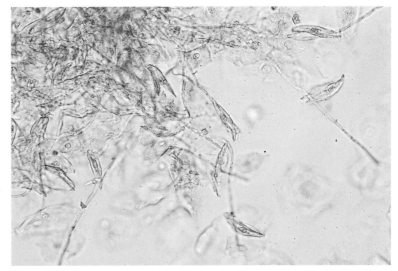

figure 1.29

This erythematous patch (left) flares out onto the thigh from the vulva. It looks as if it is extending, yet it has a sharp border. Mycelia (right) are seen in this wet preparation of skin scrapings treated with KOH, confirming the presence of a fungal infection.

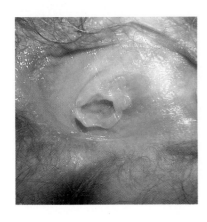

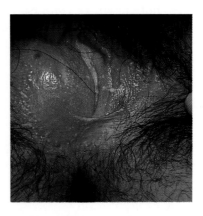

1.11

figure 1.31

This Bartholin's duct cyst occupies the characteristic site in the base of the labia minora and it extends into the vestibule and the fourchette, and laterally into the labia majora.

figure 1.30

Photograph (left) shows erythema confined to the vestibule posteriorly, just external to the hymenal ring. This is the distribution of the minor vestibular glands and of the patient's symptoms. The hymenal ring and the vagina are pink. Photomicrograph (right) shows the minor vestibular glands opening into a duct. The inflammatory infiltrate is more closely related to the duct epithelium than to that of the acini. This is characteristic of a minor vestibular gland inflammation.

Bartholin's duct or gland. Furthermore, bacterial infection of the vulva occurs nonspecifically in hair follicles or in inclusion cysts. Pyogenic granulomas also may occur. However, since such infections usually are attributed to poor hygiene, nonspecific measures such as soaks and drainage are curative (Fig. 1.32).

APOCRINE GLAND INFECTIONS

Infection of the apocrine gland system, *hidradenitis suppurativa,* is a different matter. Of unknown etiology, hidradenitis may occur in the axilla and vulva at the same time and frequently has been attributed to systemic malfunction of the apocrine gland system. The earliest lesions present as subepithelial swellings that may be firm or appear fluctuant; yet when incised, they are fleshy and do not drain well (Fig. 1.33). Extensive cases may convert the vulva into a scarred mass of intercommunicating sinuses and abscess cavities. Extensive incision and antibiotic therapy are required. Incisions should be allowed to granulate secondarily only and not closed. In contrast, Fox-Fordyce disease is a noninfectious obstruction of the apocrine gland system that results in an extremely pruritic maculopapular rash. It should be treated with oral contraceptives.

VENEREAL INFECTIONS

All of the classic venereally transmitted agents produce vulvar infections. The gonococcus is responsible for infection of Bartholin's gland. Ducrey's bacillus produces vesicles and pustules that break down, becoming ulcers. Granuloma inguinale produces ulcerative destruction of the vulva (Fig. 1.34). The chlamydial subtype responsible for lymphogranuloma venereum produces scarring, stricture and ulceration, with fenestration of the labia (Fig. 1.35). Moreover, the treponeme may be responsible for both primary and secondary vulvar manifestations, although secondary inflammations are the ones most commonly observed. Primary chancres tend to be inconspicuous in the vestibule (Fig. 1.36) and more visible on the labia (Fig. 1.37).

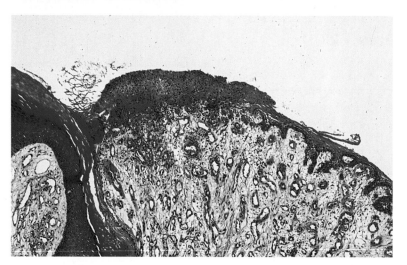

figure 1.32

A fiery-red mass (top) protrudes through the vulvar skin and is quite tender. This mass is a pyogenic granuloma. Granulation tissue (bottom) forms a mass that erodes through the overlying stratified squamous epithelium and produces an ulcerated surface covered with a fibrinopurulent exudate.

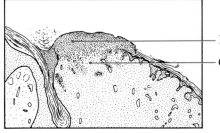

— Fibrinopurulent exudate
— Granulation

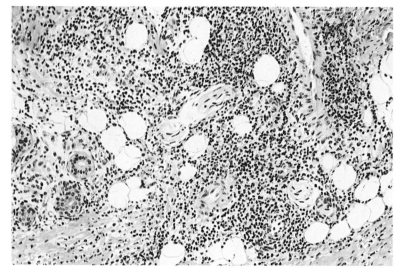

figure 1.33

A few sweat glands are as yet unaffected by this sheet of inflammation and necrosis that is infiltrating the vulvar dermis. No liquefaction is present in this example of hidradenitis suppurativa.

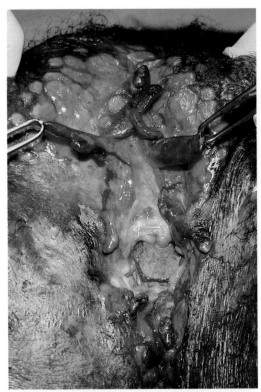

figure 1.34

Granuloma inguinale has produced extensive ulceration and destruction of the vulva. Particularly destroyed are the labia minora and the perineum. (Courtesy of Dr. D. Bard.)

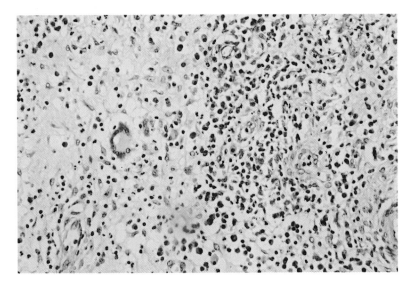

figure 1.35

This photomicrograph shows the noncaseating granulomatous reaction with occasional giant cells characteristic of lymphogranuloma venereum.

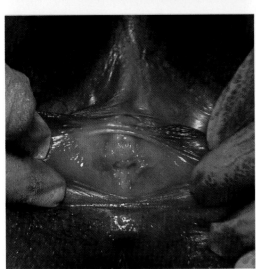

figure 1.36

Shallow red kissing ulcers are located immediately lateral to the hymenal ring. They are darkfield positive, indicative of primary treponemal infection.

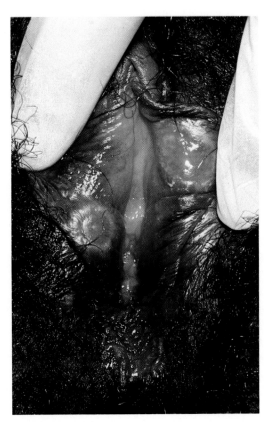

figure 1.37

These primary chancres are on the labia minora rather than in the vestibule proper and are therefore more distinguishable from the background than are those in the vestibule. (Courtesy of Dr. D. Bard.)

1.13

vulva

Amongst virally induced diseases, the most benign is molluscum. Often but not always of venereal origin, molluscum tends to occur in the intertriginous areas and on the thighs, with small punctate lesions that may be pruritic or asymptomatic (Fig. 1.38). Microscopically, intracellular inclusions that are eosinophilic in the lower epithelial layers are seen to become more basophilic in the upper layers, when the cells are cast off into the central cistern that forms the punctum of the lesion (Fig. 1.39). Molluscum is self-limited, but its cure may be hastened if the lesions are curetted.

Herpes zoster lesions occasionally occur in the vulva with the same manifestations as those seen elsewhere. Painful vesiculation erupts in the distribution of one or more nerve roots (Fig. 1.40). This is followed by secondary breakdown, scab formation, and eventual resolution. Herpes simplex lesions are less confined in distribution (Fig. 1.41). An individual who has had experience with the herpes simplex virus may be able to detect the onset of its manifestations, prior to the development of vesicles, on the basis of local tingling. In a less experienced victim, vesicles first are noticed four or more days after contact. Classically, the vesicles appear first at mucocutaneous junctions, which, in most individuals, means the inner surface of the labia minora. They may, however, occur anywhere. When the vesicles break down, they become secondarily infected and pustular, with associated swelling and pain. Therapy is supportive for all but the earliest lesions, which may benefit from acyclovir.

MISCELLANEOUS CONDITIONS

A wide variety of other disorders may result in incidental vulvar inflammation. Chicken pox in prepubertal children frequently involves both the vulva and the vagina. Crohn's disease may present as a draining sinus in the perineum. Psoriasis is of particular interest not only because it is common, but also because on the labia it may be red without the more typical silver scales (Fig. 1.42). Behçet's syndrome usually is associated with oral ulcers and iritis, as well as with vulvar ulcers. Seborrheic keratoses, which may be dramatically pigmented, must be distinguished from nevi and lentigines (Fig. 1.43). Tuberculosis and sarcoidosis also have been seen in the vulva (Fig. 1.44).

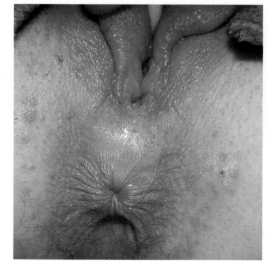

figure 1.38

To the left are typical punctate lesions; to the right, the lesions have become more inflamed. The punctate lesions are characteristic of molluscum contagiosum.

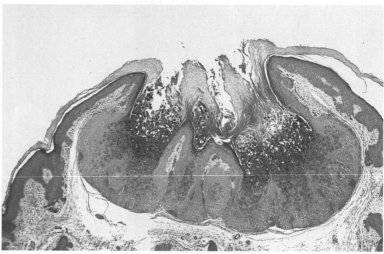

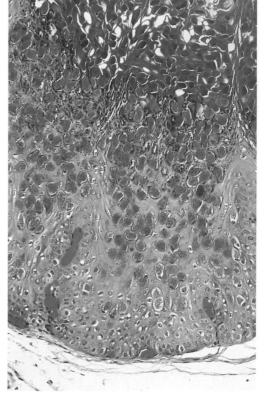

figure 1.39

The affected epithelium (top) seen in this photomicrograph of molluscum is thickened but depressed below the surface, resulting in a central cistern into which infected cells are desquamated. An eosinophilic inclusion (bottom) consisting of replicating virus is seen in the epithelial cells of the more basal layers. Near the surface, the inclusion becomes basophilic.

1.14

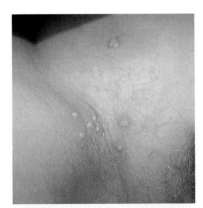

figure 1.40

In this example of herpes zoster, painful purulent vesicles are seen in the groin and on the lower abdomen in the distribution of a nerve root.

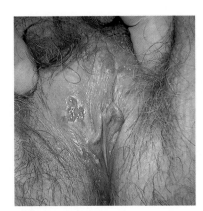

figure 1.41

In this photograph of herpes simplex, these herpetic lesions have broken down, leaving shallow ulcers. In contrast to those of herpes zoster, these lesions have no specific distribution.

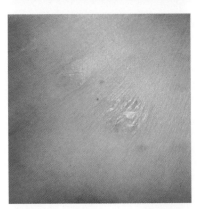 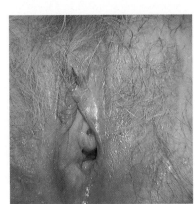

figure 1.42

A psoriatic lesion on the thigh (left) illustrates the common silver scales of this disorder. This vulvar example of psoriasis (right) may be contrasted with the lesion seen in the left-hand figure. It lacks silver scales, probably secondary to moisture.

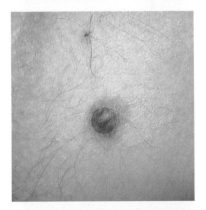 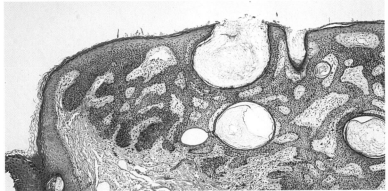

figure 1.43

Raised and pigmented, this seborrhoeic keratosis (left) can be suspected but not absolutely confirmed clinically. Seen microscopically (right), the epithelium is hyperplastic and deeply invaginated with keratin pearls. Inflammation and melanin occupy the dermis immediately beneath the lesions.

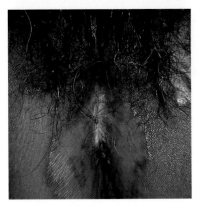 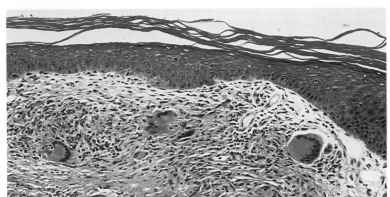

figure 1.44

Photograph of systemic sarcoidosis (left) shows changes in skin pigmentation that are characteristic of much chronic inflammation in the vulva. The whitening due to hyperkeratosis is dramatic. The noncaseating granulomas with multiple giant cells seen here (right) are found in many conditions. In this case they are consistent with the patient's systemic sarcoidosis.

Condylomata and Carcinoma In Situ

Condylomata are believed to be caused by a complex family of human papilloma viruses (HPV) divided into types based on analysis of their DNA. Designated by numbers, these types in general are associated with different manifestations.

Although the study of this subject is young and the statements made here are subject to change, in general, types 6 and 11 are believed to be responsible for the development of typical acuminate warts (Fig. 1.45). These may be single or multiple and may result in barely visible elevations of the skin or in large fungating masses (Figs. 1.46 and 1.47). They may be asymptomatic, pruritic, or painful. Microscopically, their papilliform shapes are covered with a hyperplastic squamous epithelium that not only is acanthotic, but also possesses hyperkeratosis and parakeratosis as well. Although the typical wart is not characterized by cellular atypia, mitoses may be present (Fig. 1.48). Condylomata may grow with particular rapidity during pregnancy. Extensive condylomata must be distinguished from verrucous carcinoma, a lesion with a characteristic warty form that invades locally but seldom metastasizes (Fig. 1.49). Rarely, subepithelial tumors may produce a warty external appearance (Figs. 1.50 and 1.51).

Recent interest in HPV centers around the fact that in contrast to types 6 and 11, some types of HPV do not produce typical warts but instead produce multiple flat ones that possess significant degrees of cellular atypia and appear to correspond to what previously has been diagnosed as carcinoma in situ. Clinically, these atypical warts may be reddened, hyperpigmented, or whitish, and, microscopically, they demonstrate nuclear enlargement, hyperchromatism, smudging, fragmentation, vacuolation, multinucleation and bizarre mitotic figures. Individual cells also may be dramatically koilocytotic (Fig. 1.52). Such lesions routinely are confused with carcinoma in situ and their recent recognition as a distinct entity accounts for several paradoxes of the past in which these warts were linked with the development of invasive carcinoma of the vulva. Unlike invasive carcinoma, these atypical warts are multicentric, occur primarily in young people, and occasionally regress, whereas invasive vulvar cancer is unifocal and is encountered in older women. This distinc-

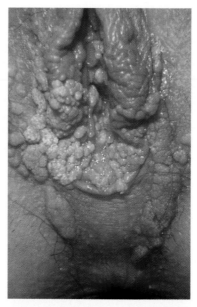

figure 1.45

These typical vulvar acuminate warts are white where moist (closer to the vaginal orifice) and brownish where dry (further away from the vaginal orifice).

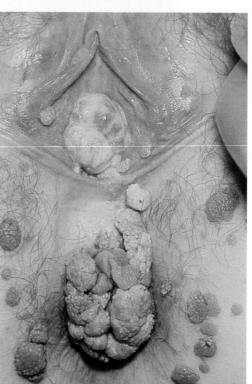

figure 1.46

These pilled-up acuminate warts are most likely to be due to HPV type 6 or 11. (Courtesy of Dr. D. Bard.)

tion is not absolute, however, because it is believed that some types of HPV produce atypical warts that do progress. Moreover, a background of condylomatous disease is characteristic of some populations of young women in whom invasive vulvar cancer is found.

The histologic demonstration of mitotic figures suggestive of aneuploidy is believed to be the hallmark of true carcinoma in situ (Fig. 1.53). Red, ulcerated, or hyperpigmented lesions and flat whitish patches are clinical characteristics of vulvar carcinoma in situ, and a biopsy should be performed on any suspicious site (Fig. 1.54). Carcinoma in situ is most likely to become invasive when seen in older individuals or in perianal sites. Local excision along with careful follow-up is the recommended therapy for any vulvar carcinoma in situ.

Vulvar Dystrophy

While carcinoma in situ is prevalent in some populations, and in some individuals may result in invasive cancer, it is not at all clear that most invasive vulvar cancer arises in such a setting. In fact, many invasive cancers appear to arise in a background of atypical hyperplastic vulvar dystrophy (Fig. 1.55). The dystrophies are poorly understood entities that have been divided on histologic grounds into lichen sclerosus and hyperplastic types. Microscopically, lichen sclerosus is characterized by loss of the rete ridges and by hyperkeratosis. There is an acellular subepithelial layer consisting of edema and collagenization, with an even deeper layer of inflammation (Fig. 1.56). Although most common in post-menopausal women, lichen sclerosus may occur in young women or even prepubertal girls (Fig. 1.57). Hyperplastic dystrophy, on the other hand, is characterized by epithelial hyperplasia with blunting and acanthosis of the rete ridges (Fig. 1.58). In contrast to the stratification seen in lichen sclerosus, subepithelial edema, scarring, and inflammation of hyperplastic vulvar dystrophy are not organized in discrete layers. Because these types frequently are mixed, however, this histologic distinction may not represent biologic reality. Lichen sclerosus presents with a parchment-like thinning of the skin and with subepithelial hemorrhage (Fig. 1.59). In some cases, hyper-

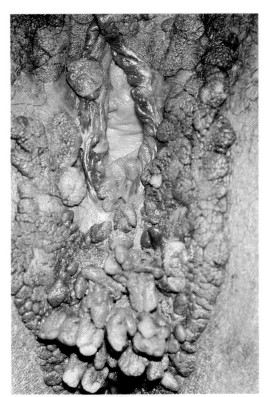

figure 1.47

These condylomata consist of both flattened and acuminate types. In addition, they are highly pigmented. Both flattening and hyperpigmentation are sometimes associated with cellular atypicality, although this is certainly not constant. (Courtesy of Dr. D. Bard.)

1.17

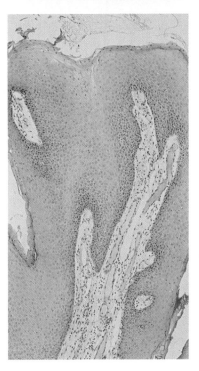
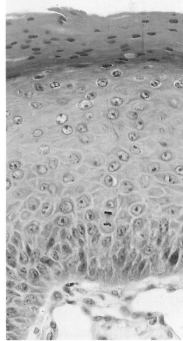

figure 1.48

The papillomatous structure of this vulvar condyloma (left) is apparent in this photomicrograph. Parakeratosis (right) is present, but there is no cytologic atypia. A single small mitotic figure is seen.

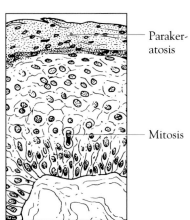

Parakeratosis

Mitosis

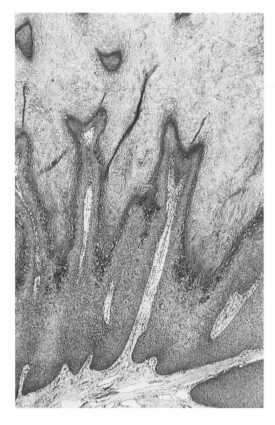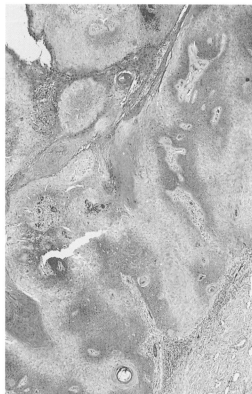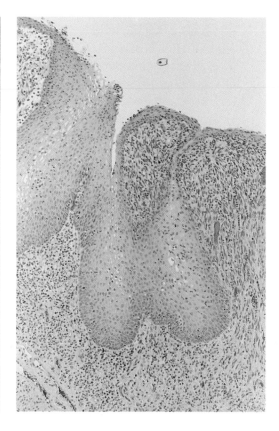

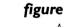

figure 1.49

Acanthotic rete pegs (left), which are seen to extend deep into the underlying tissue, characterize this verrucous carcinoma. Papillomatosis and hyperkeratosis are extreme. However, there is no destruction of the underlying tissue and, at this site, no infiltration. This verrucous carcinoma (right) is infiltrating, but all of the tumor is still contiguous with the surface mass.

figure 1.50

Both grossly and microscopically, this vulvar sarcoma with a growth pattern like that of sarcoma botryoides was initially mistaken for condylomata acuminata.

figure 1.51

A high power view of the underlying stromal neoplasm shows obvious atypicality.

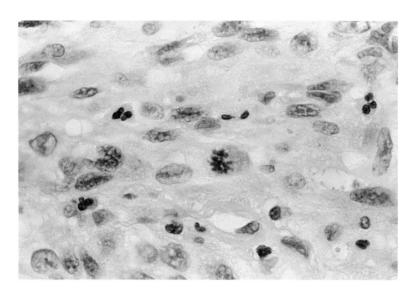

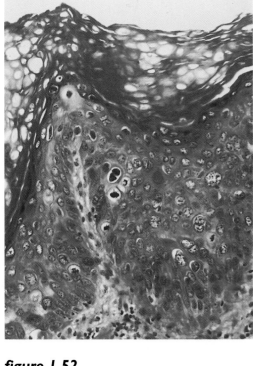
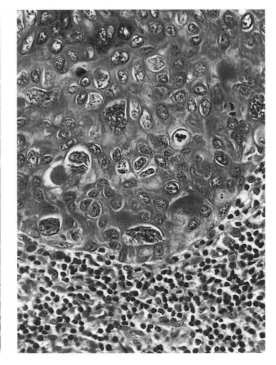
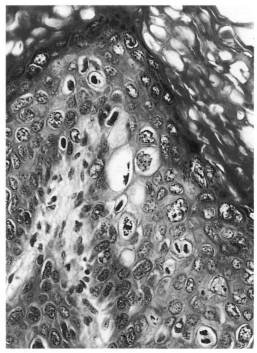

figure 1.52

Photomicrograph (left) shows that this atypical wart has significant cytologic abnormality, although the histology of the condyloma is still present. High-power view (center) shows that the nuclei are hyperchromatic, and smudged or fragmented. Some nuclei are vacuolated and some are multiple. Individual cell keratinization is present. These degenerative changes are induced by the virus. In addition to these nuclear abnormalities, koilocytosis (right) is well illustrated.

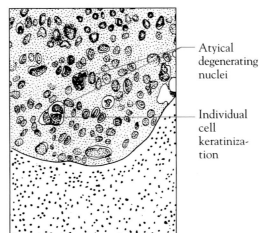

Atyical degenerating nuclei

Individual cell keratinization

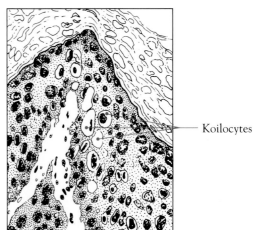

Koilocytes

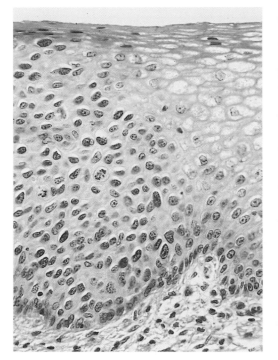
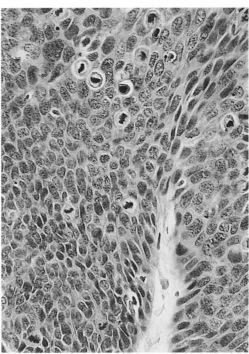

figure 1.53

In this photomicrograph of carcinoma in situ (left) the right-hand side of the field shows a normal stratified squamous epithelium. On the left-hand side the epithelium is characterized by a loss of normal cytoplasmic maturation and by cells with enlarged atypical nuclei. However, the degenerative features seen in the previous three figures are not seen here. In another example of carcinoma in situ (right), multiple atypical mitotic figures as well as atypical nuclei without degenerative features are characteristic.

vulva

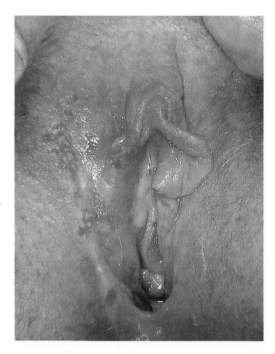 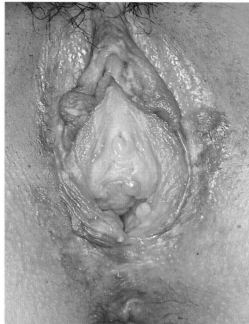 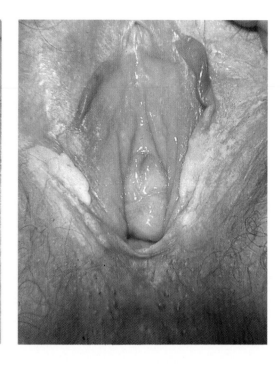

figure 1.54

Clinical characteristics of carcinoma in situ may present variously. This erythematous patch of carcinoma in situ (left) extends across the midline. It is histologically similar to Figure 1.53 (left). In the next example (center), the photomicrograph shows hyperpigmented patches located at many noncontiguous sites. In another example (right), the marked whitening of these noncontiguous patches of carcinoma in situ is due to hyperkeratosis.

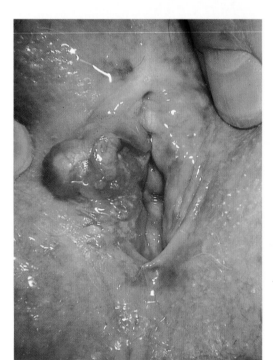 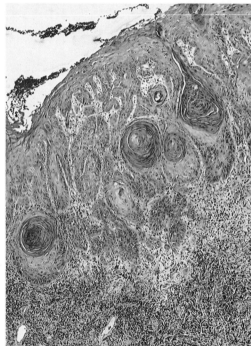 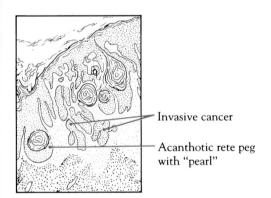

Invasive cancer

Acanthotic rete peg with "pearl"

figure 1.55

The ulcerative vulvar cancer seen here (left) is occurring in a vulva in which many of the surface structures seem inapparent due to the atrophic dystrophy. The labia and clitoris are no longer well defined. In another example (right), the far lefthand side of the field shows acanthotic rete pegs that contain prematurely keratinized pearls but there is no subepithelial infiltration. This is atypical hyperplastic dystrophy. In the right-hand side of the field, tissue infiltration by invasive cancer is occurring.

atlas of gynecologic pathology

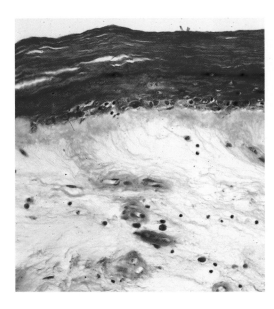

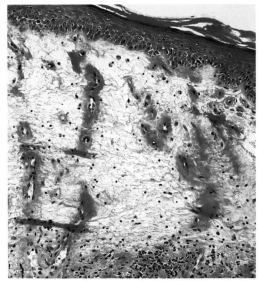

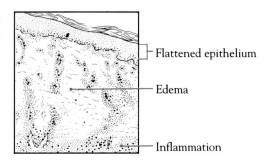

Flattened epithelium

Edema

Inflammation

figure 1.56

The epithelium in this example of lichen sclerosus (left) shows hyperkeratosis and flattening of the rete ridges. A few inflammatory cells and capillaries are scattered in the edema below. A layer of dense inflammation (right) lies below the zone of edema in this example of lichen sclerosus.

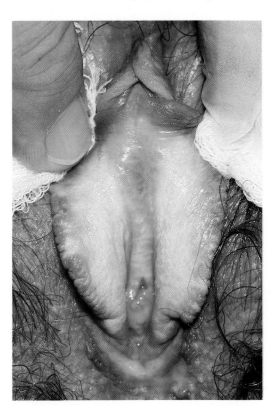

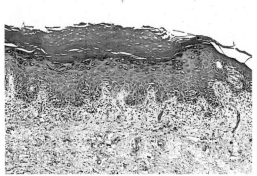

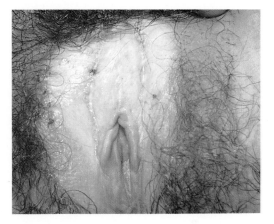

figure 1.58

Relatively normal epithelium lies to the right, but on the left it is hyperplastic and hyperkeratotic. An inflammatory infiltrate lies beneath it.

figure 1.59

This example of lichen sclerosus involves the midline above the clitoris and extends onto the labia majora. It results in occlusion of these labia and in burying of the clitoris.

figure 1.57

In this young woman, lichen sclerosis involves the inter surface of the labia minor and there is minimal involvement of the frenulum as well. (Courtesy of Dr. D. Bard.)

vulva

keratosis may produce thickened white patches. Thickening of the skin, but with the same hyperkeratosis and whitish color, is the result of hyperplastic dystrophy (Fig. 1.60).

Dystrophy often is asymptomatic, but if it is pruritic, then secondary excoriation has occurred. Atrophy and scarring may result in the obliteration of vulvar structures, occurring most dramatically in the midline. The clitoris may become covered and the fourchette narrowed due to stricturing, and secondary laceration of the outlet may occur (Fig. 1.61). Rarely occurring in prepubertal or premenopausal women, most dystrophy is found in postmenopausal women.

INVASIVE SQUAMOUS CELL CANCER

Although the dystrophies, to some minor degree, are almost ubiquitous in postmenopausal women, vulvar cancer is rare. Therefore, the dystrophies cannot be considered premalignant. However, some examples of hyperplastic vulvar dystrophy are associated with pearl formation deep in the acanthotic rete pegs (Fig. 1.62). These examples of atypical hyperplastic vulvar dystrophy do seem to provide the background from which many squamous cell cancers of the vulva arise. In fact the earliest examples of invasive vulvar cancer appear to be those in which the hypermature populations of cells in the tips of the rete pegs have protruded through the basal-cell layers into the underlying stroma (Fig. 1.63). A microinvasive stage of vulvar cancer is not well defined.

Invasive vulvar cancer is a rare disease that is found most often in the seventh and eighth decades of life. It may be exophytic (Fig. 1.64), or it may be endophytic (see Fig. 1.55), metastasizing first to the superficial and deep inguinal lymph nodes and then extending to the pelvic nodes. Histologically, it may be poorly or well differentiated, with most cases illustrating squamous cell maturation with keratin pearls. However, the spectrum of histologies is wide (Fig. 1.65). Treatment of invasive vulvar cancer is surgical with rad-

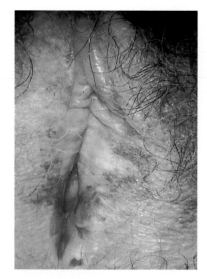

figure 1.60

In this case of hyperplastic dystrophy, the skin is whitened but has a thick appearance. Excoriation is prominent and the fourchette is becoming strictured.

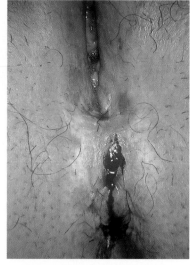

figure 1.61

This perineal tear has occurred as the result of attempts to have intercourse. The fourchette is dramatically strictured by lichen sclerosus.

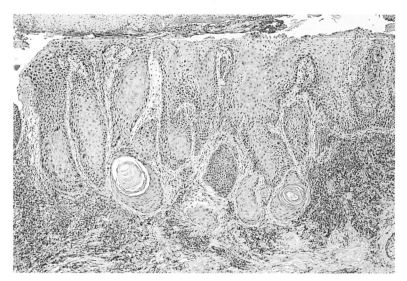

figure 1.62

In this example of hyperplastic vulvar dystrophy, the epithelium is hyperplastic and deeply acanthotic. Two of the acanthotic rete pegs contain well-developed keratin pearls.

1.22

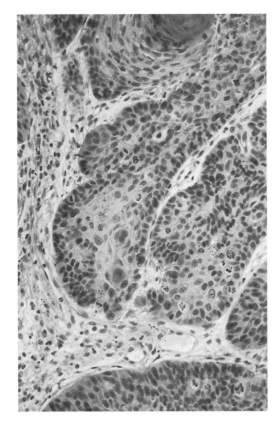

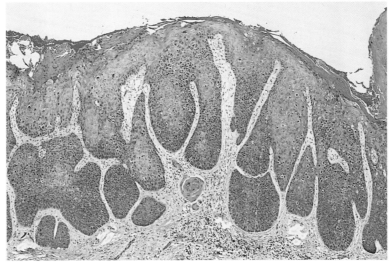

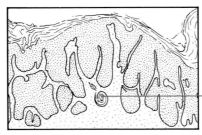

Probable early invasion

figure 1.63

This example of hyperplastic dystrophy (left) shows a few hypermature cells that seem to have broken through the epithelial basement membrane and appear to be invading the stroma. In this photomicrograph (right), most of the epithelium is a hyperplastic dystrophy, but in the center is a focus of mature squamous epithelium that probably represents early invasive cancer.

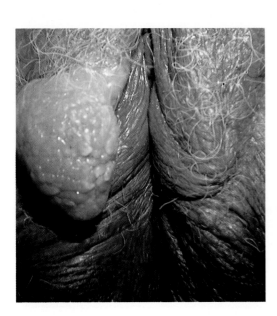

figure 1.64

This exophytic vulvar cancer is resulting in a mass that extends from the labia but little destruction of the vulva has occurred as yet. The lesion is solitary.

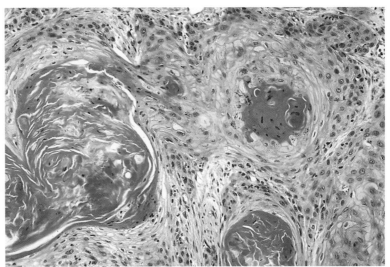

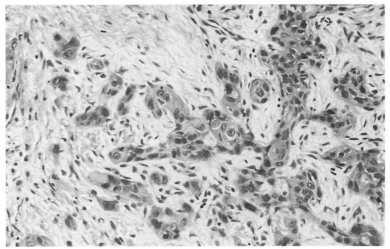

figure 1.65

The marked maturation illustrated by this keratinizing tumor (top) is typical of squamous cell cancer of the vulva. This highly undifferentiated squamous-cell cancer of the vulva (bottom) is less common than the type seen in the top figure, but it occurs consistently and pursues an aggressive course.

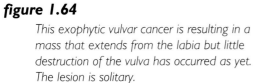

vulva

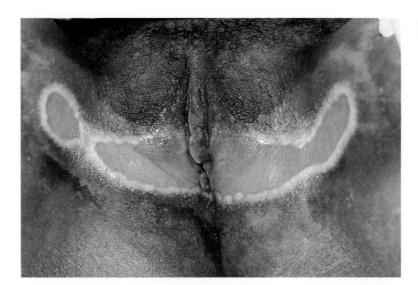

figure 1.66

These radiation burns of vulvar skin were a complication of a misplaced vaginal application of cesium. (Courtesy of Dr. D. Bard.)

1.24

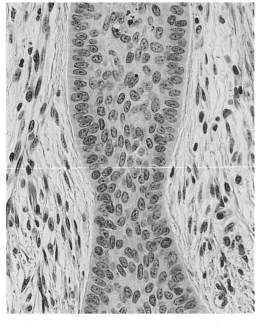

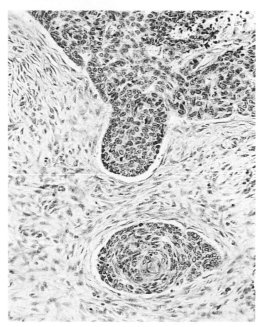

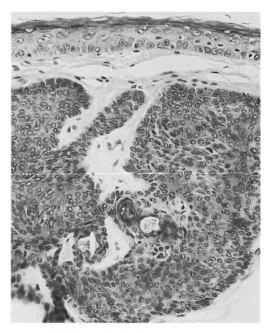

figure 1.67

A column of basal cells with well-defined palisading (left), forming a cord, extends into the soft tissue. Little destruction is apparent. In contrast, this basal-cell cancer (right) has a small focus of keratinization. However, the cells are cytologically bland.

figure 1.68

The cells in this trichoepithelioma are not very different from those seen in the basal-cell tumor, but a hair follicle is being formed in the center.

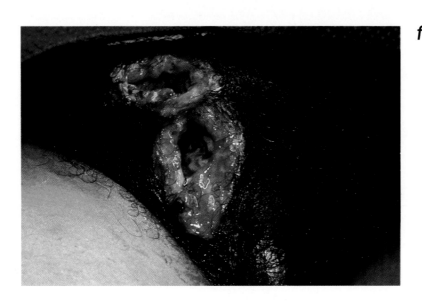

figure 1.69

This patient said she developed a "boil" that opened onto her skin and spread. (Courtesy of Dr. D. Bard.)

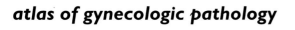

atlas of gynecologic pathology

ical removal of the vulva and groin nodes. The possible contribution of radiation therapy to the treatment of nodal disease is currently under investigation. Historically, radiation burns of the vulvar skin complicated this form of therapy (Fig. 1.66).

OTHER EPITHELIAL NEOPLASMS

Other neoplasms that arise in the surface epithelium include those producing all of the cell types of the epithelium and its appendages. Basal-cell carcinoma produces shallow ulcers with thick rolled edges. Histologically, these lesions consist of nests and cords of well-differentiated basal-type cells, with palisading at the edges of the nests (Fig. 1.67). Trichoepitheliomas, which may be nodular or ulcerated, present a histologic picture similar to that of basal-cell lesions, although they contain follicular spaces similar to hair follicles (Fig. 1.68). Furthermore, mixtures may occur (Figs. 1.69 and 1.70).

Paget's disease, in which the neoplasm reproduces cell types similar to that of the apocrine gland secretory cell, may occur in the invasive form (Fig. 1.71) or the intraepithe-

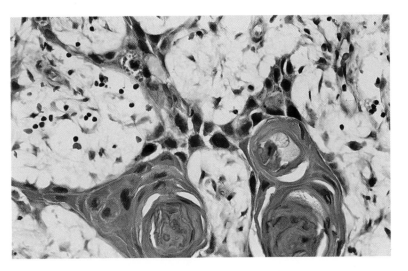

figure 1.70

Consistent with this history, the tumor had a trabecular pattern and possessed both keratin and apparent follicles.

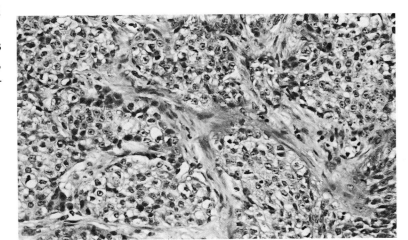

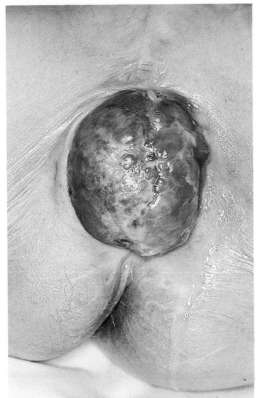

figure 1.71

A mixture of large clear apocrine-type cells along with small darker basal-type cells (top) characterizes this example of invasive Paget's disease. This large vulvar neoplasm (bottom) was histologically Paget's disease. (Courtesy of Dr. D. Bard.)

lial form (Fig. 1.72). The intraepithelial form is more common and clinically it presents as alternating white and velvety red patches in the vulvar skin (Fig. 1.73). Microscopically, the basal-cell layer is composed of collections of small dark proliferating cells interrupted by nests and acini of large clear secretory cells. The overlying squamous epithelium reveals cytologic atypia as well, and the appendages are involved by local extension. Local excision is the therapy of choice, but seldom is it totally successful as the disease extends far beyond its clinically apparent margin. Intraepithelial Paget's disease often recurs, but rarely invades the subepithelial dermis. In contrast to the intraepithelial form, invasive vulvar Paget's disease is very rare. It is a highly belligerent disease that usually is advanced at the time of diagnosis. Therapy is surgical and often not effective. The rarest histology produced by ectodermal epithelial lesions of the vulva is that characteristic of sebaceous gland cell types.

Primary tumors may arise in any of the skin appendages. Hidradenomas tend to occur between the two labia, although they may be found elsewhere (Fig. 1.74). They may or may not appear punctate, as the papillary tumor may or may not protrude through the duct orifice of the sweat gland in which it is growing (Fig. 1.75). The histology of this tumor is that of a double-cell-layered epithelium covering a complex papillary structure developing within a sweat gland. Myoepithelial cells form the irregular basal layer and both apocrine-type and eccrine-type cells form the top layer (Fig. 1.76). Simple excision is all that is required.

1.26

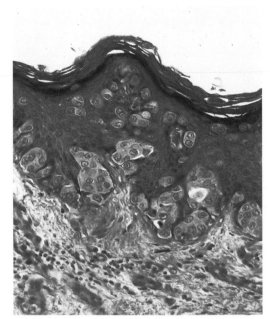

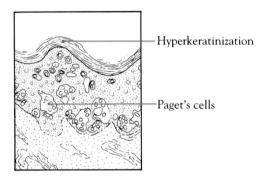

Hyperkeratinization

Paget's cells

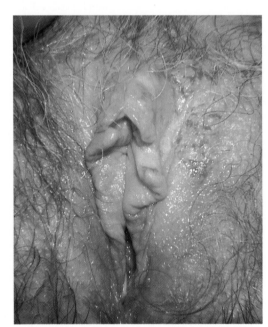

figure 1.73

White and red patches alternate in this example of intraepithelial vulvar Paget's disease. The disease appears to occupy only the upper portions of the left labia majora, extending to the midline, but microscopically it is undoubtedly more extensive than this.

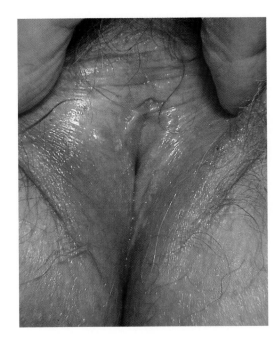

figure 1.74

This hidradenoma is a small nodule on the inner surface of the labia majora just lateral to the labia minora. This is a characteristic site.

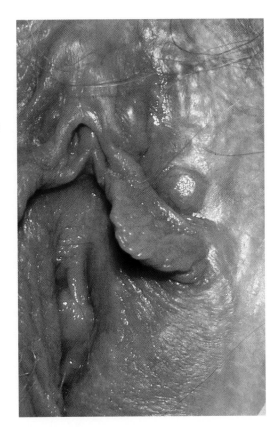

figure 1.75

Although it would take a biopsy to confirm, this is a typical punctate hydradenoma.

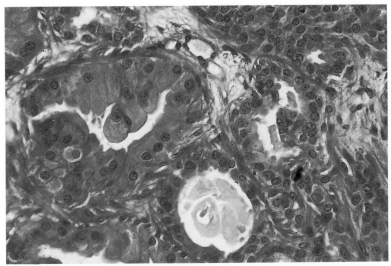

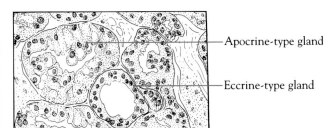

Apocrine-type gland

Eccrine-type gland

figure 1.76

The complex glandlike pattern of this hidradenoma demonstrates apocrine-type epithelium in the glands on the left and eccrine-type epithelium in those on the right. Myoepithelial cells are seen very irregularly.

vulva

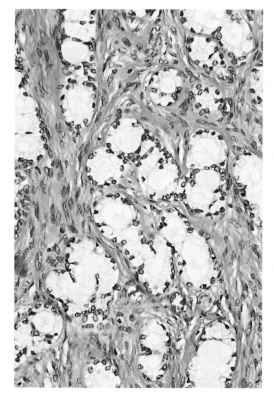

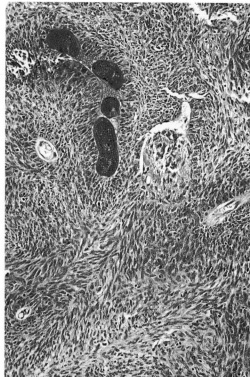

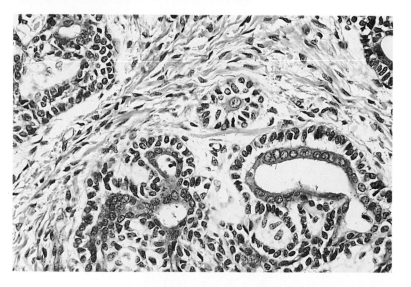

figure 1.78

This malignant tumor of Bartholin's duct (top) was composed purely of squamous-type cells. This adenocarcinoma of Bartholin's gland (center) contains multiple types of adenomatous structures, although some solid areas are present elsewhere. This Bartholin's gland tumor (bottom) is composed of cells that individually are not clearly glandular but were arranged as such and were producing a mucinous secretion.

figure 1.77

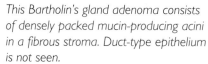

This Bartholin's gland adenoma consists of densely packed mucin-producing acini in a fibrous stroma. Duct-type epithelium is not seen.

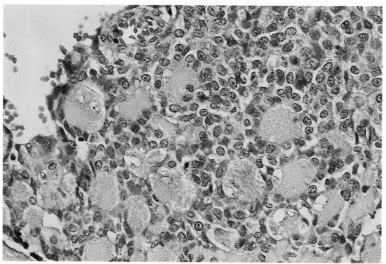

1.28

BARTHOLIN'S GLAND TUMORS

Adenomas may develop in Bartholin's gland, as well as adenocarcinomas of the mixed type similar to those seen in the salivary glands (Fig. 1.77). Although pure squamous carcinomas or adenocarcinomas are seen, more commonly these tumors are mixtures illustrating both glandlike and squamous epithelial cell types (Fig. 1.78). Developing as nodular thickenings in Bartholin's gland, they usually are large and metastatic by the time they are detected clinically. The fact that Bartholin's gland drains through lymphatics that primarily enter the pelvis rather than passing through the groin may also contribute to the development of early metastases to pelvic nodes (Fig. 1.79). Bartholin's adenitis in an older woman is a suspect diagnosis.

MELANOMA

The vulvar skin is well supplied with melanocytes and these may be responsible for benign nevi of all types (Fig. 1.80). Unfortunately, they also may be responsible for the entire spectrum of malignant melanocytic neoplasia from atypical

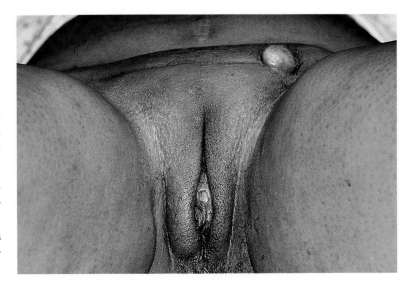

figure 1.79

This vulvar nodule is a metastasis from a Bartholin's gland carcinoma but it is possibly retrograde from the large intrapelvic mass that massively involved the left pelvic sidewall nodes. (Courtesy of Dr. D. Bard.)

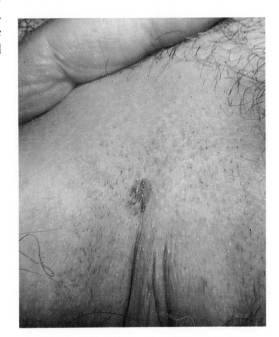

figure 1.80

A typical nevus is illustrated here but histologic confirmation is required before this can be assured.

1.29

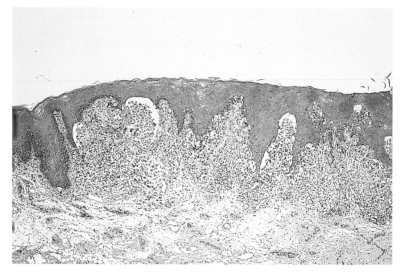

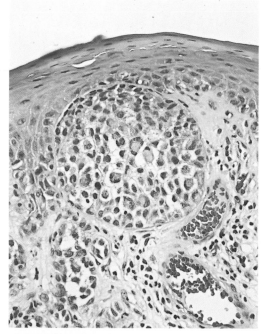

1.30

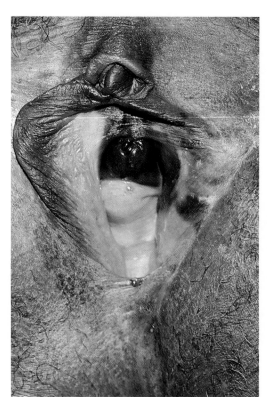

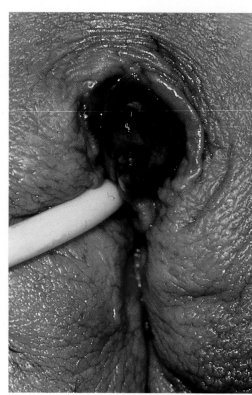

figure 1.81

Melanocytes largely confined to the papillary dermis (top left) are proliferating in situ. An associated intense inflammatory infiltrate was interpreted as an example of atypical melanocytic hyperplasia. A nest of malignant melanocytes (top right) lies immediately beneath the squamous epithelium. Tissue invasion has occurred. This is one focus in an extensive nodular melanosarcoma. This spreading melanoma (bottom left) occupies primarily the urethra and lower vagina. (Courtesy of Dr. D. Bard.) This nodular melanoma of the clitoris (bottom right) is even more ominous than usual because of it central location.

melanocytic proliferation to nodular melanosarcoma (Fig. 1.81). In general, vulvar melanoma does not differ histologically or clinically from the same disease seen elsewhere. However, the staging system has been altered somewhat to accommodate the variation in organization of the dermis encountered in the vulva. Current practice calls for vulvar melanomas to be staged on the basis of measurement of depth of invasion rather than on the histologic level to which they have extended. Melanoma is treated with a radical vulvectomy and groin dissection. Only in intraepithelial disease or in cases still confined to the papillary dermis is treatment very successful.

DERMAL TUMORS

Soft-tissue neoplasms, both benign and malignant, may arise in the vulvar dermis as elsewhere and are not specific (Figs. 1.82 and 1.83). An example is the granular-cell myoblastoma, which occasionally occurs in the vulva. As these small benign proliferations of nerve sheath cells are asymptomatic, they are usually noted only after they have produced surface irritation or breakdown. Histologically, they consist of sheets of large granular-appearing cells with small nuclei. They have a diffuse infiltrative junction with the soft tissue; thus, excision may be incomplete resulting in recurrence (Fig. 1.84). For unknown reasons, granular-cell myoblastomas tend to elicit a hyperplasia in the overlying squamous epithelium. The resulting acanthosis may be dramatic and result in the picture of pseudoepitheliomatous hyperplasia. Larger subepithelial soft-tissue tumors tend to result in fixed masses if malignant, or in pedunculated ones if benign (Fig. 1.85). All types of sarcomas have been reported in the vulvar soft tissues (Fig. 1.86). Lymphomas may present in groin nodes, and rarely other soft-tissue processes are seen (Fig. 1.87).

METASTATIC TUMOR

Metastatic cancer to the vulva may present in the subepithelial soft tissues or in the groin nodes. Intraabdominal tumors are the most common source of nodal metastases, but the endometrium is a common primary site when a subepithelial soft-tissue metastasis is present (Fig. 1.88).

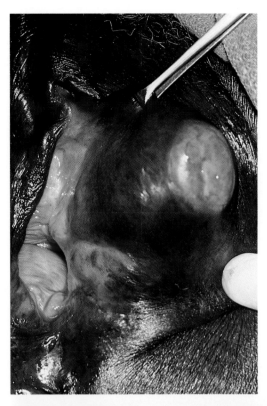

figure 1.82
This ominous appearing labial mass eroded through from beneath the surface. (Courtesy of Dr. D. Bard.)

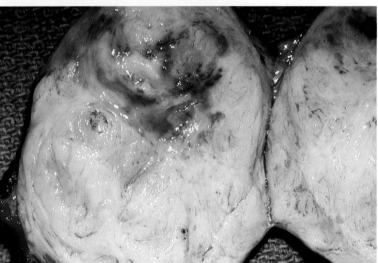

figure 1.83
Removed and cut open, the mass in the previous figure is discovered to be a benign myoma. (Courtesy of Dr. D. Bard.)

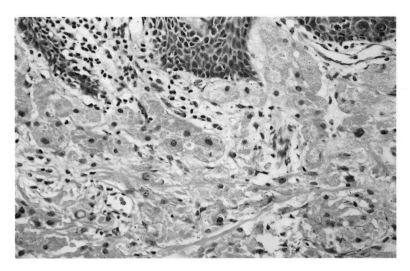

figure 1.84

Enlarged cells with granular pale-pink cytoplasm and small dark nuclei infiltrate the soft tissue beneath the epithelium in this example of a granular-cell myoblastoma. No capsule is present.

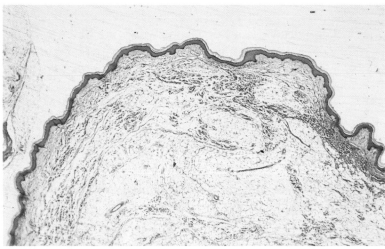

figure 1.85

Characteristic of benign soft-tissue tumors, this lipoma resulted in a polypoid pedunculated vulvar mass. No destruction of the epithelium is present.

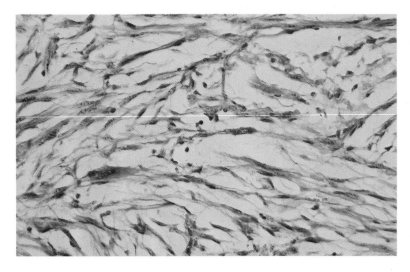

figure 1.86

This highly malignant tumor was interpreted as a fibrosarcoma. It formed an enlarging mass in the vulvar soft tissue. Atypical fibroblasts occupy the entire field.

figure 1.87

This eosinophilic granuloma is composed primarily of histiocytic cells and eosinophils.

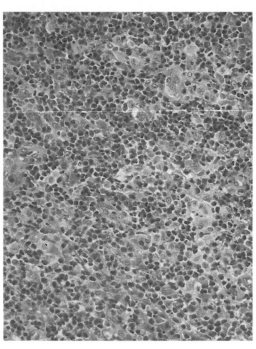

figure 1.88

The vulvar soft tissue is infiltrated with cancer that is breaking through the vulvar skin at multiple sites. The necrotic appearance of this vulva is typical of extensive metastatic cancer.

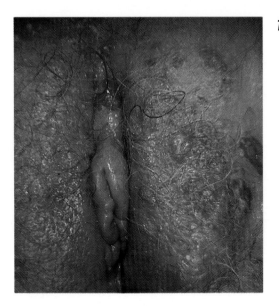

atlas of gynecologic pathology

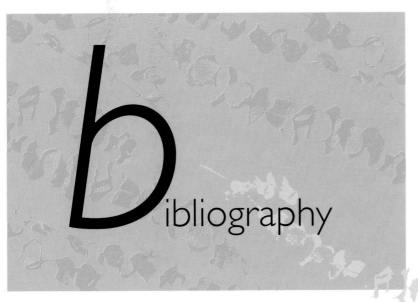

bibliography

ACOG Technical Bulletin 77. Carcinoma of the vulva. June, 1984.

Andreasson B, Nyboe J: Value of prognostic parameters in squamous cell carcinoma of the vulva. *Gynecol Oncol* 22:341, 1985.

Bock JE, Andreasson B, Thorn A, Holck S: Dermatofibrosarcoma protuberans of the vulva. *Gynecol Oncol* 20:129, 1985.

Boyce J, Fruchter RG, Kasambilides E, et al: Prognostic factors in carcinoma of the vulva. *Gynecol Oncol* 20:364, 1985.

Buscema J, Stern J, Woodruff JD: The significance of the histological alterations adjacent to invasive vulvar carcinoma. *Am J Obstet Gynecol* 137:902, 1980.

Copeland LJ, Sneige N, Gershenson DM, et al: Adenoid cystic carcinoma of Bartholin gland. *Obstet Gynecol* 67:115, 1986.

Crum CP, Liskow A, Petras P, et al: Vulvar intraepithelial neoplasia. *Cancer* 54:1429, 1984.

Davos I, Abell MR: Soft tissue sarcomas of the vulva. *Gynecol Oncol* 4:70, 1976.

Friedrich EG Jr: *Vulvar Disease, 2nd ed.* Philadelphia, WB Saunders, 1983.

Friedrich EG Jr: Vulvar dystrophy. *Clin Obstet Gynecol* 28:178, 1985.

Friedrich EG Jr: The vulvar vestibule. *J Reprod Med* 28:773, 1983.

Gardner HL, Kaufman RH: *Benign Diseases of the Vulva and Vagina,* 2nd ed. Boston, GK Hall & Co.,1981.

Hoffman JS, Kumar NB, Morley GW: Prognostic significance of groin lymph node metastases in squamous carcinoma of the vulva. *Obstet Gynecol* 66:402, 1985.

International Society for the Study of Vulvar Disease: New nomenclature for vulvar disease. *Obstet Gynecol* 47:122, 1976.

Jaramillo BA, Ganjei P, Averette HE, et al: Malignant melanoma of the vulva. *Obstet Gynecol* 66:398, 1985.

Podratz KC, Gaffey TA, Symmonds RE, et al: Melanoma of the vulva. *Gynecol Oncol* 16:153, 1983.

Sillman FH, Sedlis A, Boyce JG: A review of lower genital intraepithelial neoplasia and the use of topical 5-fluorouracil. *Obstet Gynecol Surv* 40:190, 1985.

Taylor RN, Bottles K, Miller TR, et al: Malignant fibrous histiocytoma of the vulva. *Obstet Gynecol* 66:145, 1985.

Woodruff JD, Braun L, Cavalieri R, et al: Immunological identification of papillomavirus antigen in paraffin processed condylomatous tissue. *Obstet Gynecol* 56:727, 1980.

Zucker PK, Berkowitz RS: The issue of microinvasive squamous cell carcinoma of the vulva. *Obstet Gynecol Surv* 40:136, 1985.

Vagina

chapter 2

Embryology

The vagina is a fibromuscular tube lined by a mucous membrane, the epithelium of which is derived from two sources, both mesodermal. The epithelium of the lower vagina is derived from the urogenital sinus wall, while that of the upper vagina is derived from the lining of the fused müllerian ducts. Figure 2.1 schematically demonstrates the embryologic development of the normal vagina.

By the end of the eighth week of intrauterine life, the bilateral müllerian ducts have fused in the midline to form a single structure whose tip abuts the posterior wall of the urogenital sinus. At this point, the wall of the urogenital sinus is mesoderm derived from the wolffian ducts. This is significant because it is the mesodermal wolffian duct epithelium that proliferates and differentiates into stratified squamous epithelium to form the lower part of the vagina, or the vaginal plate.

The vaginal plate and the müllerian duct are patent from early in development, and it is this patency that is associated with the conversion of columnar müllerian duct epithelium into stratified squamous epithelium by squamous metaplasia. Between 21 and 26 weeks of gestational age, stromal proliferation around the müllerian duct results in development of the cervix, producing functional obstruction at the level of the external os. Epithelial conversion stops here, resulting in the development of a squamocolumnar epithelial junction.

Normal Anatomy

The anatomy of the fully formed vagina is illustrated in Figure 2.2. Although it is extremely elastic and distensible, the vagina normally is only a potential space that, in cross section, is H-shaped in the lower portion of the canal and more of a simple slit in the upper portion (Fig. 2.3). In the individual whose uterus is directed anteriorly, the vagina normally is

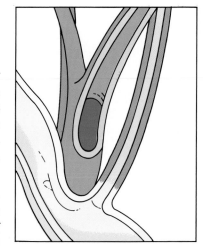

(a) 8 weeks

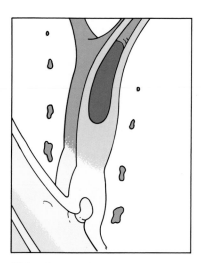

(b) 9 weeks

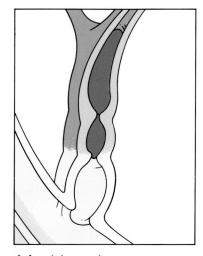

(c) 16 weeks

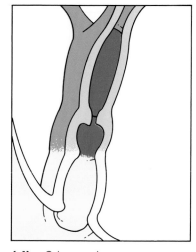

(d) 21 weeks

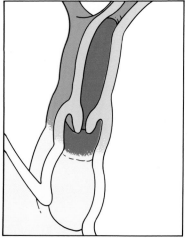

(e) 26 weeks

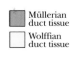 Müllerian duct tissue
 Wolffian duct

☐ Wolffian duct tissue
☐ Urogenital sinus tissue

figure 2.1

*Fused müllerian ducts touch the urogenital sinus wall between the wolffian ducts causing the wall to bulge **(a)**. Contact between müllerian duct tissue and urogenital sinus tissue induces growth of the vaginal plate; at this point the wolffian ducts have disappeared **(b)**. The septum between the vaginal plate and the müllerian duct breaks, resulting in a continuous vaginal canal **(c)**. At 21 weeks, the cervix is developing **(d)** and is formed at 26 weeks of age **(e)**. Note that for the purposes of this drawing, the orientation of the developing uterus in relation to the other structures has been modified.*

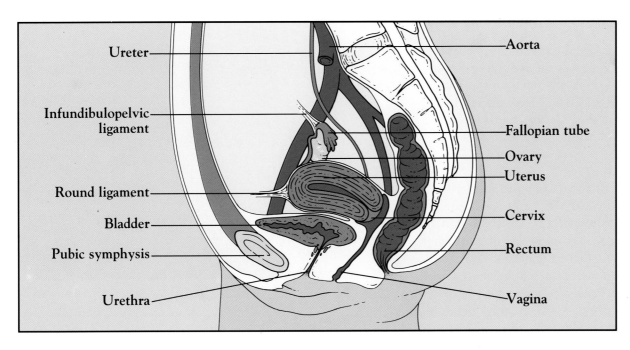

figure 2.2

Normal anatomy of the female urogenital tract. This drawing shows the basic anatomical relationships between the vagina and other pelvic structures, although individual variation is to be expected.

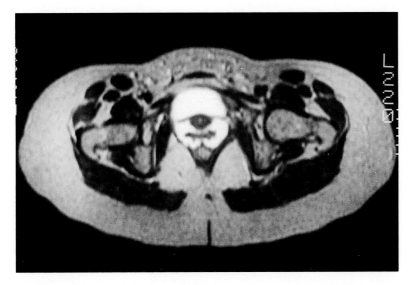

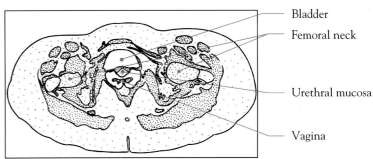

figure 2.3

Axial MRI of the normal vagina shows a section taken at the level of the femoral neck. The urinary bladder is very bright in signal intensity on this T2-weighted image. Posterior to the bladder, the urethra is demonstrated as a rounded structure whose bright center represents the urethral mucosa. The vagina, which exhibits a flattened configuration, is immediately posterior to the urethra.

directed posteriorly (Fig. 2.4). If the uterus is retroverted, however, the vaginal axis may be more directly cephalad (Fig. 2.5). When prolapse occurs, the vaginal axis is often rotated anteriorly, and successful repair is associated with restoring a posterior axis (Figs. 2.6 and 2.7). The cervix enters the vagina in its anterior wall so that the anterior vaginal wall is usually about 2.5 cm shorter than the posterior wall, which is approximately 9.5 cm long.

The epithelium of the vagina is supported by a loose reticular stroma. An inner circular layer and an outer longitudinal layer of smooth muscle are the most apparent components of the vaginal wall, although these layers are not distinct but are intermingled. Large numbers of elastic and collagen fibers also contribute to the vaginal wall.

The stratified squamous epithelium of the vagina is dramatically sensitive to estrogen. Newborn females exposed to high levels of maternal hormone will have thick highly differentiated vaginal epithelia, although this will begin to regress as maternal hormone levels decline (Fig. 2.8). A much thinner epithelial membrane exists in the premenarcheal child, and, with the development of endogenous estrogen levels at puberty, the epithelium again becomes thick and well differentiated (Fig. 2.9). In the mature woman, the vaginal mucous membrane is pale pink and arranged in rugae that run circumferentially around the vagina. These folds are broken up by grooves to produce a pebbly appearance (Fig. 2.10).

The stratified squamous epithelium in the vagina of a mature woman does not normally keratinize, but reflects an estrogen environment with the development of a superficial cell layer (Fig. 2.11). This development is to some extent counteracted by progesterone so that superficial cell development is inhibited during the progestational phase of the menstrual cycle and during pregnancy. Lactation also may be associated with a relatively immature epithelium.

When menopause occurs and estrogen production drops or ceases, the epithelium becomes quite thin and atrophic (Fig. 2.12). A typical appearance is that of a few layers of flattened cells with nuclei that are dark, dense, and still relatively large on top of two or three basal-cell layers (Fig. 2.13). With estrogen administration, this bilaminar appearance is converted to one that is more normal. Postmenopausal epithelium, which may become even more atrophic, is very subject to trauma and inflammation. If adjacent surfaces experience epithelial ulceration, then adhesions or even vaginal obliteration or obstruction may develop. If prolapse of the vagina occurs, then the mucous membrane is subject to drying and trauma (Fig. 2.14). The protective response to prolapse is the development of a granular zone, along with true keratinization (Fig. 2.15).

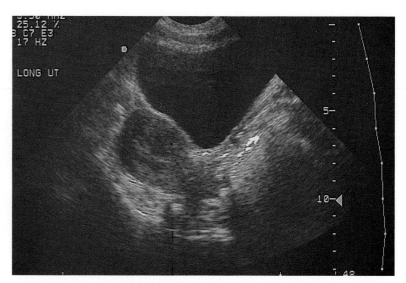

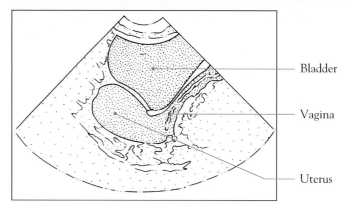

Bladder

Vagina

Uterus

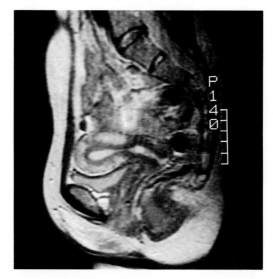

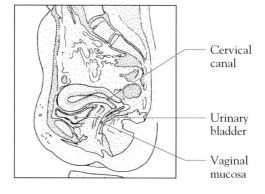

Cervical canal

Urinary bladder

Vaginal mucosa

figure 2.4

Logitudinal transabdominal ultrasound of the normal vagina (top) displays the uterus through a distended urinary bladder. A dense linear echo produced by the opposing mucosal surfaces denotes the lumen of the vagina. Sagittal MRI of the normal vagina (bottom), a proton density image, shows the vaginal mucosa as a bright linear signal posterior to the urinary bladder. The cervix invaginates posteriorly into the fornices of the vagina.

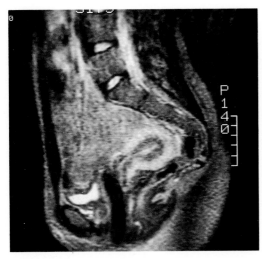

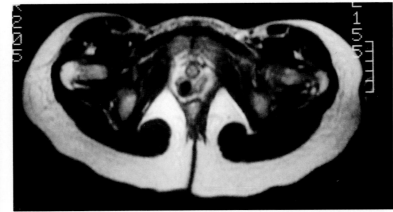

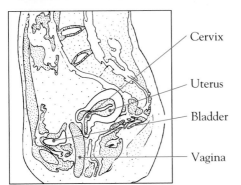

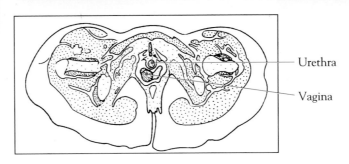

Cervix

Uterus

Bladder

Vagina

Urethra

Vagina

figure 2.5

Sagittal MRI of the normal vagina. (left). A tampon placed within the vagina for purposes of localization. The absence of mobile protons in the tampon is reflected as a signal void. The uterus is retroverted. The cervical and endometrial mucosa are the areas of high signal intensity in this

T2-weighted image. Axial MRI of the normal vagina (right) with the T1-weighted section taken at the level of the femoral neck. The vagina is marked by a tampon, which is displaced to the right of midline. The urethra is seen anteriorly as a round structure.

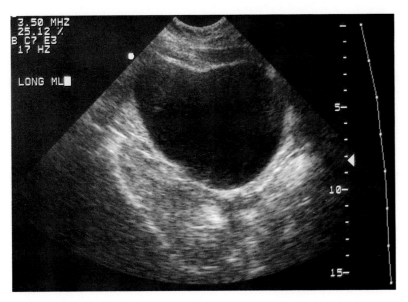

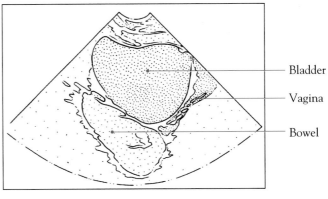

Bladder

Vagina

Bowel

figure 2.6

Longitudinal, transabdominal ultrasound of the vagina post hysterectomy. A distended urinary bladder allows visualization of pelvic structures. The vagina is seen as a curvilinear density parallel to the posterior wall of the bladder. The retrovesical space is filled by the rectum in the

absence of the uterus. Compare the axis of this postoperative vagina with the normal vagina in Figure 2.4. This vagina is not as posterior to the urinary bladder nor is it as deep as the normal vagina.

vagina

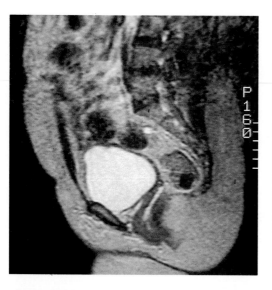
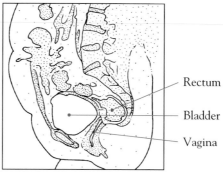

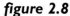

figure 2.7

Sagittal MRI of the vagina post hysterectomy displays the urinary bladder as a bright signal on this T2-weighted image. The vaginal mucosa has similar signal intensity posterior to the bladder. The gas filled rectum is identified superior to the vagina. Again, the vaginal axis could be more posterior.

Rectum

Bladder

Vagina

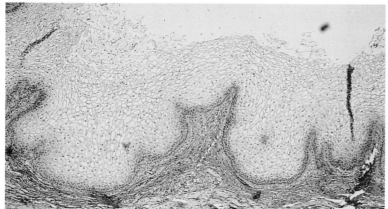

figure 2.8

Photomicrograph of a normal newborn vagina shows how the squamous epithelium is dramatically thickened and folded associated with the high levels of maternal hormone. Superficial and intermediate cell layers are prominent. The stromal tissues are cellular and well defined.

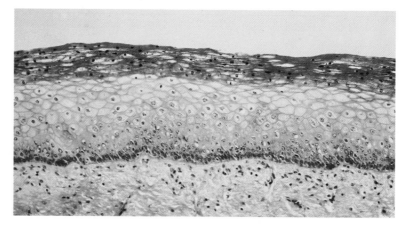

figure 2.9

Photomicrograph of normal vaginal epithelium shows well-developed stratified squamous epithelium, with striking differential staining of the intermediate and superficial cell layers, indicating adequate estrogen production. A well-developed basal cell layer is present and the epithelium is supported by a loose stroma.

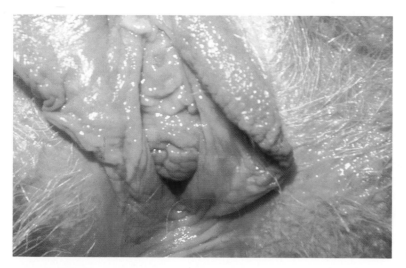

figure 2.10

Photograph of normal vaginal epithelium shows a portion of the anterior vaginal wall protruding between the labia minora, immediately beneath the urethra. Primary transverse rugae are broken up by vertical grooves, giving the epithelium a rough appearance.

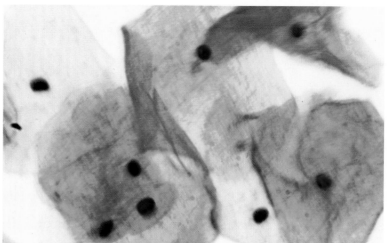

figure 2.11

These superficial cells were shed from the surface of a vaginal epithelium well supported with estrogen. They are large, flat and polyhedral, with small dark pyknotic nuclei. (Courtesy of Dr. Yener Erozan.)

atlas of gynecologic pathology

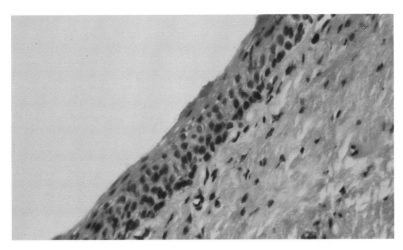

Basal and parabasal cells
Flattened eosinophilic cells

figure 2.12

Photomicrograph depicting postmenopausal atrophy shows epithelium that is dramatically thinner than that of Figure 2.9. It has a bilaminar appearance with basal-type and parabasal-type cells forming the lower layer and flattened cells with marked cytoplasmic eosinophilia suggesting maturation, forming the top layer. These cells are not as flattened as those found on the surface of the normal epithelium and the nuclei remain large.

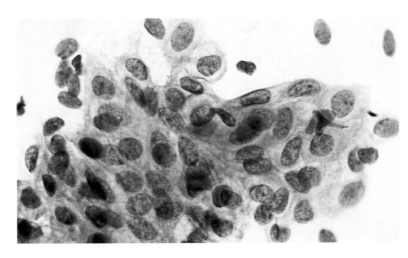

figure 2.13

These cells were shed from the surface of an atrophic postmenopausal epithelium. They are rounder than the ones seen in Figure 2.11 and their nuclei remain large and vesicular. (Courtesy of Dr. Yener Erozan.)

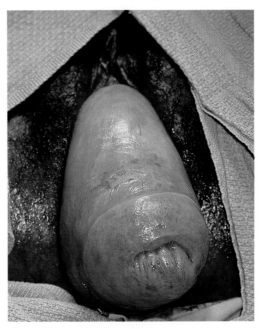

figure 2.14

This exposed vaginal mucosa is only slightly stained after exposure to Schiller's reagent. The well estrogenized vagina is stained dark brown by this reagent. (Courtesy of Dr. D. Bard.)

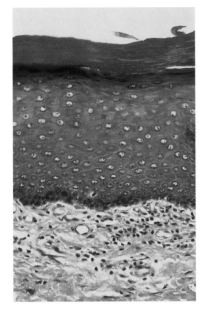

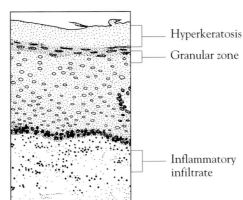

Hyperkeratosis
Granular zone
Inflammatory infiltrate

figure 2.15

Photomicrograph of vaginal prolapse in which the vaginal mucous membrane was prolapsed entirely through the introitus. A subepithelial inflammatory infiltrate demonstrates the resulting irritation. The development of a granular zone, along with extensive hyperkeratosis on the epithelial surface, indicates the protective response.

Congenital Anomalies

Congenital anomalies of the vagina are varied. If the müllerian ducts do not develop properly and they fail to migrate to the urogenital sinus, then the vagina will not develop and the vestibule will exist as a cul-de-sac, or a blind pouch (Fig. 2.16).

This lack of development may be relatively complete or it may occur on one side, as when there is a unilateral failure of the wolffian ducts to develop. Since the müllerian duct uses the wolffian duct as a guide for its migration into the pelvis, the unilateral absence of a wolffian duct will cause the müllerian duct on that side to fail to reach the urogenital sinus.

The resulting vaginal anomaly will take the form of a blind pouch on the affected side, separated from the unaffected side by a longitudinal septum. The blind side of this septum will be lined by mucus-secreting epithelium, since, in failing to reach the urogenital sinus, the blind pouch has never achieved the patency required for conversion of müllerian duct epithelium to stratified squamous epithelium. In addition, there may be a urologic anomaly on the same side as the vaginal anomaly. The unilateral form of this congenital anomaly, although much more common than the bilateral form, may or may not be detectable, whereas the bilateral defect usually is discovered in the postpubertal adolescent who presents with amenorrhea.

In the case where both müllerian ducts have reached the urogenital sinus but have failed to fuse with one another, two vaginas will form, one on each side of a complete longitudinal septum (Fig. 2.17). This finding may be associated with a doubling of the upper tract as well. At the point where the urogenital sinus component of the vagina meets the müllerian duct component, transverse septa may develop, partially or completely obstructing the vaginal canal (Fig. 2.18). As occurs with unilateral failure of the müllerian duct to open into the lower canal, the upper surface of the transverse septum will be lined by mucus-secreting epithelium. Both transverse vaginal septa and more complete forms of vaginal atresia may be associated with dilatation of the upper genital tract due to fluid collections (Fig. 2.19).

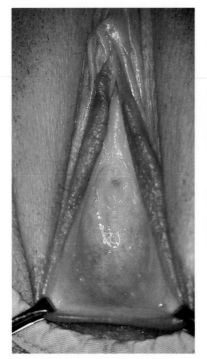

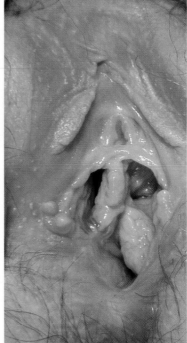

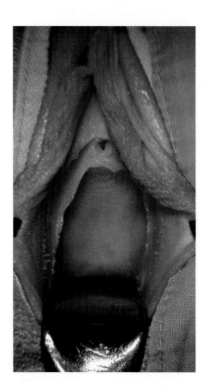

figure 2.16
Photograph of congenital absence of the vagina in which the vestibule, of urogenital sinus origin, exists as a blind pouch with no vaginal orifice. The vulva is formed normally. (Courtesy of Dr. John Rock.)

figure 2.17
In this photograph of a double vagina, the müllerian ducts have failed to fuse, resulting in two canals with an intervening longitudinal septum. Both vaginas open normally into the posterior wall of the vestibule, and the vulva is formed normally.

figure 2.18
The complete transverse septum pictured here is located at the junction of the urogenital (lower) portion and the müllerian duct (upper) portion of the vagina. (Courtesy of Dr. John Rock.)

2.8

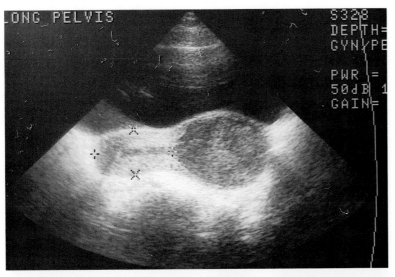

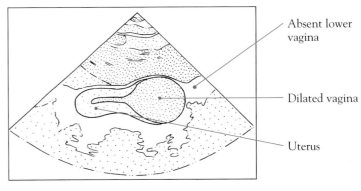

Absent lower vagina

Dilated vagina

Uterus

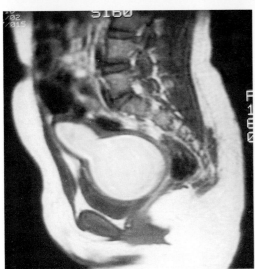

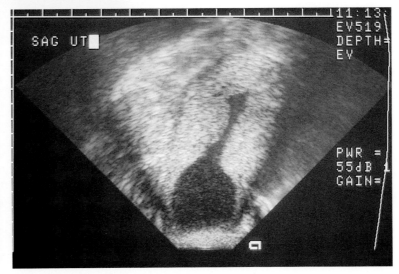

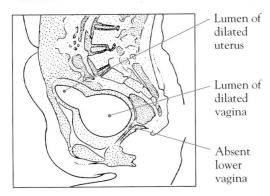

Lumen of dilated uterus

Lumen of dilated vagina

Absent lower vagina

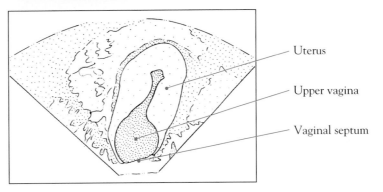

Uterus

Upper vagina

Vaginal septum

figure 2.19

Transabdominal longitudinal ultrasound image (top) of vaginal atresia with hematocolpos. The plane of the uterine cavity is parallel to the posterior wall of the bladder. The endometrium is hypoechoic, indicating the presence of minimal intrauterine fluid. The upper vagina is expanded by a heterogeneous mass. Sagittal T1-weighted MRI (lower left) of vaginal atresia with hematometrocolpos. The uterus and upper vagina are expanded by a mass with densely bright signal intensity signifying blood. The lower vagina is not visualized, compatible with vaginal atresia. Sagittal endovaginal ultrasound (lower right) of vaginal septum with hydrometrocolpos. The probe is placed within the lower vagina, visualizing the expanded upper portion. The fluid, which is filling the expanded upper vagina, is filled with particulate material representing debris. This fluid collection is continuous with that within the uterus.

Similarly, the posterior wall of the urogenital sinus, which forms the hymenal membrane, may fail to cavitate partially or completely, resulting in hymenal variation (Fig. 2.20). Complete obstruction of the canal is associated with fluid collection above the level of the obstruction and with mass formation. Endometriosis also is a common sequela.

des exposure

Alterations in vaginal development also will occur in the presence of prenatal exposure to diethylstilbestrol (DES). Empiric results suggest that DES exposure inhibits normal development in the following ways:

1. By inhibiting development of the vaginal plate such that the müllerian duct component of the vagina is lower in the adult canal than it would be otherwise.
2. By preventing transformation of the mucus-secreting columnar cell epithelium such that the adult female will still have mucus-secreting-type columnar epithelium in her vagina, a condition that is termed adenosis and which rarely occurs spontaneously (Fig. 2.21).
3. By inhibiting organization of the subepithelial stroma that forms the cervix and the walls of the rest of the genital canal, resulting in developmental anomalies of the upper vagina, cervix, uterus, and fallopian tubes.

The clinical results of these developmental anomalies may include one or all of the following:

1. The lower vaginal canal will have a smaller than normal caliber.
2. The vaginal mucosa, where affected by adenosis, will look and feel much rougher and will be erythematous.
3. The vaginal mucosa, where metaplasia is occurring, will be pink and red.
4. Rather than the development of clear cut fornices and a cervix, the upper vagina will consist of irregular folds of mucosa that obliterate the fornices and give the os a hooded appearance (Fig. 2.22).

2.10

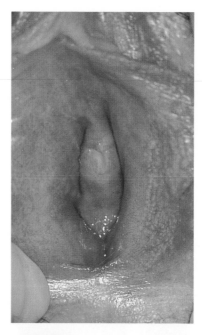

figure 2.20

This hymenal membrane contains no perforations, producing a picture similar to that of Figure 2.16 (congenital absence of the vagina). In this case, however, pelvic examination reveals normal internal genitalia. Again, the vestibule is formed normally. (Courtesy of Dr. John Rock.)

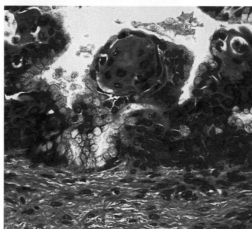

figure 2.21

Photomicrograph of vaginal adenosis in which a single cell layer of mucinous epithelium is being lifted off of the underlying stroma and replaced by squamous metaplasia. The metaplasia is still immature.

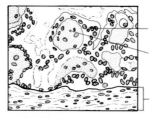

Mucinous epithelium

Metaplastic squamous epithelium

Stroma

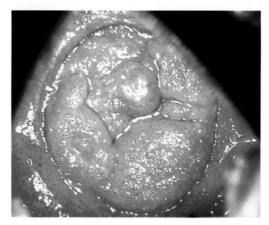

figure 2.22

This deformed cervical structure is typical of vaginal adenosis. The epithelial surface seems pebbly and erythema is present. The columnar mucus-secreting epithelium is thin and inflamed. The vaginal fornices are poorly formed. (Courtesy of Dr. Warren Patow.)

CLEAR CELL ADENOCARCINOMA

Vaginal adenosis gradually is replaced by squamous metaplasia, a repair process that usually is completed by close to the end of the second decade of life although sometimes not until later. This repair process appears to be important, since it is the persisting vaginal müllerian duct epithelium that is thought to be at increased risk for the development of clear cell adenocarcinoma—a tumor known for many years preceding the use of DES, but whose incidence was found to be dramatically increased in women with adenosis resulting from prenatal exposure to DES. Beginning in the latter first decade of life, the incidence of clear cell adenocarcinoma rises to a peak between the ages of 15 and 20, with occasional cases late in the third decade.

Although there is histologic variability in these tumors, two main patterns may be distinguished. The first is that of clear cells with vacuolated or empty cytoplasm, which may be arranged in sheets, cords, papillae, or glandular spaces (Fig. 2.23). The second is composed of a similar type of cell arranged in single cell layers of epithelium, with prominent nuclei that appear to project as pegs (Fig. 2.24). This appearance is heightened if the cytoplasmic membrane of the cell is disrupted and only a bare nucleus exists, as is often the case. This pattern is termed the hobnail pattern and is best described as the projection of bare nuclei from the epithelial surface into the lumen of glandlike spaces.

To date, clear cell adenocarcinoma has been treated most effectively by radical surgery. Salvage rates are approximately 90% for individuals without node involvement and 50% for individuals with node involvement.

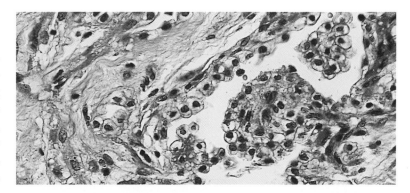

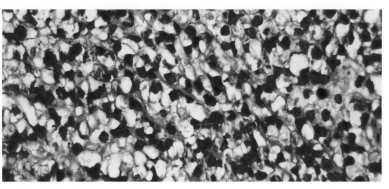

figure 2.23

Photomicrographs taken from tumor specimens of clear cell adenocarcinoma. In one specimen (top) clear cells line the glandular spaces and papillae. In the other specimen (bottom) clear cells form a solid sheet of tumor with large atypical nuclei.

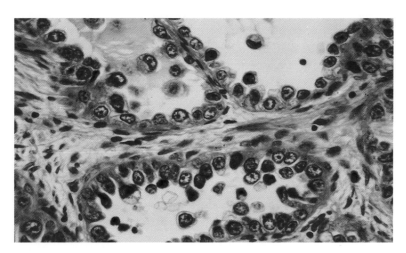

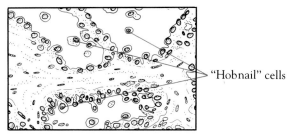

"Hobnail" cells

figure 2.24

Photomicrograph of clear cell adenocarcinoma showing tumor composed of glandular spaces lined by a single cell layer. The cytoplasm of these cells is either lightly vacuolated or clear, but the prominent feature of these cells is their atypical nuclei that appear to project as pegs into the lumen of the gland.

vagina

Cystic Masses

There are several types of vaginal cysts, probably the most common of which is the inclusion cyst secondary to trauma (Fig. 2.25). This structure is usually solitary in an episiotomy repair, and although it may be noticed by the patient, it usually is asymptomatic. The stratified squamous epithelium that lines this cyst often has been altered by the pressure of the accumulated material (desquamated surface squames), and, on histologic examination, does not appear to be fully developed. Simple excision suffices for treatment.

DEVELOPMENTAL CYSTS

Other vaginal cysts include those secondary to either müllerian or wolffian duct remnants in the vaginal wall. Either of these types of epithelial remnants may secrete fluid into an enclosed space resulting in the formation of small or large cysts. Müllerian duct remnants are commonly lined by epithelium typical of that found elsewhere in the genital canal, specifically, in other müllerian duct derivatives (Fig. 2.26). Gartner's or wolffian duct cysts may also contain ciliated epithelium typical of that found in the genital canal, but these cysts tend to possess a low cuboidal cell epithelium with a prominent basement membrane (Fig. 2.27). Gartner's cysts are described as occurring classically in the anterolateral vaginal wall, but they, as well as müllerian duct cysts, may occur anywhere in the vaginal wall (Fig. 2.28). They are routinely asymptomatic and should be ignored unless they are large. Surgical excision of these structures can sometimes become considerably more formidable than anticipated, as they may extend into the broad ligament and involve important structures. Cystoceles have been mistaken for Gartner's cysts (Fig. 2.29).

The congenital anomaly discussed earlier, in which the müllerian duct unilaterally fails to reach the urogenital sinus, presents as a cyst when the cul-de-sac protrudes into the normally formed vaginal compartment.

INFLAMMATORY CYSTS AND ENDOMETRIOSIS

Varicosities may appear as cysts in the suburethral area and may be confused with other suburethral cysts, such as urethral diverticulae or Skene's duct abscesses (Fig. 2.30). Varicosities, however, are most likely to arise in pregnancy, while urethral diverticula and Skene's duct infections often are associated with urinary symptoms (Fig. 2.31).

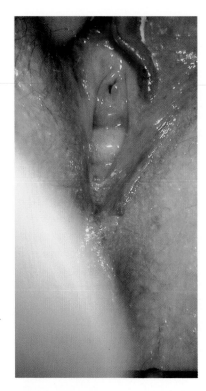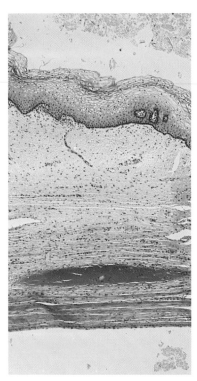

figure 2.25

An inclusion cyst (left) occupies the site of a previous episiotomy repair. This clear cystic tumor is an incidental finding. The introitus is slightly inflamed but there are no symptoms. Tissue sample from an inclusion cyst (right) shows an overlying normal squamous epithelium that is separated from the cyst below by dense stroma and scarring. The cyst is lined by a flattened squamous epithelium that is altered by the pressure within the cyst.

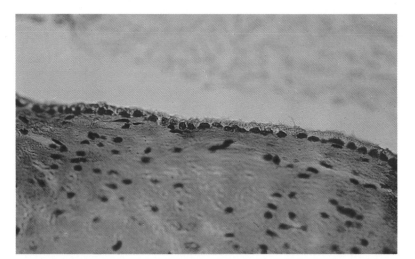

figure 2.26

A single layer of mucinous cells lines the vaginal cyst in this photomicrograph. The similarity of these cells to those that line the endocervix suggests that this cyst is a müllerian duct remnant.

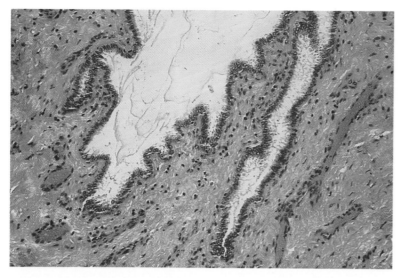

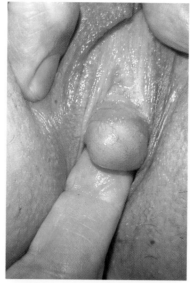

figure 2.27

Photograph of a Gartner's cyst (left) shows a single cell layer of well-defined cuboidal epithelium lining the cyst; the epithelial appearance is more consistent with that of a wolffian duct remnant. Immediately inside the hymenal ring, this cystic structure (right) is in the upper lateral wall of the vagina. Although the location of this cyst is classically Gartner's, this position is not absolutely diagnostic.

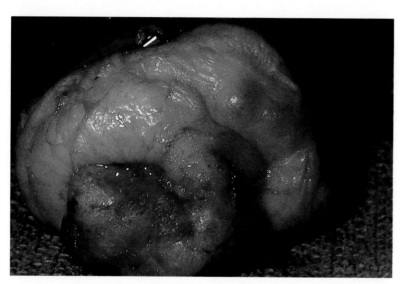

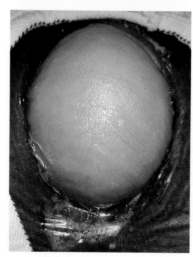

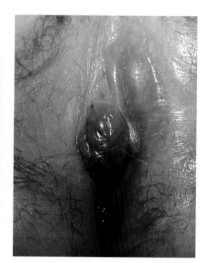

figure 2.28

These vaginal cysts are in the fornix, anterior-lateral to the cervix. This is a classic location for Gartner's duct cysts. (Courtesy of Dr. D. Bard.)

figure 2.29

This large cystic structure protruding through the vaginal introitus was initially presumed to be a Gartner's cyst. More careful examination revealed only cystocele. The normally rugose vaginal wall has been stretched and flattened.

figure 2.30

A singular vulvar varicosity lies between the labia minora and majora, on the patient's left. Multiple vaginal varicosities arising in the suburethral plexus of veins protrude through the introitus like a urethrocele.

figure 2.31

Photograph of a urethral cyst (left) shows a bulging mass immediately beneath the urethra. The mass is soft and may result in a urethral discharge when palpated. The overlying squamous epithelium is intact. A cystic structure (right) is filled with pus. This Skene's duct abscess, when palpated, may or may not result in the expression of pus through the orifice of the duct. Usually it is tender.

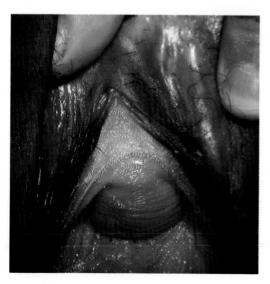

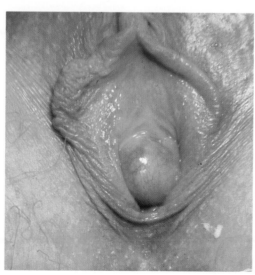

vagina

Multiple cystic blebs found all over the vaginal mucosa may constitute vaginitis emphysematosa (Fig. 2.32). This condition of uncertain origin consists of subepithelial cystic spaces lined by giant cells, and it occurs most often in patients who are critically ill.

Endometriosis may occur in the vagina as a penetrating growth from the cul-de-sac of Douglas or as a spontaneous development in peritoneal remnants in a rectovaginal septum. It also may occur following implantation in an episiotomy repair. The result usually is a painful mass, although velvety erythematous patches also are possible (Fig. 2.33).

Endometriosis beneath the surface epithelium may result in the formation of endometriomas, which appear as blue cystic elevations of the vaginal mucosa (Fig. 2.34). Dyspareunia is a common symptom and, while drug therapy may be efficacious, surgery is often required.

Inflammatory Conditions

VAGINITIS

Although the common vaginal infections are associated with their characteristic discharges, the vagina itself presents a nonspecific pattern of erythema when inflamed. Monilial infection characteristically produces a thick white discharge consisting of clumps of epithelial cells and fungi (Fig. 2.35). Hyphae may be dramatic.

In contrast, infection with Trichomonas produces a discharge that is yellow-green, bubbly, and filled with free-swimming trichomonads. Trichomonas infection is similar to and most commonly confused with Gardnerella vaginitis (Fig. 2.36).

Tampons may produce nonspecific erythema or acute ulcerations (Fig. 2.37). The ulcers tend to be sharply demarcated, and, although not uncommon, they usually are only evanescent. Histologically, they are typical ulcers occurring with a dense inflammatory response and with associated granulation (Fig. 2.38). Granulation tissue is also seen in the vaginal vault as a result of healing post-hysterectomy and, in that setting, may be confused with a prolapsed fallopian tube (Fig. 2.39).

CONDYLOMATA

Histologically, condylomata in the vagina are not significantly different from those seen elsewhere, although grossly they are more likely to be whitish in the moist environment of the vagina than on the vulva, where they tend to be dry and brown (Fig. 2.40). The features seen most frequently are the

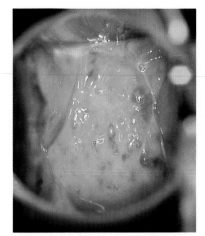

figure 2.32

Multiple subepithelial blebs can be seen in this photograph of vaginitis emphysematosa. The site of the blebs is erythematous but the rest of the vaginal mucosa is uninflamed.

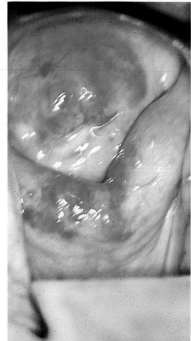

figure 2.33

In this photograph of endometriosis, both the cervix and the vaginal mucosa demonstrate velvety erythematous patches that bleed easily when touched; they also bleed spontaneously, cyclically. The rest of the vaginal mucosa is uninflamed.

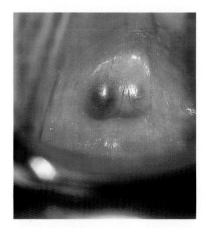

figure 2.34

In this patient with endometriosis, elevating the cervix reveals two dark-blue cystic structures in the posterior fornix of the vagina. They do not bleed visibly, but they are tender and result in dyspareunia. The rest of the vagina is healthy.

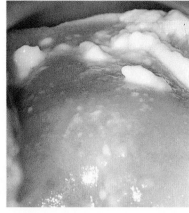

figure 2.35

This photograph of a monilial infection shows the vagina to be reddened and coated with large clumps of thick white discharge that resembles soft cheese, to which it is often compared. (Courtesy of Dr. John Hawkinson.)

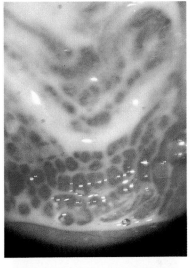

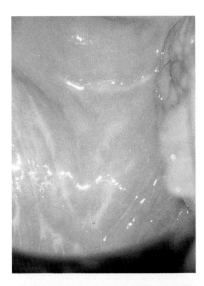

figure 2.36

A thick frothy discharge (left) fills the vaginal vault, with intense erythema of the vaginal wall visible where the discharge thins. Numerous large and small bubbles characterize this Trichomonas infection. The thin watery discharge in this case of Gardnerella vaginitis (right) is strongly contrasted with that of the lefthand figure. Bubbles are not a prominent feature and the vagina is less erythematous. (Courtesy of Dr. John Hawkinson.)

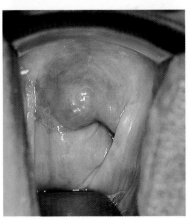

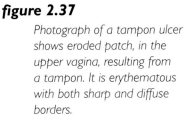

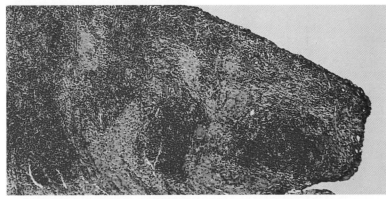

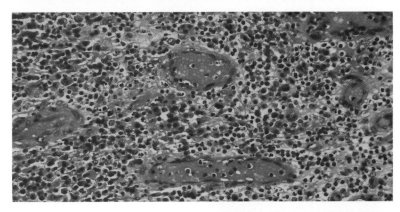

figure 2.38

Photomicrograph (top) shows granulation tissue in the base of a tampon ulcer, with dense inflammatory infiltrate. Both responses are typical following injury from any source. This tissue from a tampon ulcer (bottom) consists of a loose edematous stroma with a dense, acute, and chronic inflammatory infiltrate supporting multiple fine capillaries, with endothelial cell proliferation. This is typical of granulation tissue from any source.

2.15

figure 2.37

Photograph of a tampon ulcer shows eroded patch, in the upper vagina, resulting from a tampon. It is erythematous with both sharp and diffuse borders.

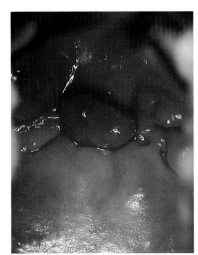

figure 2.39

An erythematous protruding mass is seen in the postoperative incision site in the vaginal vault. Normal vaginal mucosa is below. Microscopically, this mass is granulation tissue but, grossly, it is also consistent with a prolapsed fallopian tube.

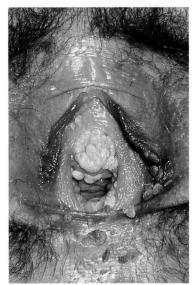

figure 2.40

Photograph of condylomata shows white acuminate warts occupying the vestibule and the vagina, while the ones on the perineum below the fourchette are brown. The fact that they are multiple is typical.

vagina

classic ones of papillomatosis, acanthosis, parakeratosis, and hyperkeratosis (Figs. 2.41 and 2.42). Condylomata with cytologic atypia, however, may be seen as well. These condylomata have normal maturational patterns with perhaps some papillomatosis, but they show marked individual cell atypicality in the form of nuclear changes, consisting of enlargement, hyperchromatism, smudging, vacuolation, fragmentation, multiple forms (Fig. 2.43), and koilacytosis.

Furthermore, patterns exist in which there are multiple atypical mitoses in addition to these other atypicalities, and it is presumed that such patterns represent transitions between condylomata and true intraepithelial neoplasia. It is becoming increasingly apparent that different types of condyloma viruses are responsible for these different histologies.

Vaginal Cancer

Currently, some types of condyloma viruses are believed to be responsible for malignant transformation in the lower genital canal, and, when this occurs, then vaginal intraepithelial neoplasia exists. The gross appearance of these entities may be variable, but some combination of inflammation and hyperkeratosis usually results in thickened red and white patches that may be single or multiple (Fig. 2.44).

Intraepithelial neoplasia in the vagina may have a variety of histologies from an almost pure basal-cell type or parabasal-cell type to a more differentiated form with hyperkeratosis (Fig. 2.45). In either case, the epithelium lacks organization and the cells possess nuclear atypia, both characteristic of malignancy. Vaginal intraepithelial neoplasia may be treated with local chemotherapeutic agents or by local excision; although in either case, it tends to be multicentric and may recur.

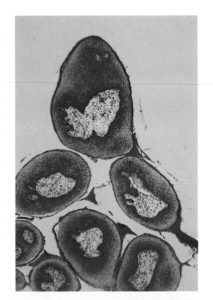

figure 2.41

Photomicrograph of condylomata shows multiple papillae dramatically illustrating the papillomatous character of this viral infection. Despite this evidence of proliferation, the epithelium is well organized.

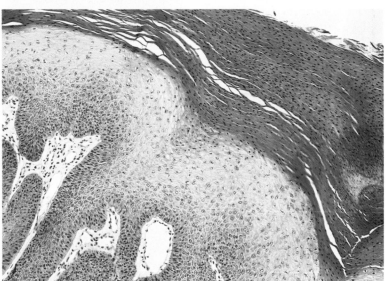

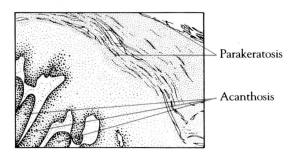

Parakeratosis

Acanthosis

figure 2.42

Photomicrograph in which two other histologic features of condylomata are prominent: parakeratosis and acanthosis. Again, the epithelium is well organized.

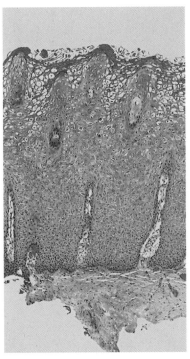
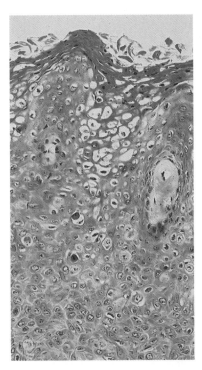
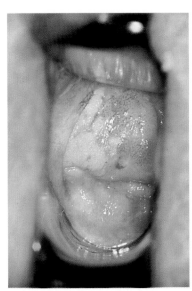

2.17

figure 2.44

This well-demarcated lesion in the upper vaginal vault looks granular and consists of alternating white and erythematous patches. It is a typical example of vaginal carcinoma in situ. (From Novak and Woodruff, 1979.)

figure 2.43

Low-power view (left) of flat condyloma with atypia shows a thickened vaginal epithelium demonstrating less dramatic acanthosis and papillomatosis. The epithelium, however, also is less well organized and when intermediate cells appear they are koilocytotic. A higher power view of the same epithelium (right) shows koilocytosis as well as nuclear atypia consisting of hyperchromatism with smudging, focal vacuolation, multinucleation, and fragmentation. There is little hyperkeratosis or parakeratosis.

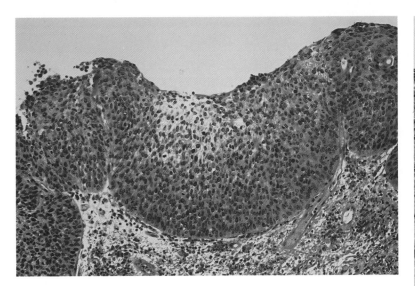
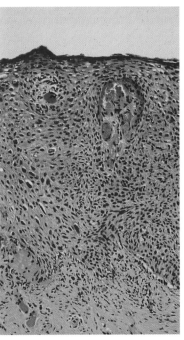

figure 2.45

This example of carcinoma in situ (left) is composed primarily of basal-type cells, although there is some cytoplasmic maturation in the central portion of the picture. The tumor will look red, clinically. This example of carcinoma in situ (right) shows more cytoplasmic maturation with abortive surface keratinization that may give the tumor a white appearance. In both examples, the capillaries reach high in the epithelium, in the papillae between the rete ridges.

Although cytology usually is an effective means of detecting the intraepithelial disease, tragic examples of advanced vaginal cancer continue to occur (Fig. 2.46). While less frequently observed today, both prolapse and pessaries have been associated histologically with the development of vaginal cancer. Prolapse is believed to result in an irritation of the vaginal mucous membrane, which predisposes to the development of malignancy (Fig. 2.47). Invasive vaginal cancer, histologically similar to the cervical disease, is largely of the epidermoid variety and usually illustrates little maturation (Fig. 2.48). In approximately 15% of all cases, maturation with keratinization does occur. The prognosis for vaginal cancer is poorer than it is for cervical cancer. This is presumed to be based on the fact that the vaginal wall is sufficiently thin so that the disease extends beyond the wall at a relatively early stage. MRI may be very helpful in delineating the extent of the tumor (Figs. 2.49 and 2.50). Cases that are high in the canal metastasize to the pelvic lymph nodes, while those that are lower may spread to the inguinal nodes as does vulvar disease. Some cases spread to both sites and therefore present a particularly complex problem. In Figure 2.51, the FIGO staging for vaginal carcinoma is presented along with very approximate five-year salvage rates, assuming radiation therapy.

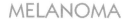

2.18

MELANOMA

Histologically, vaginal melanomas are typical of melanomas occurring at any site, and they have a particularly poor prognosis, since almost all are advanced at the time of diagnosis (Fig. 2.52).

Focal collections of melanocytes, seen occasionally in the vagina, are presumed to be the source of these very rare vaginal melanomas (Fig. 2.53). They are of uncertain origin, they may be single or multiple, and biopsies should be obtained.

SUBEPITHELIAL SOFT-TISSUE NEOPLASMS

Although many types of subepithelial soft-tissue tumors are seen in the vagina, individually, each type is quite rare. Not clearly a neoplasm, the vaginal polyp nevertheless may be confused with neoplasia. Single or multiple polypoid structures may protrude into the vaginal space (Fig. 2.54). The epithelium of these structures is intact and the supporting stroma contains enlarged atypical cells. Features such as nuclear vacuolation suggest degeneration and do not represent malignancy (Fig. 2.55). Vaginal polyps are most common in postpubertal premenopausal women and require only excision.

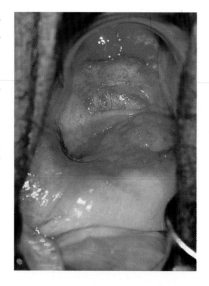
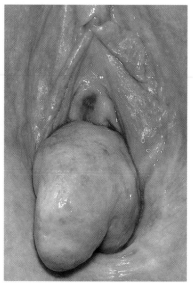
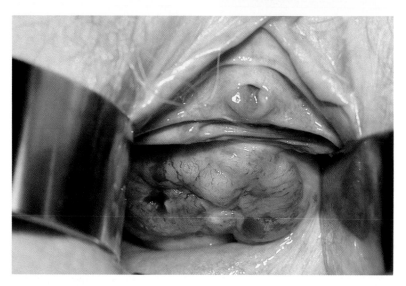

figure 2.46

In this gross clinical photograph (top left) the ulceration in the posterior wall of the vagina is an invasive vaginal cancer. Its endophytic growth pattern has resulted in significant penetration of the vaginal wall, although the tumor mass is still small. The cervix is everted and looks inflamed, but it is uninvolved. This unusually exophytic tumor (top right) is a primary vaginal carcinoma. (Courtesy of Dr. D. Bard.) This nodular vaginal carcinoma (bottom) occupies most of the anterior wall of the vagina. (Courtesy of Dr. D. Bard.)

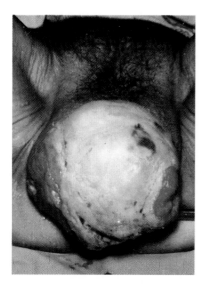

figure 2.47

Although prolapse is associated with the development of vaginal cancer, the multicentric invasion seen in this case of vaginal cancer is unusual.

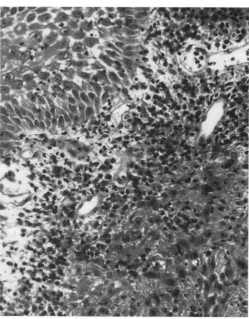

figure 2.48

These photomicrographs were obtained from three different cases of invasive vaginal cancer. In one case (upper left), the tumor is composed of basal-type cells. They form a sheet of undifferentiated epidermoid cancer infiltrating beneath the normal epithelium. In another case (lower left), the vaginal cancer depicted does not achieve complete differentiation, but intermediate-type cells are formed. The pattern is infiltrative. In the third case (lower right), although the tumor is composed primarily of basal-type cells, maturation in some areas is dramatic, with focal keratinization and pearl formation.

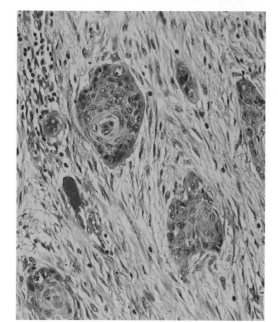

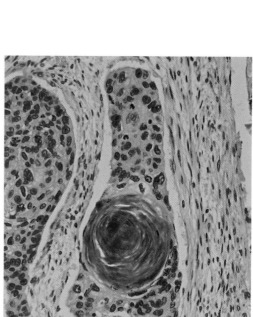

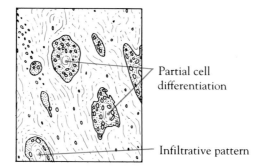

Partial cell differentiation

Infiltrative pattern

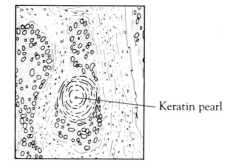

Keratin pearl

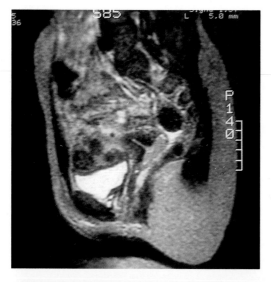
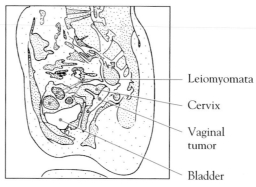

figure 2.49

Sagittal MRI of a vaginal carcinoma exhibits a soft tissue mass filling the posterior half of the vagina. The mass does not extend into the cervix, which is identified by the bright endocervical mucosa. There are multiple leiomyomata in the uterus, which are low in signal intensity on this T2-weighted image.

Leiomyomata

Cervix

Vaginal tumor

Bladder

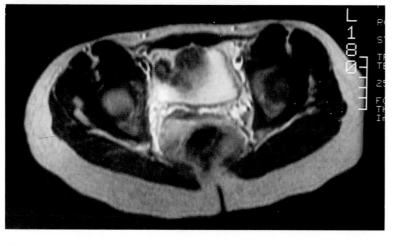
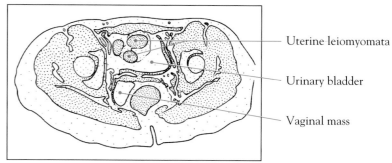

Uterine leiomyomata

Urinary bladder

Vaginal mass

2.20

figure 2.50

Axial MRI of a vaginal carcinoma with the T2-weighted image taken at the level of the femoral head shows the urinary bladder partially indented by uterine leiomyomata from the anteverted uterus small

bowel loops. Posterior to the urinary bladder, the right vaginal fornix is filled by a soft tissue mass. This mass appears confined to the vagina and does not extend into the rectum or pelvic sidewall.

FIGO Staging System for Carcinoma of the Vagina

STAGE	CRITERIA	FIVE-YEAR SALVAGE RATES (with radiation therapy)
0	Intraepithelial	—
I	Limited to vaginal wall	80%
II	Extends to subvaginal tissue but not to pelvic side wall	50%
III	Extends to pelvic side wall	30%
IV	Extends beyond true pelvis or involves mucosa of bladder or rectum	5%
IV **a**	Adjacent organs	—
IV **b**	Distant organs	—

figure 2.51

Table of FIGO staging of carcinoma of the vagina. Note that as the vaginal wall is very thin, even small vaginal cancers will become stage II cases, in contrast to cervical tumors of comparable size.

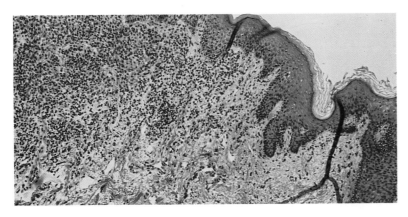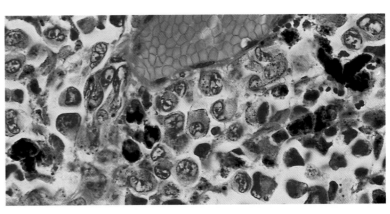

figure 2.52

Low-power photomicrograph (left) of malignant melanoma showing the edge of a collection of proliferating melanocytes. They are poorly organized and infiltrating beneath the vaginal epithelium. A higher power view of the same specimen (right) shows significant nuclear atypia associated with large amounts of both intracellular and extracellular melanin.

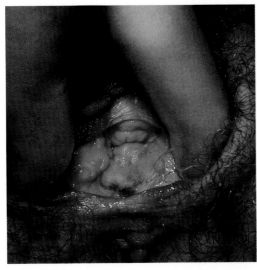

figure 2.53

In this case of vaginal melanosis, the pigmented spots in the posterior vaginal wall are unusual, although this is not an unusual site for them. Although often benign, biopsies should be taken to rule out malignant melanoma.

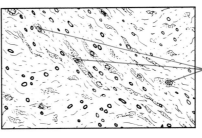

figure 2.54

Photograph of a vaginal polyp shows polypoid structure (grasped by the Kelly clamp) with an intact squamous epithelium showing no evidence of erosion or erythema.

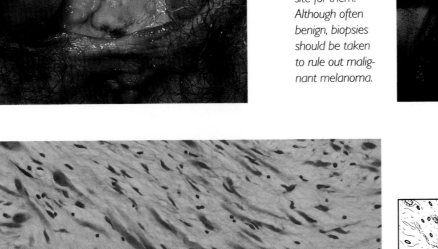

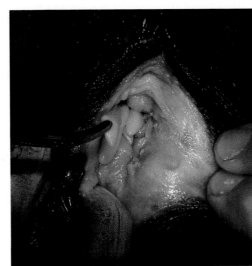

Large atypical cells

figure 2.55

A histologic section of a vaginal polyp shows that significant cytologic atypia exists. Both nuclei and cytoplasm are enlarged, however, and there is smudging and vacuolation of the nuclei suggesting degeneration.

vagina

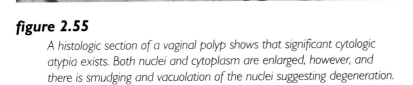

Polypoid lesions occurring in infancy may be embryonal rhabdomyosarcomas, grossly presenting as sarcoma botryoides. In such cases, small but atypical rhabdomyoblasts proliferate beneath the epithelium forming a so-called cambium layer and raising the epithelium into multiple polypoid projections (Fig. 2.56). The epithelium usually is intact but often it is thinned and inflamed and may be invaded by tumor cells (Fig. 2.57). Classically, treatment of this entity has been surgical, although multiagent chemotherapy may become more important in the future. It also should be noted that a similar gross appearance is typical of almost any subepithelial tumor in small children, and occasionally germ-cell tumors such as the endodermal sinus tumor will occur in this clinical setting. The classic histologic finding in the endodermal sinus tumor is the Schiller-Duvall body (Fig. 2.58). These tumors also usually produce large quantities of γ-feto-protein. Currently, treatment of endodermal sinus tumors consists of multiagent chemotherapy.

Both myomas and leiomyosarcomas may occur in the vagina and result in protruding vaginal masses that are detected only after they have become large (Figs. 2.59 and 2.60). The histologic variations that are seen in muscle tumors of the uterus are also seen in those tumors that occur in the vagina. Initial treatment consists of the surgical excision required to make the diagnosis. Both low-grade and high-grade stromal sarcomas as well as mixed lesions may be seen, and they too are similar to those seen elsewhere in the genital canal (Figs. 2.61 and 2.62).

Sarcomas typical of other soft-tissue sites (such as fibrosarcomas, lymphomas, as well as undifferentiated sarcomas) also occur in the vagina (Figs. 2.63 to 2.66).

Most of these tumors are asymptomatic until large, and their histology is not unique to the site. The photomicrograph in Figure 2.67 is from a very rare example of an adenomatoid tumor found in the vaginal wall.

METASTATIC CANCER

Metastatic cancer in the vagina is not uncommon when malignancy occurs elsewhere in the pelvis. In cases of endometrial cancer or choriocarcinoma, the suburethral site is a classic one for the production of vaginal masses, but metastases also are seen in the cul-de-sac and elsewhere. The vaginal vault is a frequent site of recurrence following surgical therapy for pelvic cancer (Fig. 2.68).

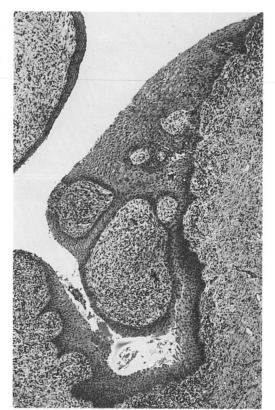

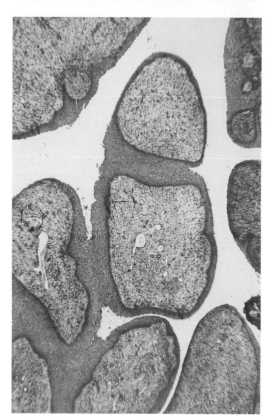

figure 2.56

Photomicrograph of sarcoma botryoides shows cellular proliferation that is particularly dense immediately beneath the surface epithelium (top). This cambium layer is seen to result in nodular elevation of the surface epithelium. The photomicrograph shows proliferating sarcoma cells having produced such exuberant growth that polypoid masses project into the vaginal lumen (bottom). With additional edema, these become the grapelike protrusions of sarcoma botryoides.

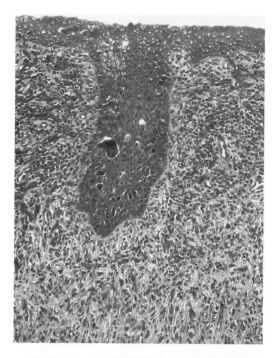

figure 2.57

In the sarcoma botryoides seen here, proliferating sarcoma cells not only form a dense subepithelial layer, but they also have focally invaded the epithelium, which remains intact.

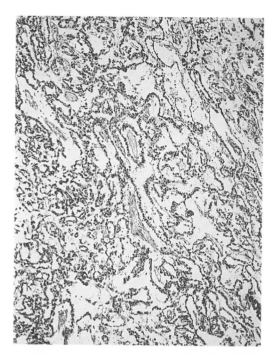

figure 2.58

Photomicrograph of endodermal sinus tumor shows complex folds of embryonic endoderm as the major feature of this tumor. A capillary within an endodermal fold forms a Schiller-Duvall body in the center of the field.

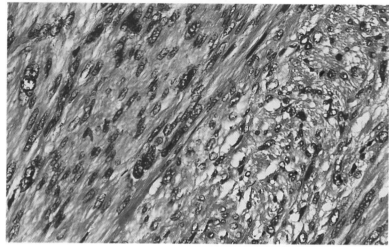

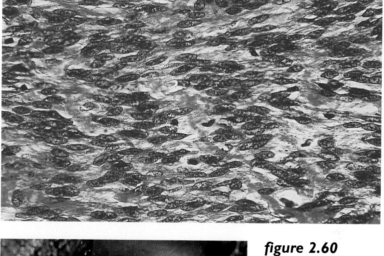

2.23

figure 2.59

Photomicrograph of a bizarre myoma shows cytologic atypia similar to that seen in Figure 2.55 (vaginal polyp) and typical of that seen in bizarre myomas in the uterus.

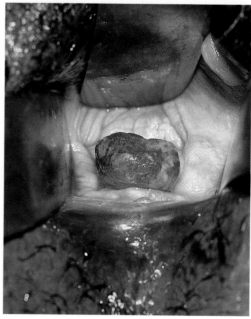

figure 2.60

This leiomyosarcoma in the vaginal wall (top) possesses mitoses and lacks fully normal differentiation. This malignant tumor (bottom) in the posterior vaginal wall is a leiomyosarcoma. (Courtesy of Dr. D. Bard.)

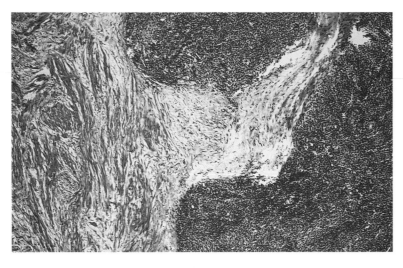

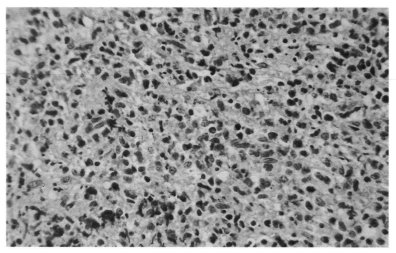

figure 2.61

Photomicrograph of stromatosis in which this low-grade stromal sarcoma is seen to possess an infiltrative pattern (left). There is no inflammation and no tissue destruction. On higher power (right), highly vascular stromal tissue, with little atypicality, is present.

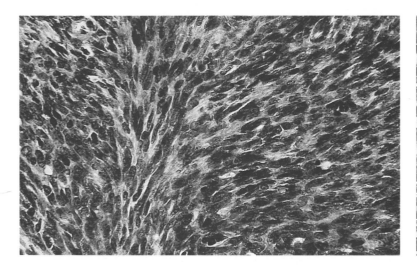

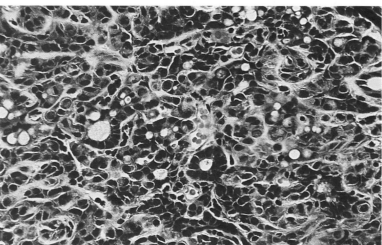

figure 2.62

The stromal sarcoma seen in this photomicrograph (left) is similar to
the stromatosis seen in Figure 2.61, but in this case there is more
cytologic atypia and there are atypical mitoses. In one field of this
tumor (right) epithelial elements are present. The pattern is that of
nests and cords.

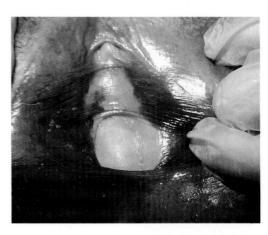

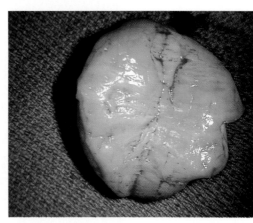

figure 2.63

Gross clinical photograph of a vaginal fibroma (left) shows a firm mass in the vaginal
wall covered with an intact epithelium, producing a nodular protrusion into the vaginal
canal. When removed (right), the tumor is
found to be encapsulated and homogenous.
These features suggest a benign process
but they do not necessarily predict cell type.

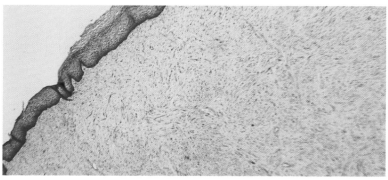
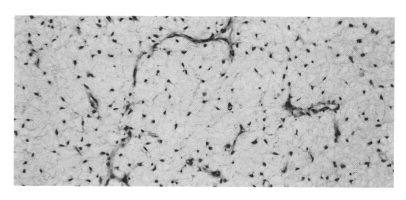

figure 2.64

Low-power view of a vaginal fibroma (left) shows an intact squamous epithelium covering a homogenous mass of proliferating fibroblasts. On

higher power (right), proliferating capillaries are seen to form a delicate pattern in the otherwise uniform mass.

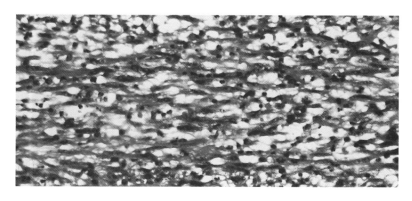
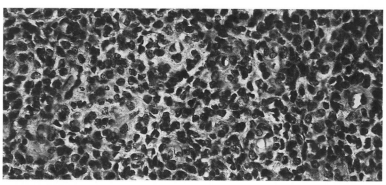

figure 2.65

Photomicrograph of a fibrosarcoma shows that this tumor also is composed of fibroblasts but they are large and atypical.

figure 2.66

Although the undifferentiated sarcoma shown in this photomicrograph arose in the vaginal wall, this tumor is not unique to the vagina.

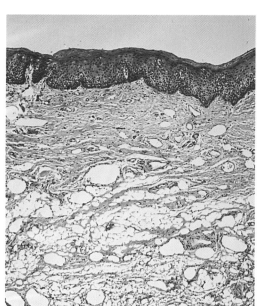

figure 2.67

Photomicrograph showing an extremely rare example of an adenomatoid tumor in the vaginal wall. Cystic spaces are lined with both cuboidal-type and mesothelial-type cells, and there is a minimal stromal response.

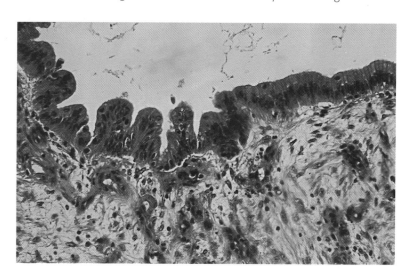

figure 2.68

This mucinous metastatic tumor appeared in the vaginal vault following surgical therapy for pseudomyxoma peritonei. The histology of this low-grade tumor is illustrative of the primary process consisting of cytologically benign mucinous epithelium.

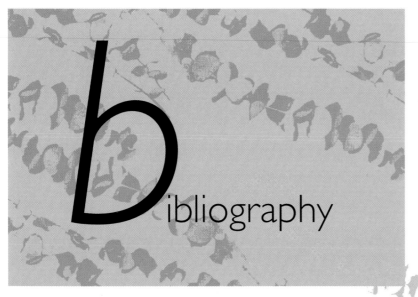

bibliography

Barnes AB: Diethylstilbestrol in gynecology and infertility. In Taymor ML, Nelson JH (eds.): *Progress in Gynecology.* New York, Grune & Stratton, 1983.

Davos I, Abell MR: Sarcomas of the vagina. *Obstet Gynecol* 47:342, 1976.

Forsberg JG: Cervicovaginal epithelium: Its origin and development. *Am J Obstet Gynecol* 115:1025, 1973.

Gardner HL, Kaufman RH: *Benign Diseases of the Vulva and Vagina.* St. Louis, CV Mosby Co., 1969.

Herbst AL, Ulfelder H, Poskanzer DC: Adenocarcinoma of the vagina: Association of maternal stilbestrol therapy with tumor appearance in young women. *N Engl J Med* 284:878, 1971.

Jones HW Jr., Rock JA: *Reparative and Constructive Surgery of the Female Genital Tract.* Williams & Wilkins, Baltimore, 1983.

Norris HJ, Taylor HB: Melanomas of the vagina. *Am J Clin Pathol* 46:420, 1966.

Norris HJ, Taylor HB: Polyps of the vagina—A benign lesion resembling sarcoma botryoides. *Cancer* 19:227, 1966.

Novak ER, Woodruff JD: *Novak's Gynecologic and Obstetric Pathology.* WB Saunders, Philadelphia, 1979.

Sternberg WH, Clark WH, Smith RC: Malignant mixed müllerian tumor (mixed mesodermal tumor of the uterus). *Cancer* 7:704, 1954.

Terruhn V: A study of impression moulds of the genital tract of female fetuses. *Arch Gynecol* 229:207, 1980.

Woodruff JD, Parmley TH: Epidermoid carcinoma of the vagina. In Evans TN, Hafez ESE (eds.): *Human Vagina.* Amsterdam, Elsevier-North Holland, 1978.

Woodruff JD, Parmley TH: Vaginal tumors, benign and malignant. In Evans TN, Hafez ESE (eds.): *Human Vagina.* Amsterdam, Elsevier-North Holland, 1978.

Cervix

development and histology

During the second trimester of pregnancy, the stroma, in that portion of the wall of the müllerian duct which will become the cervix, begins to differentiate (Fig. 3.1). This results in a relative increase in its structural rigidity. Injection studies suggest that in association with this increase in structural rigidity, the endocervical canal ceases to be functionally patent to the external environment. Meanwhile, the vagina enlarges and envelops the lower pole of the developing cervix, thus producing the fornices.

As the cervical body develops the adult form and as the endocervical canal ceases to be in contact with the vaginal milieu, the columnar epithelium of the müllerian duct lining the endocervix ceases to be converted to a squamous epithelium. The result is a junction of vaginal squamous epithelium and endocervical columnar epithelium at the external os of the cervix (Figs. 3.2 and 3.3). The squamous epithelium is multicell-layered and stratified (Fig. 3.4). A basal layer consists of small dark cells with prominent nuclei and only a little basophilic cytoplasm (Fig. 3.5). Above this layer, parabasal cells develop additional basophilic cytoplasm. Above the parabasal cells, glycogen is synthesized in the intermediate cell layer. As routine processing removes glycogen, the cells are clear in H & E sections. They also demonstrate flattening and intercellular bridges (Fig. 3.6). The most superficial cells are highly flattened and contain small dark pyknotic nuclei. Their cytoplasm contains less glycogen and more structural protein, and consequently is eosinophilic.

In the endocervical canal, the epithelium is composed of a single cell layer of columnar mucin-producing cells. Undifferentiated reserve cells are occasionally seen along the basement membrane. These are the source of epithelial renewal (Fig. 3.7). The endocervical epithelium is thrown into complex folds that result in the formation of a papillary frondlike surface (Fig. 3.8), which becomes less complex and flatter, higher in the canal. The normal endocervix is viewed grossly in Figure 3.9.

The stromal tissue which differentiates into the body of the cervix includes that portion of the embryonic mesoderm containing both the wolffian and müllerian ducts. Consequently, remnants of the wolffian duct may or may not persist in the wall of the adult cervix. Most often these remnants

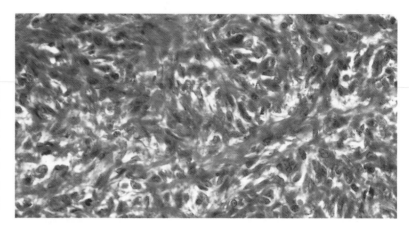

figure 3.1

Eosinophilic fibrillar bands in the developing cervical wall consist of collagen and elastic fibers. This cervical stroma is becoming adultlike in the second trimester.

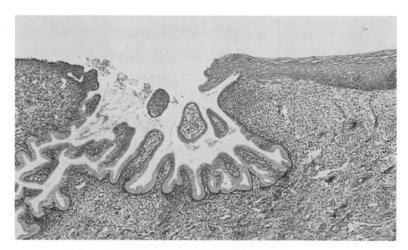

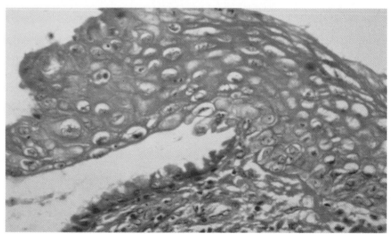

figure 3.2

The squamous epithelium (top) extends to the right, while the mucinous epithelium lines the cleft to the left. Slight darkening of the stroma of the papillary frond to the left and of the stroma just beneath the squamocolumnar junction indicates an inflammatory infiltrate. A higher power view (bottom) shows the details of the squamocolumnar junction. There is some blunting of the columnar cells of the mucinous epithelium, as well as increased cytoplasmic eosinophilia. Both are consistent with the underlying inflammation.

consist of a few tubules lined by cuboidal cells with clear-cut cell borders and a prominent basement membrane (Fig. 3.10). Occasionally, a sufficient number of tubules is present as to suggest that proliferation has occurred; if that is the case, the term *mesonephric adenoma* is used (Fig. 3.11). Even if remnants of the wolffian duct are not present, the site of its course is clearly discernible in the cervix, as the cervical stroma is separated into two laminae at this level. The external or deeper lamina consists of fairly well delineated smooth muscle and firm connective tissue, while the most superficial lamina is a loose, reticular layer. In the endocervix, this looser layer is the lamina propria that contains the papillary fronds and the intervening clefts (Fig. 3.12). The line of demarcation between the two laminae is approximately 5 mm from the surface, in many cases. However, prenatal DES may significantly alter cervical development (Fig. 3.13).

Cervical Eversion

The bilaminar organization of the cervical wall is important, because when the cervix hypertrophies in response to sex steroids, the inner lamina hypertrophies more. As a result, endocervical tissue tends to pout through the external os, producing an eversion of the mucus-secreting epithelium into the vaginal environment. This occurs most prominently in the newborn, at puberty, and at the time of the first pregnancy.

When endocervical mucus-secreting epithelium is everted into the vagina, it is damaged by the high acidity found there. The damage is expressed by a subepithelial inflammatory infiltrate and by alteration of the mucin-producing epithelial cells (Fig. 3.14), which change from tall cells with clear or faintly eosinophilic cytoplasm to cuboidal ones with a smaller amount of eosinophilic cytoplasm. Subsequently, a repair process is initiated—that of squamous metaplasia. Undifferentiated reserve cells along the basement membrane proliferate and produce a layer of basal-type cells that elevate the mucin-producing epithelium (Fig. 3.15). Further proliferation results in a four- to five-cell layer of parabasal-type cells, before the mucinous epithelium is lost (Fig. 3.16). The epithelium that results from this process may remain an immature squamous-type epithelium or it may

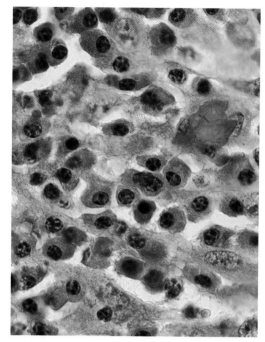

figure 3.3

The inflammatory response in the normal transformation zone (top) is characterized by a heavy influx of plasma cells. IgG antibodies are a prominent part of the local immune response. In this case (center), the endocervical mucous-secreting epithelium is less damaged because no eversion was present and there is little inflammation at the site of the squamocolumnar junction. This colposcopic view (bottom) illustrates an acute squamocolumnar transition that might give rise to a picture such as that seen in the center slide. (Courtesy of Dr. D. Bard.)

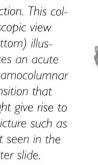

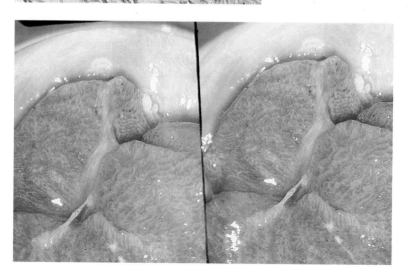

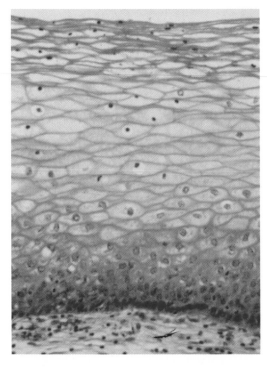

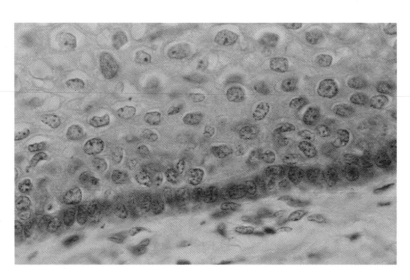

figure 3.4

Approximately three cell layers of parabasal-type cells with eosinophilic cytoplasm overlie the single cell layer of basal-type cells. Above these cells, the intermediate cells have a clear cytoplasm and well-defined cell membranes. Their nuclei are small and dark, and become progressively so, as the surface is approached.

figure 3.5

The basal-cell layer, a single cell layer with parabasal cells above it, is well defined. In the top of the photograph, the cytoplasmic clearing indicates that glycogen production is beginning.

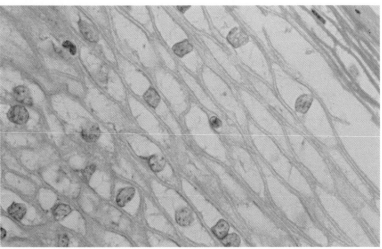

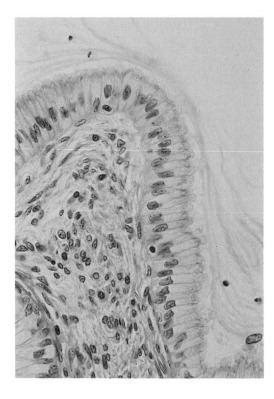

figure 3.7

A single cell layer of tall, columnar, mucin-producing cells lines this endocervical surface. Two indifferent cells are seen in the base of this strip of columnar epithelium.

figure 3.6

Large amounts of glycogen have been removed from their intermediate cells, leaving them apparently "clear." Their cell borders are thick and attached by intercellular bridges. Nuclei become less prominent, as one goes from the parabasal layer (in the lower left) to the surface (in the upper right), where the flattened cells are eosinophilic rather than clear.

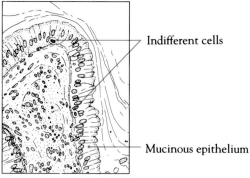

Indifferent cells

Mucinous epithelium

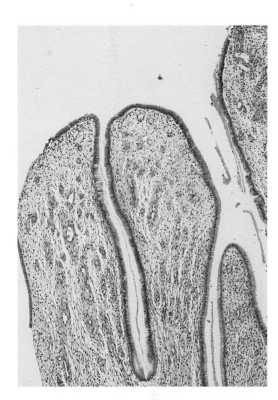

figure 3.8

The endocervical surface is thrown up into papillary fronds lined by a single cell layer of columnar mucin-producing cells.

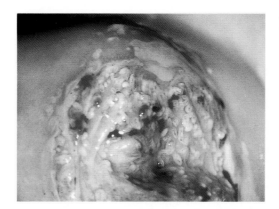

figure 3.9

The normal endocervix is seen grossly. It is significantly everted, and metaplasia is occurring. (Courtesy of Dr. John Hawkinson.)

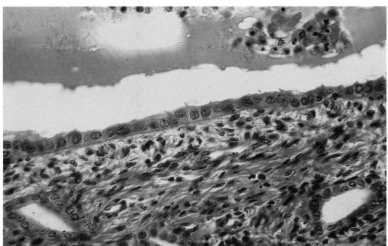

figure 3.10

A single cell layer of cuboidal cells rests on a clearly defined basement membrane in this mesonephric duct remnant. Three tubules lie below the main duct.

3.5

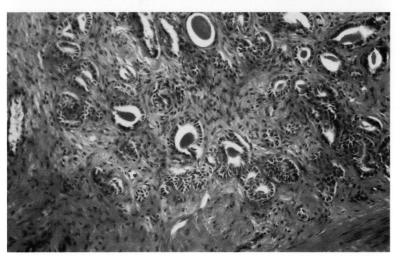

figure 3.11

The pattern of multiple tubules, seen here, is termed a mesonephric adenoma. The eosinophilic intraluminal secretion is typical.

cervix

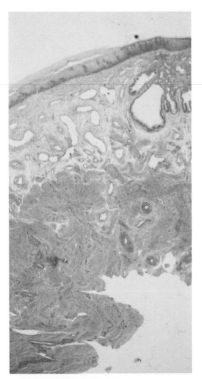
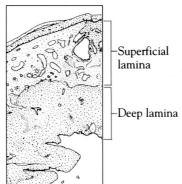

Superficial lamina

Deep lamina

figure 3.12

As seen in this photomicrograph, the most superficial lamina of the cervix is loose and vascular. It contains the endocervical clefts, but extends beneath the squamous epithelium (to the left), well out onto the vaginal portion of the cervix. The deeper lamina is denser and contains more muscle and collagen.

3.6

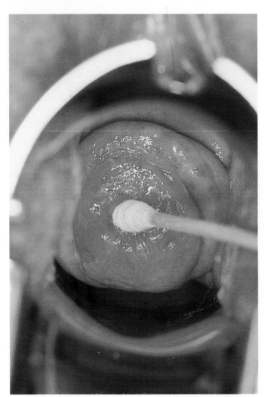
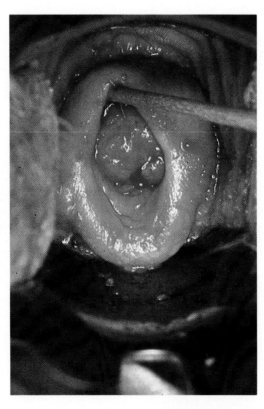

figure 3.13

The body of the cervix (left) is flattened so that the vaginal mucosa forms a collar around it. Red endocervical epithelium extends out onto the cervix and vagina. In this case (right), almost no cervical body exists. A vaginal collar contains an orifice, the endocervix. (Courtesy of Dr. D. Bard.)

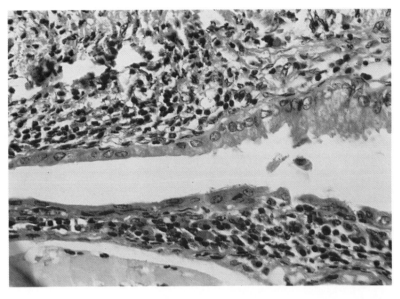

figure 3.14

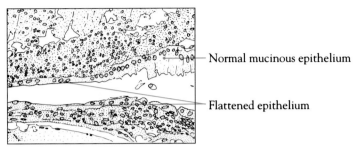

Normal mucinous epithelium, without an underlying infiltrate, lines the cleft to the right and above. To the left and above, the mucinous epithelium is flattened with an underlying infiltrate; the cytoplasm is eosinophilic. Below, the cleft is lined by even more flattened eosinophilic epithelium, and the underlying infiltrate is more intense.

—— Normal mucinous epithelium

—— Flattened epithelium

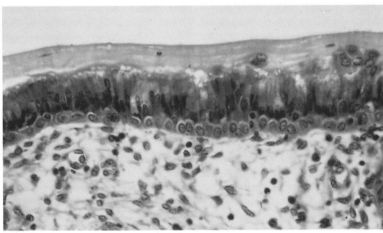

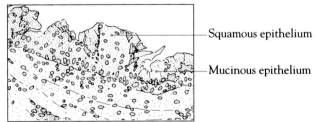

figure 3.15

This mucinous epithelium (left) is elevated by a single cell layer of basal-type cells that represent the initial stage of squamous metaplasia. Benign squamous metaplasia (right) is covering this eversion.

Although it lacks opacity, no distinctive vascular pattern is seen. (Courtesy of Dr. Joseph Buscema.)

figure 3.16

Focally, the basal cell layer is overlain by maturing squamous cells. The mucinous epithelium is elevated and is eventually lost at these sites.

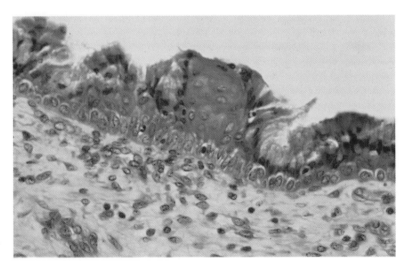

—— Squamous epithelium

—— Mucinous epithelium

cervix

possess cells with both mucin-producing and squamous differentiation (Fig. 3.17). Eventually, however, it becomes a mature stratified squamous epithelium, not unlike that found on the adjacent ectocervix, although a line of demarcation may be apparent late in the process (Fig. 3.18). When a mature stratified squamous epithelium has developed, the subepithelial inflammation clears.

The repair process that transforms the mucus-secreting epithelium into a squamous epithelium occurs in a band or zone around the external os referred to as the transformation zone (Fig. 3.19).

Newborn eversion is largely repaired by age 10, while pubertal eversion is largely repaired by the middle of the third decade of life, if no subsequent eversion occurs. The eversion that is produced by the first pregnancy may require additional years to repair.

Squamous metaplasia occurs across the tips of the papillary fronds of the endocervix because the toxic vaginal environment does not penetrate down into the clefts (Fig. 3.20). Therefore, the metaplasia tends to cover over the clefts, thus resulting in mucus-secreting epithelium trapped beneath the squamous epithelium, and in the formation of inclusion, or nabothian, cysts (Fig. 3.21).

When pregnancy occurs, the cervix hypertrophies dramatically, with the internal lamina affected more so than the external one. The clefts become deep and prominently filled with mucin (Fig. 3.22). Almost ubiquitously, microscopic foci of endometrial-type tissue are found within the endocervix, with ciliated epithelium often a prominent feature of these foci. When pregnancy occurs, these foci may demonstrate a decidual reaction (Fig. 3.23). The postpartum cervix experiences epithelial loss, and stromal hemorrhage may result in the presence of demonstrable hemosiderin for months after delivery (Fig. 3.24).

Oral contraceptives produce a hypertrophy and an eversion of the cervix similar to that produced by pregnancy. These drugs are particularly responsible for the development of microcystic mucoid metaplasia, or microglandular hyperplasia. While this epithelial alteration can occur in the absence of a history of oral contraceptives, it is most dramatic in its presence. A combination of both squamous and mucinous metaplasia may be seen. Secretory vacuoles develop within the mucin-producing cells and seem to be trapped. As they expand, the cells rupture, and adjacent vacuoles may

3.8

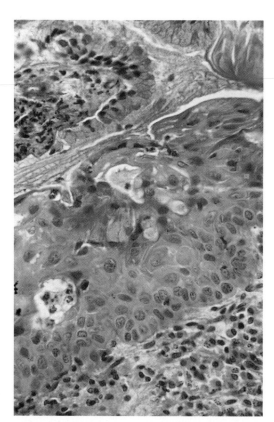

figure 3.17

An immature squamous epithelium replacing the original mucinous epithelium continues to contain cells with mucinous differentiation. Where these break down, cystic spaces containing cellular debris develop.

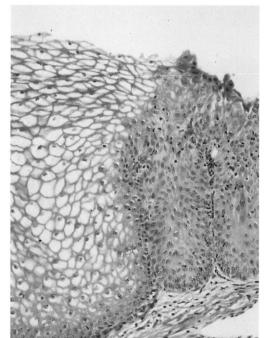

figure 3.18

To the left, mature squamous epithelium is present. To the right, immature squamous epithelium exists as the result of the metaplastic replacement of preexisting mucinous epithelium. Eventually, maturation will occur on the right, and the demarcation will be inapparent.

form a common cystic space within the epithelium, which is filled with mucin, cellular debris, and inflammatory cells. Alternatively, the mucin may extravasate into the surrounding stroma, resulting in mucinification and inflammation (Fig. 3.25). When the combination of steroids found in oral contraceptives produces the type of enlarged atypical nuclei characterizing the Arias-Stella reaction, the resulting cytologic atypicality may lead to an erroneous diagnosis of adenocarcinoma (Fig. 3.26).

Cervical Infection

One of the functions of the cervix is to separate two biologically different environments. The lower genital canal is infested with a large number of different types of microbiological flora, while the endometrial cavity is sterile. Many of the defense mechanisms that produce this separation are found in the cervix, and thus the cervix is the site of many different types of infection. Attention has already been called to the inflammation that occurs in the everted endocervix (Fig. 3.27). While not in itself infectious, this inflammation may be exaggerated by superimposed bacterial infection. Specific histologies have not been identified in association with most bacterial infections. Tuberculosis is, of course, a conspicuous exception.

NONVIRAL INFECTIONS

Nonspecific inflammation is believed to be responsible for the development of cervical polyps. These polypoid masses of endocervical tissue, on a thin or thick stalk, extend from the wall of the endocervix, down the cervical canal (Fig. 3.28). If the endocervical tissue reaches as far as the external os, then the mucus-secreting epithelium on its surface will exhibit the same metaplastic repair that occurs when an eversion exists (Fig. 3.29).

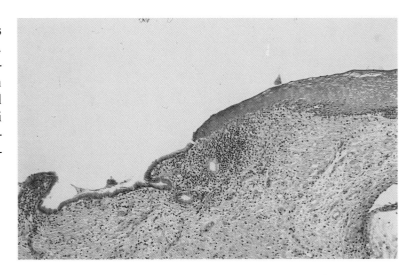

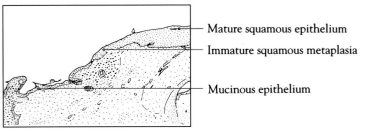

Mature squamous epithelium
Immature squamous metaplasia
Mucinous epithelium

figure 3.19

From left to right, this transformation zone illustrates mucinous epithelium lining the endocervix, immature squamous epithelium occupying the zone being transformed, and mature squamous epithelium covering the ectocervix. Note that the stromal darkening, which indicates inflammation, is largely confined to the transformation zone.

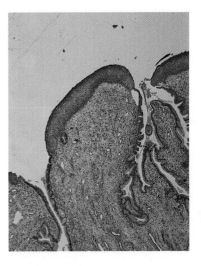

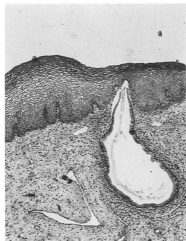

figure 3.20

The mucinous epithelium on the tip of this papillary frond has been replaced by squamous epithelium; the epithelium in the clefts is unchanged. The inflammation producing the transformation has cleared.

figure 3.21

Only remnants of an endocervical cleft persist beneath this squamous epithelium, which is extended across the tips of two adjacent papillary fronds.

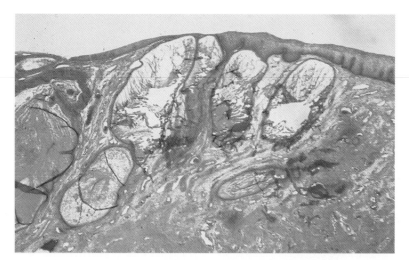

figure 3.22

The endocervical clefts seen in this pregnancy are dramatically expanded and filled with mucin. This development is striking, especially in comparison to Figures 3.2 (top), 3.12, and 3.20.

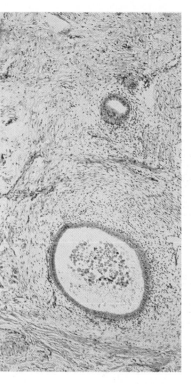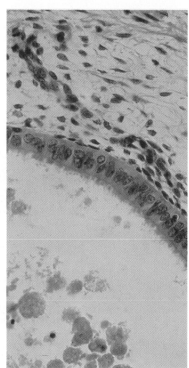

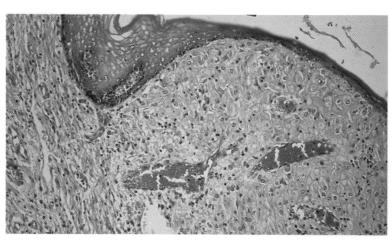

figure 3.23

The focus of endometriosis seen here (left) is deep within the cervical stroma, an atypical site. A higher power view (center) shows both epithelium and stroma. Within the lumen of the gland, large hemosiderin-laden macrophages indicate that bleeding has occurred. A sheet of decidualized stroma (right) occupies a typical site immediately beneath the squamous epithelium in this example of the cervix during pregnancy.

figure 3.24

Two months postpartum, large hemosiderin-laden macrophages still occupy the cervical stroma.

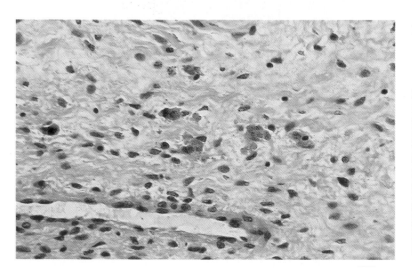

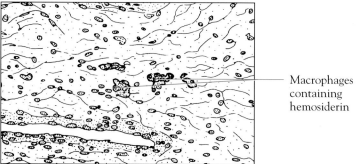

Macrophages containing hemosiderin

atlas of gynecologic pathology

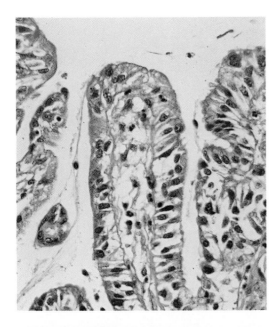

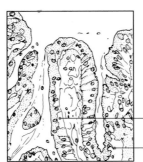

Intraepithelial cystic space

Mucin in stroma

figure 3.25

Intracellular vacuoles are coalescing into larger intraepithelial cystic spaces at several sites. In some places, the mucin is extravasating into the stroma.

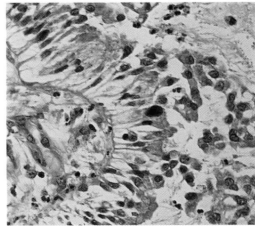

figure 3.26

In the center of this photomicrograph, a single nucleus is dramatically enlarged and atypical. This is an example of an Arias-Stella-type reaction in microglandular hyperplasia.

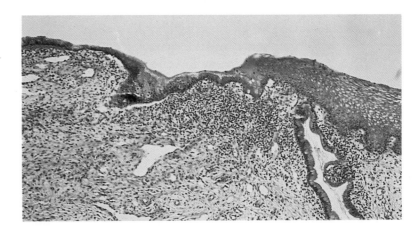

figure 3.27

An inflammatory infiltrate lies below the mucinous epithelium immediately adjacent to the squamous epithelium. The stroma, higher in the endocervix and below the mature squamous epithelium, is uninflamed.

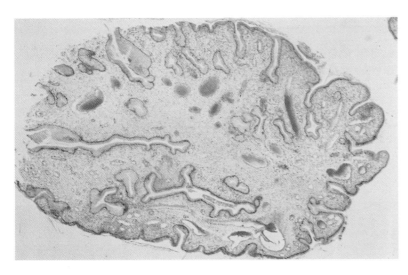

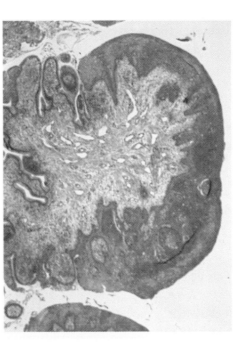

figure 3.29

This polyp protruded into the vaginal space; its exposed tip is covered with a metaplastic squamous epithelium.

figure 3.28

The endocervical polyp seen in this photomicrograph demonstrates the characteristic polypoid shape, stromal edema, and vascular injection.

Follicular cervicitis, in which prominent lymphoid follicles with germinal centers occur, has been attributed to infection by chlamydia, while other chlamydial organisms are thought to be responsible for lymphogranuloma venereum (Fig. 3.30). In some parts of the world, schistosomiasis is a prominent cause of cervical infection (Fig. 3.31).

VIRAL INFECTIONS

All of the epithelium of the lower genital canal, but particularly the immature squamous metaplasia of the transformation zone, are subject to infection with venereally transmitted viruses. While the prominent intranuclear inclusions produced by the herpesvirus in cytologic preparations are well known, the histology of herpesvirus infection, short of ulcer formation, is less well identified. In contrast, extensive descriptions of the various histologies associated with different types of human papilloma virus (HPV) are available.

Different types of HPV may be identified by using DNA hybridization techniques. While this technology is new and rapidly changing, it appears that different types of the virus are responsible for different histologies. HPV infections may be associated with very little alteration in the epithelium (Fig. 3.32), or they may possess all of the classic features of condylomata acuminata, i.e., papillomatosis, hyperkeratosis, acanthosis, and parakeratosis. Alternatively, they may demonstrate a variety of forms that show relatively dramatic atypicality (Fig. 3.33). In some cases they are characterized by koilocytosis, with little nuclear atypia beyond that of degeneration (Fig. 3.34). However, they can be characterized primarily by nuclear atypicality, including enlarged hyperchromatic smudged nuclei, empty or fragmenting nuclei, bizarre forms, and multiple nuclei. Mitoses suggesting polyploidy are present (Fig. 3.35). These atypical flat condylomata merge with similar lesions, which, in addition to the above features, contain disorganized basal layers with loss of cytoplasmic maturation and atypical mitotic figures suggesting aneuploidy (Fig. 3.36). These lesions may represent a transitional stage between HPV infection and true cervical intraepithelial neoplasia (CIN).

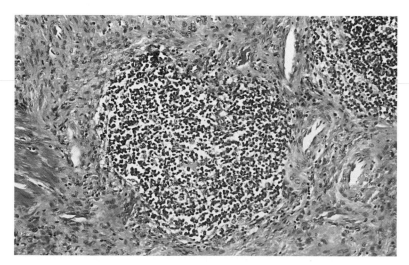

figure 3.30

One of several lymphoid follicles found in this cervix. Elsewhere, inflammation is intense. This is an example of follicular cervicitis.

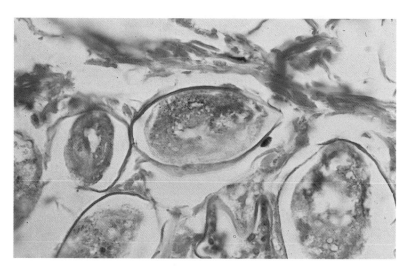

figure 3.31

Multiple encysted forms of schistosoma are embedded in scar. Calcium deposition is beginning.

Cervical Cancer

PREINVASIVE CANCER (CIN)

Cervical intraepithelial neoplasia, or preinvasive cancer, presents as a histologic spectrum consisting of a malignant squamous epithelium that displays varying amounts of cytoplasmic maturation in the upper layers of the epithelium (Figs. 3.37 and 3.38). The nuclei are typically malignant, with significant pleomorphism, and clumping or margination of chromatin; atypical mitotic figures are present. The basal cell layer is not identified as a single cell layer.

If cytoplasmic maturation begins in the bottom one-third of the epithelium, the lesion is traditionally viewed as CIN I. Among many such cases, however, are those condylomata with atypical mitotic figures described above; these are distinguishable from fully developed CIN. If cytoplasmic maturation occurs only in the topmost layers, then the lesion is a CIN III; if none occurs, then it is carcinoma in situ, although, it is not biologically different from CIN III (Fig. 3.39). Indeed, Richart (1973) has shown that all CIN are most accurately viewed as a single disease. In contrast to benign metaplasia described above, CIN does not confine itself to the tips of the papillary fronds, but instead extends into the intervening clefts; this should be distinguished from true invasion (Fig. 3.40).

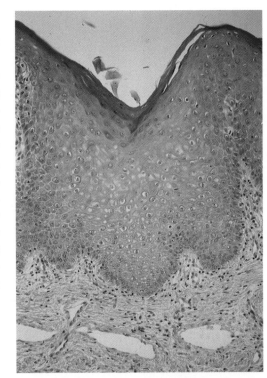

figure 3.32

This cervical condyloma (top) is characterized by epithelial hyperplasia and hyperkeratosis, but almost no cytologic atypia. More atypicality (bottom) characterizes this cervical condyloma, but it is not dramatic. Papillomatosis, acanthosis, and minimal koilocytosis are present.

INVASIVE CERVICAL CANCER

The earliest stages of invasive cervical cancer are referred to as *microinvasion*, a process which itself occurs in stages. Initially, a tongue of tumor still attached to the overlying epithelium protrudes through the basement membrane. Characteristically, it consists of a population of cells, which possess the cytoplasmic differentiation that imparts to them motility; such a tongue of invasive tumor will elicit a significant inflammatory reaction (Fig. 3.41). Subsequently, nests of tumor cells completely isolated from the overlying epithelium will develop. Characteristically, these microcarcinomas exhibit a growth pattern that results in the production of large masses of cervical tumor before much additional extension occurs, although metastases to pelvic nodes are characteristic (Fig. 3.42).

In some cases, however, the growth pattern consists of the production of additional satellite lesions before any significant mass develops at the site of the original invasion. If this growth pattern persists, the result is an infiltrative picture of lymph-vascular space involvement (Fig. 3.43). This type of growth is associated with a higher than average likelihood of nodal metastases (Fig. 3.44).

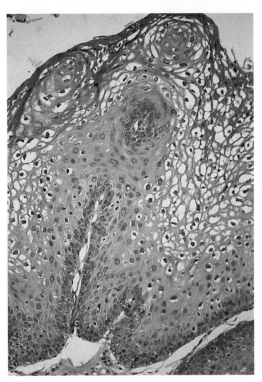

SPECIFIC HISTOLOGIC TYPES

The histology of cervical cancer is more varied than is often assumed. If the tumor consists of basal- or parabasal-type cells, it is referred to as small-cell-type cancer (Fig. 3.45). If the tumor shows maturation to the level of intermediate-type cells, it is referred to as large-cell nonkeratinizing cancer (Fig. 3.46). Only about 15% of cervical cancers illustrate significant keratinization, and these are referred to as large-cell keratinizing types. Extensive sampling of large tumors will frequently reveal heterogeneity in the degree of differentia-

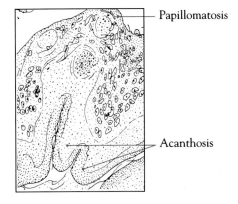

Papillomatosis

Acanthosis

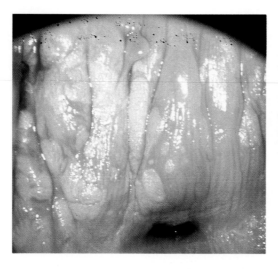

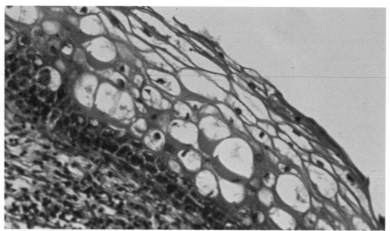

figure 3.33

These flat warts may have a variety of histologies. (Courtesy of Dr. Joseph Buscema.)

figure 3.34

Dramatic koilocytosis is the main feature of this condyloma. The nuclei are fragmenting.

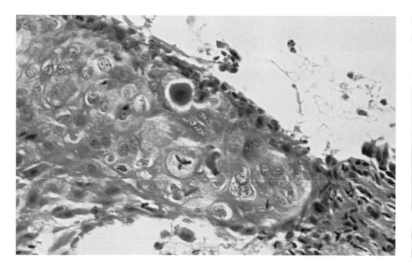

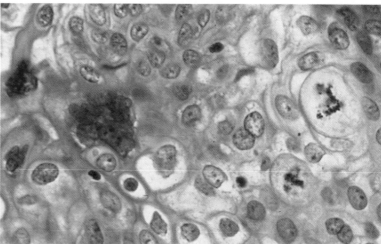

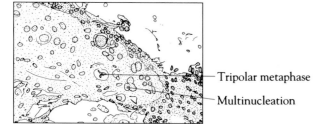

— Tripolar metaphase
— Multinucleation

figure 3.35

In addition to individual cell keratinization and nuclear atypicality (left), there are tripolar metaphase figures suggesting polyploidy. Multinucleation is present. The multinucleation and large bizarre mitotic figures (right) suggest polyploidy.

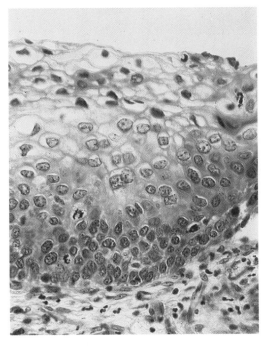

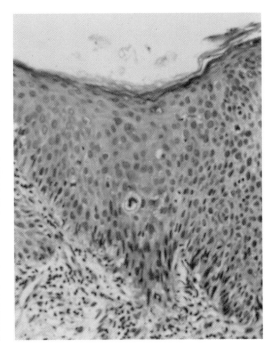

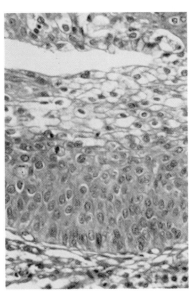

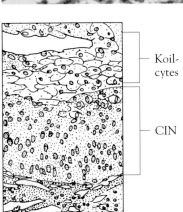

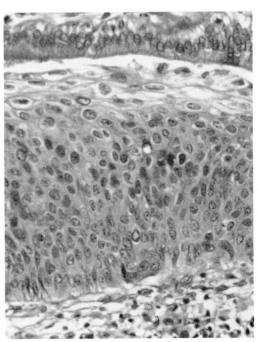

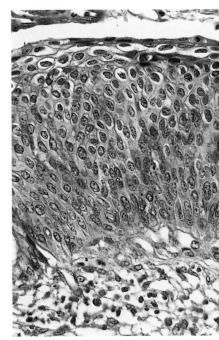

figure 3.36

Although koilocytosis, multinucleation, and nuclear degeneration (left) suggesting HPV infection are present in the upper layers of this epithelium, the lower layers are characterized by disorganization, the absence of cytoplasmic maturation, and atypical mitotic figures suggesting aneuploidy. Hyperkeratosis and nuclear degeneration (right) suggest HPV infection, particularly to the left. Atypical mitotic figures, in the absence of epithelial organization or cytologic maturation, suggest CIN.

figure 3.37

These large white plaques in the transformation zone are most compatible with CIN. (Courtesy of Dr. Joseph Buscema.)

Koil-cytes

CIN

figure 3.38

In this photograph (left), approximately 50% of the total epithelial thickness is replaced with CIN. The upper cell layers are koilocytotic, suggesting a previous HPV infection. Less than one-third of this epithelium (center) possesses cytoplasmic maturation. Classically, this is a more advanced CIN than the previous view. Only the top two or three cell layers (right) show cytoplasmic maturation. These three figures, all from different sites in the same case, illustrate the biologic unity of CIN.

cervix

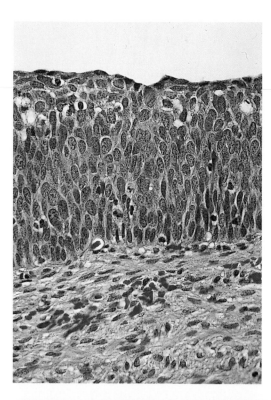

figure 3.39

The only hint of cytoplasmic maturation present in this example of carcinoma in situ is the flattened topmost cell layer.

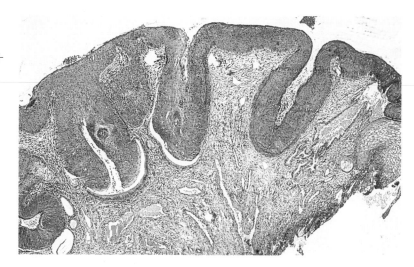

figure 3.40

Papillary fronds are separated by CIN extending into the intervening clefts.

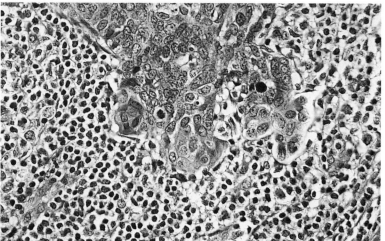

figure 3.41

Three tongues of cells with relative cytoplasmic eosinophilia extend from the overlying basophilic epithelium into the underlying stroma. An intense inflammatory reaction is present.

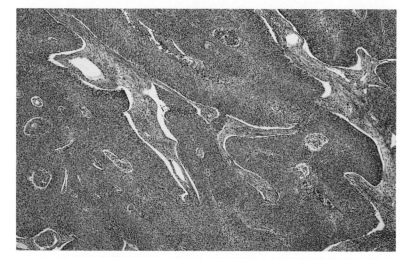

figure 3.42

A solid tumor has replaced most of the cervical stroma, resulting in a large tumor mass. The tumor is a small-cell type.

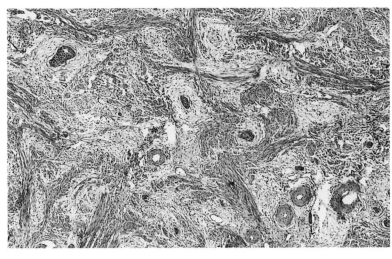 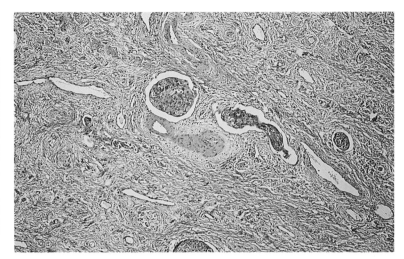

figure 3.43

The tumor (left) is widely infiltrating throughout the cervical stroma, but there is little tumor mass. Multiple apparent lymph-vascular channels (right) are filled with infiltrating tumor, but there is little tumor mass.

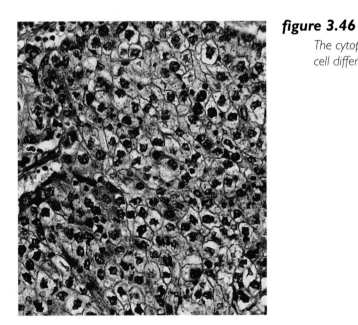 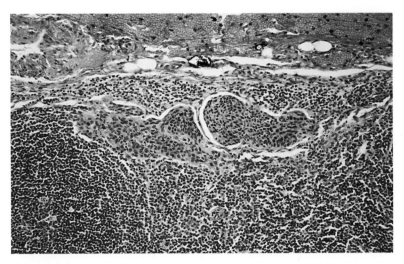

figure 3.44

Metastatic small-cell-type cancer occupies the peripheral sinus of this pelvic lymph node. It has not yet begun to extend into the node.

figure 3.45

This cervical cancer is composed of basal- and parabasal-type cells. Mitoses are frequent.

figure 3.46

The cytoplasm of these cells is clear and consistent with intermediate cell differentiation. This is a large-cell nonkeratinizing-type tumor.

cervix

tion (Fig. 3.47). When a tumor of any cell type invades anew, it again develops the population of eosinophilic, apparently mature cells seen with the original microinvasion.

When cervical cancer has invaded less than 3 mm from the overlying basement membrane, pelvic node metastases is unlikely; however, in an invasion of 3 to 5 mm, particularly in cases of infiltrative lymph–vascular space involvement, the incidence of metastases to the pelvic nodes may reach 10%. A more significant invasion that is still confined to the cervix is associated with a 15 to 30% incidence of nodal disease. In general, the incidence of para-aortic node involvement is one third to one half that of the pelvic nodes at any given stage of the disease. Grossly, squamous cell cancers of the cervix may present in the exophytic or endophytic forms of classic pathologic descriptions (Fig. 3.48). Endophytic forms tend to result in so-called barrel-shaped cervices and probably represents more aggressive disease. MRI shows much promise as a method for detecting gross extent of tumors in the pelvic soft tissues (Fig. 3.49).

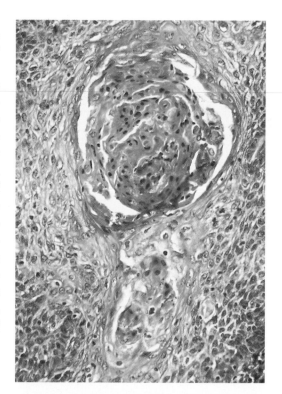

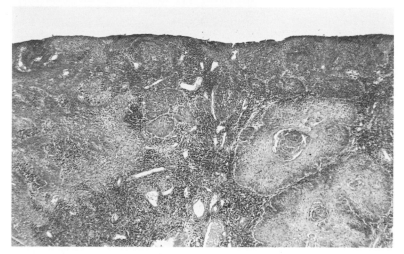

figure 3.47

A well-developed keratin "pearl" characterizes this example of large-cell keratinizing tumor (top). A lower power view of the same tumor (bottom) shows that, in other fields, the degree of cellular differentiation varies. A small-cell population occupies the left side of the field and the large-cell keratinizing component is on the right.

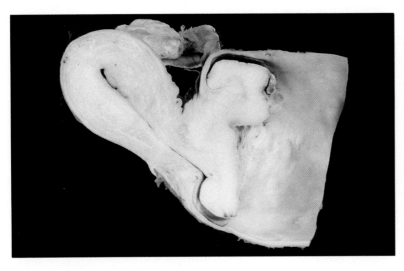
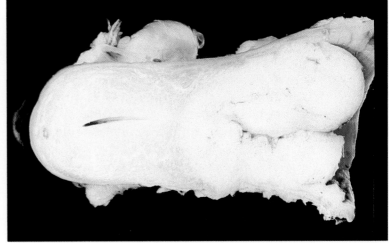

figure 3.48

A large exophytic mass (left) dilates the upper vagina. Despite its broad extent, it has a relatively small attachment to the anterior lip of the cervix. This mass (right) does not extend throughout the vagina, *but occupies and dilates almost the entire cervix as well as extending up into the myometrium. (From Tuck and Fletcher, 1985.)*

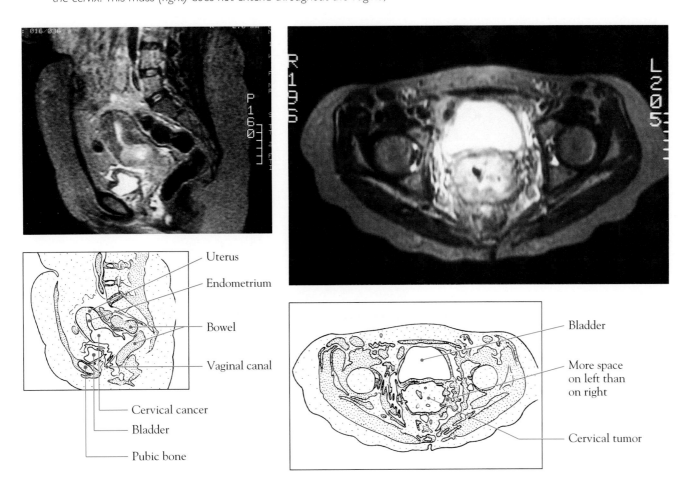

Uterus

Endometrium

Bowel

Vaginal canal

Cervical cancer

Bladder

Pubic bone

Bladder

More space on left than on right

Cervical tumor

figure 3.49

Saggital T2-weighted MRI of cervical carcinoma (left). The endometrial cavity is continuous with a large bright signal mass that involves the whole cervix. The mass extends to the upper half of the vagina, obliterating the vaginal canal. The lower half is identified as a bright linear echo designating the vaginal canal. Axial T2-weighted MRI *of cervical carcinoma (right) viewed through the cervix shows a bulky mass replacing the whole thickness of the cervix. There is marked necrosis within the mass. The right paracervical region is partially obliterated, suggesting extension from the mass.*

cervix

Other cell types occur in cervical cancer. Here, as elsewhere in the lower genital canal, a well-differentiated verrucous carcinoma may be seen (Fig. 3.50). The small-cell cancer mentioned above is composed of basal- and parabasal-type cells, but a true small-cell lesion occasionally is seen in the cervix. It is composed of cells with a small amount of basophilic cytoplasm and a small dense nucleus (Fig. 3.51). Whether or not the examples of this lesion reported in the past correspond to the lesions with neurosecretory granules described below is problematic. As elsewhere in the body, these may be highly aggressive lesions, and some may be examples of primary lymphomas.

Invasive cancers composed of well-differentiated basal-type cells resembling basal-cell carcinomas of the skin develop in the cervix. The infiltrating cells produce solid cords and nests that penetrate the underlying cervical stroma, but usually they are not very extensive. These adenoid basal tumors are discovered incidentally in most cases (Fig. 3.52). A histologically similar lesion is one in which cystic spaces fill with an eosinophilic material developing in the epithelial cords. These usually are more extensive tumors and are termed adenoid cystic (Fig. 3.53). On a stage-for-stage basis, they are as aggressive as other cervical cancers. Some examples of these or similar small-cell tumors have suggested carcinoids. Neurosecretory granules have been identified ultrastructurally in some cases.

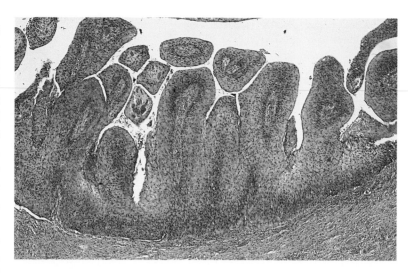

figure 3.50

Although the cervix and upper vagina were replaced by tumor, this warty growth is composed of well-differentiated squamous epithelium and is only locally invasive, although deeply set.

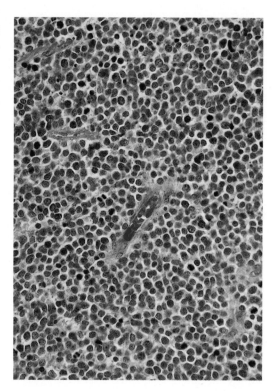

figure 3.51

This small-cell cancer is composed entirely of undifferentiated small cells more typical of the lymphoma than of cervical cancer. It is clinically primary.

3.20

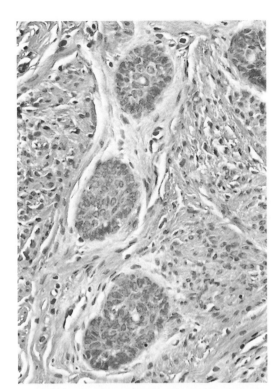

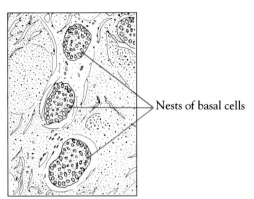

Nests of basal cells

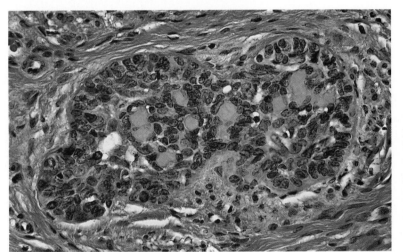

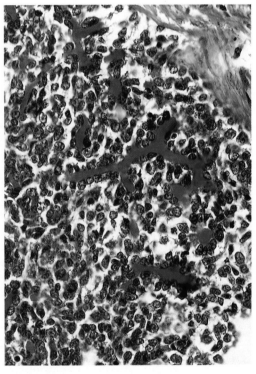

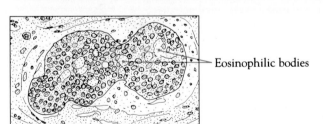

Eosinophilic bodies

figure 3.53
Small eosinophilic collections (left) produce a folliculoid pattern in this cervical cancer. The cells are basal in type. There is little tissue destruction in the tumor. The eosinophilic material (right) forms anastomosing cords among the basal-type cells.

3.21

cervix

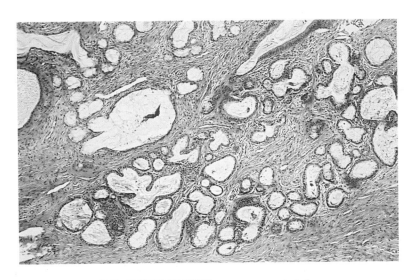

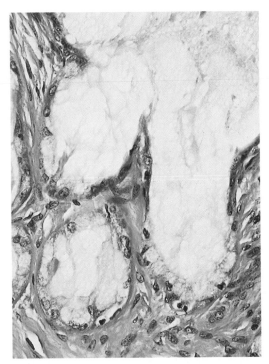

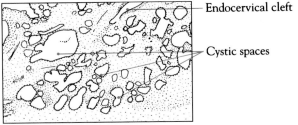

Endocervical cleft

Cystic spaces

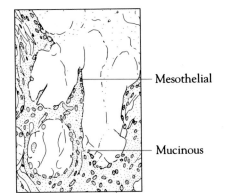

Mesothelial

Mucinous

figure 3.54

Multiple crowded cystic spaces (left) associated with a minimal amount of reactive stroma lie at the base of an otherwise normal endocervical cleft. This focus of adenomatous hyperplasia was incidental, as is routine. Both columnar, mucinous, and flattened mesothelial-type cells (right) line the cystic spaces in this focus of adenomatous hyperplasia.

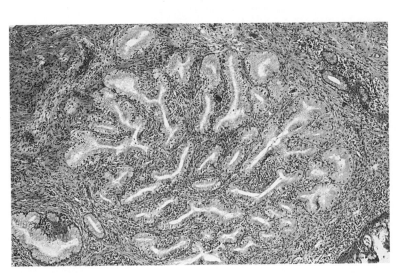

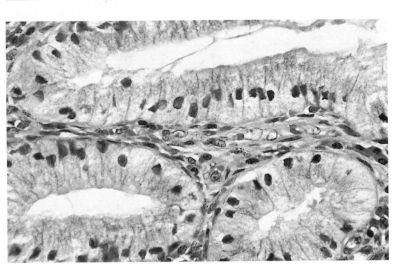

figure 3.55

This crowded collection of endocervical clefts (left) appears to represent an adenomatous proliferation of endocervical epithelium. There is associated inflammation. The epithelium (right) is only mildly atypical.

The nuclei are somewhat hyperchromatic and tend to be elevated from the basal portion of the cells.

atlas of gynecologic pathology

endocervical alterations

METAPLASIA, HYPERPLASIA, AND NEOPLASIA

Metaplasia, hyperplasia, and neoplasia also are seen in the endocervical epithelium. The most common metaplasia is probably that of ciliated or endometrial-type epithelium in endocervical glands. The microcystic mucoid metaplasia or microglandular hyperplasia associated with oral contraceptives has been mentioned. Among hyperplasias, perhaps the most common is adenomatous hyperplasia of the endocervix. This common lesion, without clinical significance, is presumed to be of hormonal origin. It consists of proliferation of the endocervical epithelium with cystic dilatation of the clefts and an associated stromal reaction (Fig. 3.54). The epithelium of the hyperplastic glands is made up of cuboidal, mucin-producing cells, as well as flattened mesothelial-type cells. The pattern is similar to that seen in adenomatoid tumors elsewhere in the genital canal. Occasionally, endocervical clefts and glands are sufficiently crowded as to suggest the formation of an adenoma, although the clinical significance of such a lesion is unknown. The epithelium is normal or only slightly atypical in these cases (Fig. 3.55). An unusual papillary proliferation, also of unknown significance, has been seen in the cervix (Fig. 3.56).

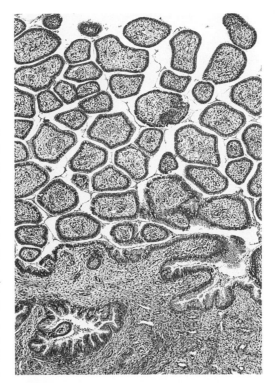

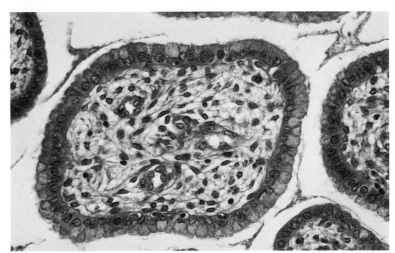

figure 3.56

The endocervix (top) is composed of proliferating papillae containing a stromal core. There is no evidence of extension into the underlying tissue. The epithelium over the papillae (bottom) is minimally undifferentiated. Some of the cells have a goblet-type appearance. The stroma is cellular and appears to be participating in the proliferative process.

ADENOCARCINOMA

Malignant neoplasia occurs in the endocervical epithelium as well. There are epidemiologic studies suggesting that adenocarcinoma of the cervix is an estrogen-related disease similar to endometrial or ovarian cancer, but there is histologic evidence that it develops in a background similar to that of epidermoid cancer of the transformation zone. Atypical endocervical cells, with nuclear changes similar to those seen in a squamous epithelium infected with HPV, have been seen, and viral DNA has been identified in some cervical adeno-carcinomas (Fig. 3.57). Early adenocarcinomas of the endocervix are often associated with coexisting CIN (Fig. 3.58). While examples of endocervical carcinoma are seen that are extremely superficial and presumably still *intraepithelial* (Fig. 3.59), criteria for distinguishing in situ, microinvasive, and fully developed invasive adenocarcinoma, have been difficult to establish (Fig. 3.60).

3.24

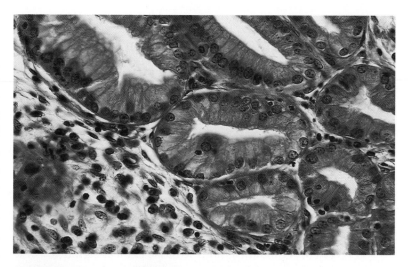

figure 3.57

A large, multinucleated cell (top) occupies this endocervical gland. Multinucleation and nuclear smudging (bottom) characterize these endocervical cells.

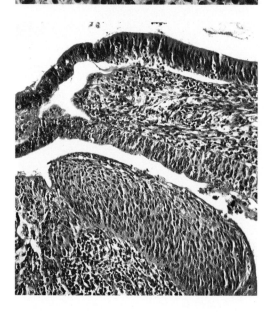

figure 3.58

Malignant glandular epithelium lines the papillary frond above, while a focus of typical CIN is seen below.

Histologically, endocervical adenocarcinoma may resemble any of the adenocarcinomas seen in the upper genital canal. Mucinous (Fig. 3.61), endometrial (Fig. 3.62), serous (Fig. 3.63), clear-cell (Fig. 3.64), papillary (Fig. 3.65), and mixed types have been identified. Among the mixed epithelial types, those with a component of squamous epithelium are the most dramatic (Fig. 3.66), while others, such as combinations of mucinous and endometrial-type epithelium, are more common. A particularly well differentiated form of the mucinous endocervical adenocarcinoma has been singled out by some, but its clinical behavior is as aggressive as the others. Undifferentiated forms are also common (Fig. 3.67).

While early adenocarcinomas tend to be multicentric, they are not commonly seen. This is because endocervical cancer is detected less readily by routine screening procedures than the more common cervical cancer, presumably because it occurs higher in the endocervical canal. Consequently, adenocarcinomas are more advanced by the time they are diagnosed. There is no evidence that on a stage-for-stage basis they behave any more malignantly than epidermoid carcinomas arising in the transformation zone.

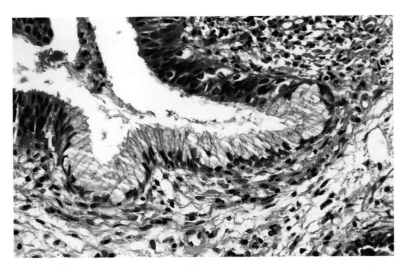

figure 3.59

The malignant glandular epithelium seen in continuity with the benign mucinous epithelium in this endocervical cleft is presumably still in situ, though it is not apparent how it would differ histologically if it were not.

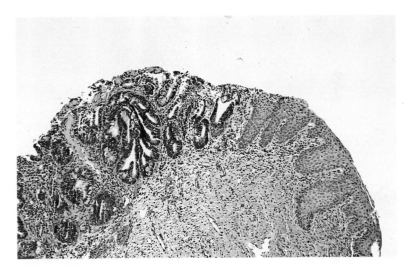

figure 3.60

This adenocarcinoma is quite superficial and still confined to that portion of the cervix which contains the clefts. The degree of arborization of the glands and the amount of tissue reaction suggest invasion; however, no definite conclusion is possible.

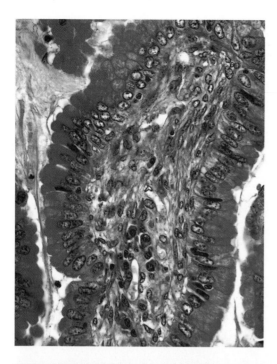

figure 3.61

The epithelium is clearly mucinous, but this cervical adenocarcinoma was deeply invasive. Nuclear atypicality is apparent.

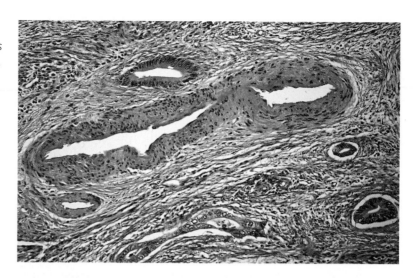

figure 3.62

This endocervical adenocarcinoma is composed of endometrial-type epithelium, forming glands. In addition, it is demonstrating the same infiltrative growth pattern illustrated in Figure 3.43.

3.26

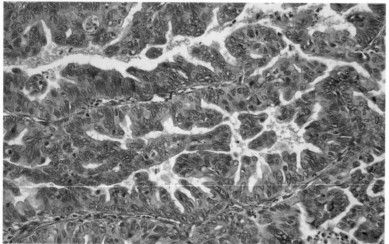

figure 3.64

This is a typical clear cell cancer as seen in the vagina, endometrium, and ovary.

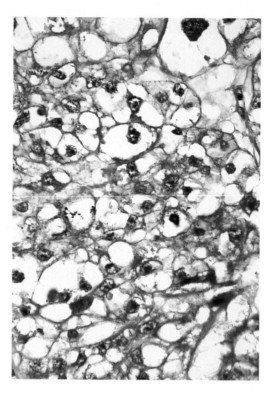

figure 3.63

This finely papillary serous tumor is characteristic of lesions seen higher in the genital canal.

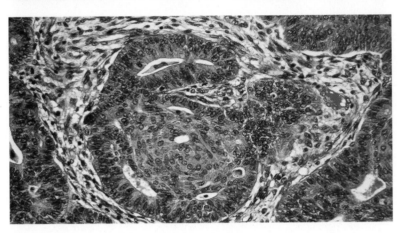

figure 3.65

This papillary lesion has a variety of cell types.

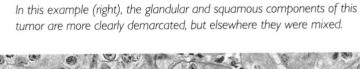

figure 3.66

This endometrioid tumor (left) contains a squamous component that produces a pattern similar to the adenoacanthoma in the endometrium.

In this example (right), the glandular and squamous components of this tumor are more clearly demarcated, but elsewhere they were mixed.

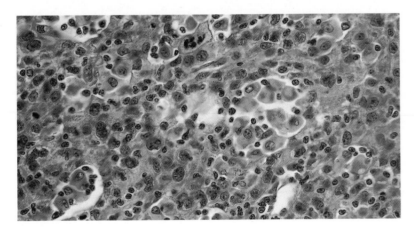

figure 3.67

Foamy cytoplasm and relatively large cells characterize this undifferentiated lesion (left). The very distinctive appearance (right) produced by

the large amount of foamy cytoplasm in this undifferentiated tumor has resulted in the term glassy-cell carcinoma.

cervix

Other Cervical Neoplasms

MELANOMA

Melanomas are only rarely seen in the cervix. Apparently, they arise in cervical nevi (Fig. 3.68), which are also rare. It is not clear what type of aberrant embryology results in the presence of these neural crest cells in the cervix. Melanomas, of course, are highly malignant tumors, and in this site they are likely to be advanced by the time they have broken through the surface and have been recognized (Fig. 3.69). Treatment is surgical, initially.

SARCOMA

Among the sarcomas, all of the histologic types known to occur in the genital canal have been described, at least on occasion, in the cervix. When embryonic sarcomas produce sarcoma botryoides in infants, they develop in the lower vagina. However, in older children and in teenagers, they develop in the upper vagina and cervix. Classically these lesions are diagnosed late. Although they have been treated by radical surgery in the past, chemotherapy may have some usefulness in the future. Leiomyomas of the routine type, cellular leiomyomas, and leiomyosarcomas have been described in the cervix (Fig. 3.70). Their histology is not different from that of the same lesions seen elsewhere in the genital canal, but the malignant forms of this tumor are almost invariably diagnosed late because of their subepithelial site of origin. They are treated surgically, when they can be treated at all.

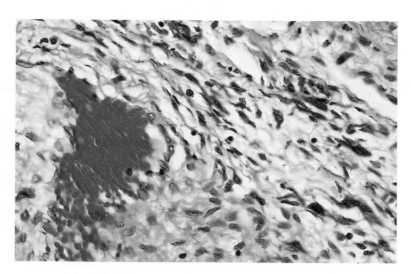

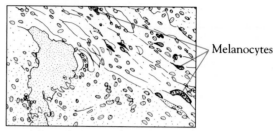
Melanocytes

figure 3.68

Melanocytes in profusion occupy the stroma in this cervical nevus. The lesion was grossly pigmented. (Courtesy of Dr. Belur Bhagavan.)

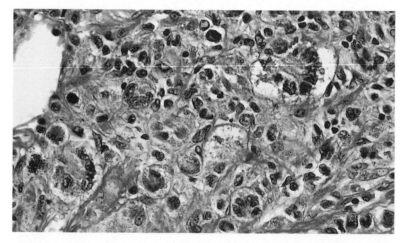

figure 3.69

Several clear-cut rosettes are seen in this malignant melanoma. (Courtesy of Dr. Belur Bhagavan.)

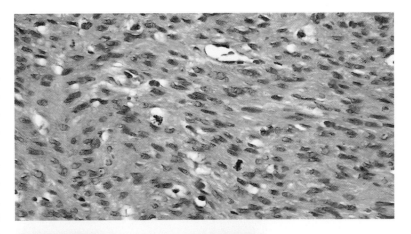

MIXED MESODERMAL TUMORS

Stromal sarcomas of all grades have been described in the cervix (Fig. 3.71). Some endocervical polyps are characterized by stromal hyperplasia. More aggressive stromal sarcomas arise in the soft tissue of the cervical wall. Mixed mesodermal tumors arising in the cervix tend to present as polypoid lesions, and whenever large polyps are observed in the cervix, either descending from the endometrium or arising from the cervix itself, the possibility of mixed mesodermal tumor should be considered. The low-grade ones, such as adenofibroma and adenosarcomas, present symptoms before they have progressed too far and thus are treated successfully with surgery (Fig. 3.72). Similar outcomes are unlikely with high-grade mixed mesodermal tumors. All histologic types are found in the cervix, and, apart from grade, their histology seems to have no bearing (Fig. 3.73). Treatment is surgical.

metastatic tumors

Metastatic tumors also occur in the cervix (Fig. 3.74). The most common example is endometrial malignancy that extends into the cervix directly at the level of the epithelium or, alternatively, in the subepithelial stroma. It may metastasize to the endocervix from the endometrium in a skip manner that suggests multicentric origin. Occasionally, multicentric origin may be the true explanation for this appearance.

Occasionally, ovarian disease is metastatic to the cervix. Usually, this occurs when ovarian tumors extend through the cul-de-sac into the posterior cervical wall. More rarely, distant neoplasms involve the cervix and produce infiltrative patterns.

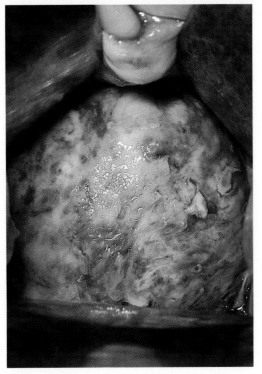

figure 3.70

Smooth muscle cells, with large atypical nuclei (top), characterize this leiomyosarcoma. A mitotic figure is present. This alarming looking tumor (bottom) was a benign leiomyoma. (Courtesy of Dr. D. Bard.)

cervix

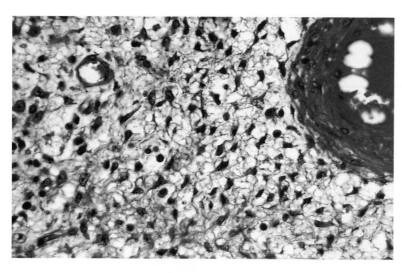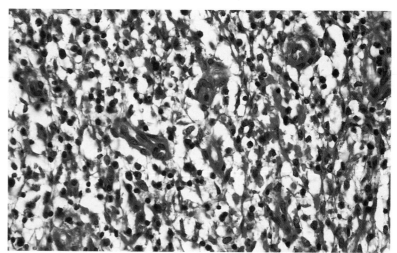

figure 3.71

This stromal sarcoma (left) is composed of large atypical cells in an edematous stroma. A greater degree of cellularity (right) is apparent in this lesion. The cells are smaller, and there is less edema.

3.30

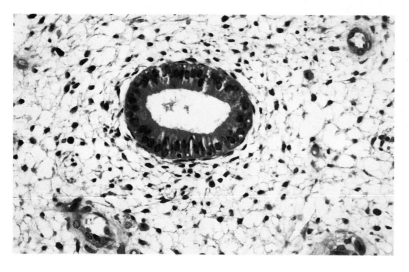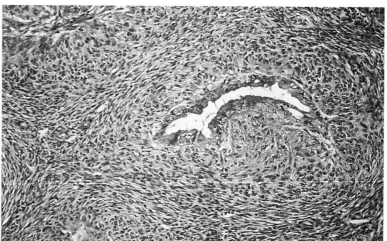

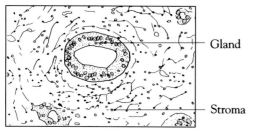

Gland

Stroma

figure 3.72

The epithelium in this mixed tumor appears benign, but it is embedded in a sarcoma similar to that seen in Figure 3.71 (left). The apparently benign glands were sparse in this tumor.

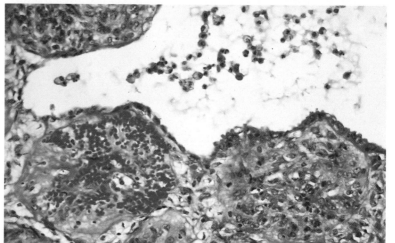

figure 3.73

This mixed tumor (top) contains malignant epithelium and stroma. There is a focus of poorly differentiated cartilage. Both clear-cut and less well-defined foci of cartilage (bottom) are seen in this mixed tumor.

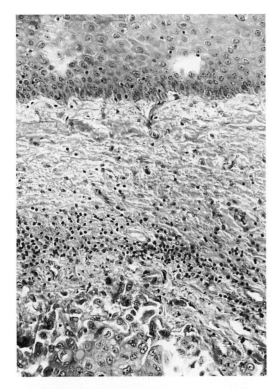

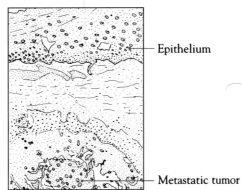

Epithelium

Metastatic tumor

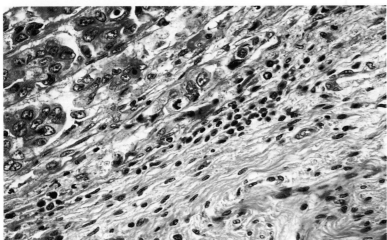

figure 3.74

The subepithelial location of this metastatic cancer (top) is typical of lesions from distant sites. A higher power view (bottom) shows poorly differentiated cancer metastatic from the pelvis.

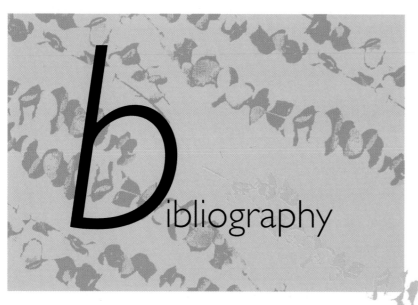

bibliography

Aalders JG, Abeler V, Kolstad P: Stage IV endometrial carcinoma: A clinical and histopathological study of 83 patients. *Gynecol Oncol* 17:75, 1984.

Blaustein A: *Interpretation of Biopsy of Endometrium.* New York, Raven Press, 1980.

Boronow RC: Endometrial cancer: The emergence of therapeutic individualization. In Taymor ML, Nelson JH (eds.): *Progress in Gynecology.* New York, Grune & Stratton, 1983.

Boronow RC, et al: Surgical staging in endometrial cancer: Clinical-pathologic findings of a prospective study. *Obstet Gynecol* 63:825, 1984.

Creasman WT, Boronow RC, Morrow CP, et al: Adenocarcinoma of the endometrium: Its metastatic lymph node potential. *Gynecol Oncol* 4:239, 1976.

Fox H: The endometrial hyperplasias. *Obstet Gynecol Annu* 13:197, 1984.

Gambrell RD Jr., Bagnell CA, Greenblatt RB: Role of estrogens and progesterone in the etiology and prevention of endometrial cancer: Review. *Am J Obstet Gynecol* 146:696, 1983.

Hammond CB, Ory SJ: Conservative therapy of endometriosis. In Taymor ML, Nelson JH (eds.): *Progress in Gynecology.* New York, Grune & Stratton, 1983.

Hendrickson MR, Kempson RL: *Surgical Pathology of the Uterine Corpus.* Philadelphia, WB Saunders Co., 1980.

Hertig AT, Norris HJ, Abell MR: *The Uterus.* Baltimore, Williams & Wilkins Co, 1973.

Kurman RJ, Norris HJ: Evaluation of criteria for distinguishing atypical endometrial hyperplasia from well-differentiated carcinoma. *Cancer* 49:2547, 1982.

Mahboubi E, Eyler N, Wynder EL: Epidemiology of cancer of the endometrium. *Clin Obstet Gynecol* 25:5, 1982.

Noyes RW, Hertig AT, Rock J: Dating the endometrial biopsy. *Fertil Steril* 1:3, 1950.

Tuck JL, Fletcher CDM: *Royal Colege of Surgeons of England Slide Atlas of Pathology.* Reproductive System, London, Gower Medical Publishing Ltd., 1985.

endometrium

chapter 4

Early Growth and Development

The endometrium develops from both the epithelium of the müllerian duct and the stroma of its wall, and correspondingly consists of both stroma and an epithelium (Fig. 4.1). In the developing uterus, at about 20 weeks of gestational age, smooth muscle begins to differentiate in the future myometrium. Early in the third trimester the endometrial stroma is distinguishable from myometrium, although it is not dramatically developed (Fig. 4.2); the endometrial epithelium at this time forms only a few small glands. By term, approximately 5% of endometria will have developed sufficient responsiveness to steroids that they become decidualized in response to high maternal hormone levels, but later slough after delivery when maternal hormones are no longer present. Approximately one-third of newborn endometria show lesser degrees of secretory change, while about two-thirds are either proliferative or inactive.

During the prepubertal years, the endometrium is low with rudimentary glands but its stroma may be distinguished easily from myometrium (Fig. 4.3). With the onset of estrogen production at puberty, the endometrium becomes mature and proliferative (Fig. 4.4). The stroma of proliferating endometrium consists of small cells that resemble fibroblasts cut parallel and perpendicular to their long axis (Fig. 4.5). They are suspended in a fine reticular network of fibers. The epithelium of proliferating endometrium is columnar, with oval basal nuclei oriented perpendicular to the basement membrane (Fig. 4.6). In addition, there are scattered

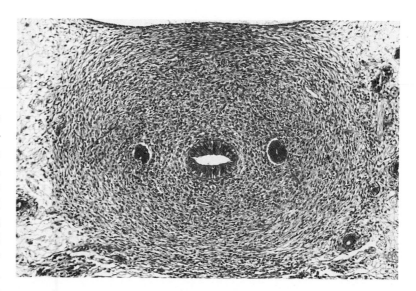

figure 4.1

Photomicrograph taken at about nine weeks gestational age shows the epithelium of the müllerian duct lying between the two disappearing wolffian ducts. All three are embedded in a common mass of mesodermal stroma.

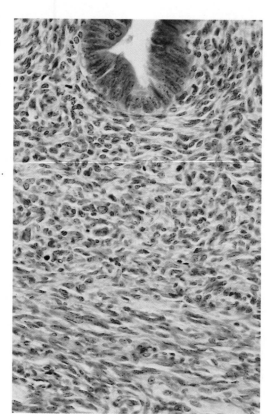

figure 4.2

The endometrial epithelium above is supported by a loose cellular stroma. Below, muscle is beginning to differentiate from the common mesenchyme.

4.2

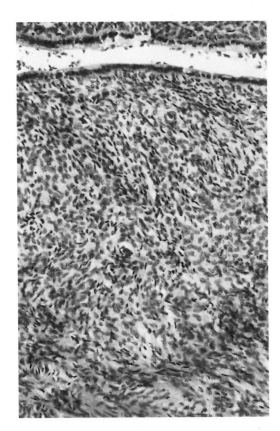

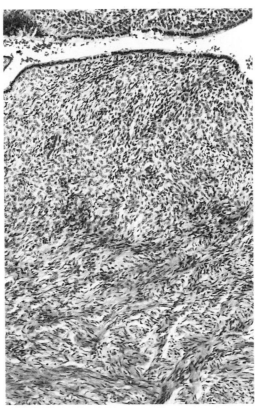

figure 4.3

Low, flat epithelium (left) is supported by minimal endometrial stroma in this prepubertal uterus. The myometrium below (right) is clearly distinguishable from the endometrial stroma above. Glands are sparse.

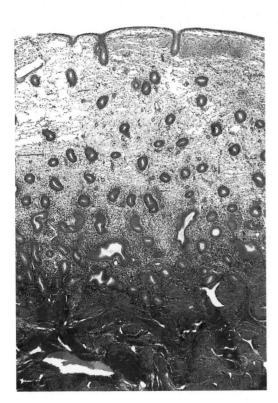

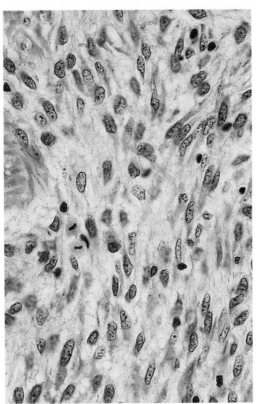

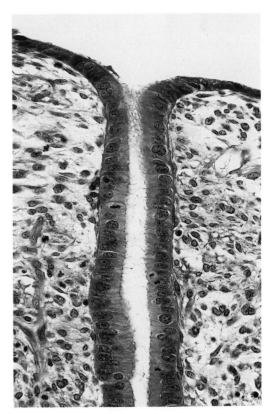

figure 4.4

Photomicrograph of a proliferative endometrium that is composed of straight tubular glands in a homogeneous stroma.

figure 4.5

Stromal mitoses are present in this proliferating stroma, which is composed of fibroblastic-type cells. The nuclei seen here and in the following two figures have mildly atypical features, which may make the diagnosis of individual cell atypicality a challenge.

figure 4.6

In this photomicrograph, a straight tubular gland at the surface of a proliferative endometrium is lined with columnar epithelium containing mitoses.

endometrium

ciliated cells (Fig. 4.7). Because estrogen, which induces growth in the endometrium, does so more effectively in the epithelium than in the stroma, during the anovulatory cycles characteristic of adolescence the epithelium tends to outgrow the stroma. Epithelial hyperplasia may result (Fig. 4.8) but is rapidly resolved when ovulation begins.

the Normal Cycle in the Endometrium

PRE- AND POSTOVULATORY CHANGES

During the estrogenic phase of the normal cycle, mitotic figures are prominent in both epithelium and stroma. In the midportion of the phase there is an increase in stromal edema, but it is not sufficiently distinctive as to be helpful in recognition. The epithelial cells tend to become taller, and the epithelium becomes pseudostratified (Fig. 4.9). Ciliated cells, distinguished by their round nuclei and adjacent cytoplasmic clearing, may become even more prominent. As this phase progresses, the entire endometrium thickens and the straight glands become taller and somewhat more tortuous. Yet ultrasonically, fully developed preovulatory endometrium is still relatively thin (Fig. 4.10).

Immediately preovulation, a small amount of progesterone production begins, which will be amplified post-ovulation; this results in the beginning of glycogen production in the basal portion of the epithelial cells. With routine histologic processing, the glycogen is removed from the cells so that apparent clear vacuoles are visualized in the sections. On about the second postovulatory day (day 16 of the cycle), significant numbers of these subnuclear vacuoles are first identified in the middle zone of the functional portion of the endometrium. These vacuoles are generalized by the third post-ovulatory day, and on the fourth through fifth day they slip by the nucleus to the luminal edge of the cell (Fig. 4.11). By the fifth postovulatory day, the nuclei have moved back down on the basement membrane and there are no mitoses seen in epithelium or stroma. The glycogen vacuoles are then secreted by an apocrine mechanism (Fig. 4.12). Glycogen is present in glandular lumina maximally on day 20 to 21 of the cycle, at which time the epithelial cells, having lost substance, are beginning to shorten (Fig. 4.13). On day 21 to 22, there is a sudden increase in the amount of stromal edema, and secretions in the glandular lumina become inspissated (Fig. 4.14). These changes may be thought of as facilitating implantation, which occurs classically on day 20.

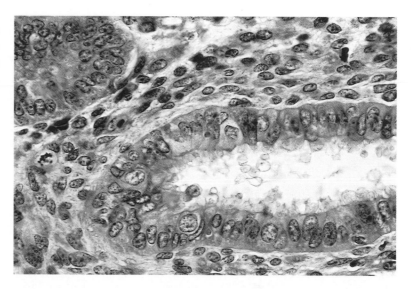

figure 4.7

Several ciliated cells characterized by eosinophilic luminal edges and perinuclear cytoplasmic clearing are seen in the epithelium of this gland.

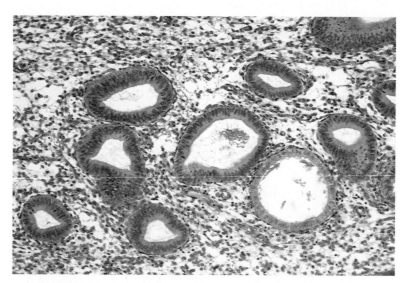

figure 4.8

The glands seen in this photomicrograph are somewhat dilated and crowded, and the one on the bottom right is lined by an eosinophilic epithelium that is composed of ciliated cells.

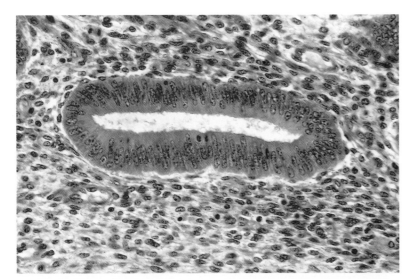

figure 4.9

This proliferative gland is lined by pseudostratified epithelium containing mitoses.

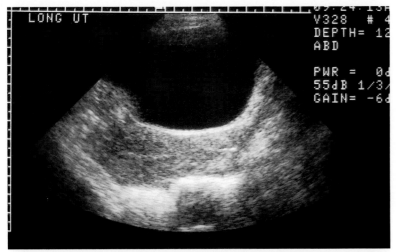

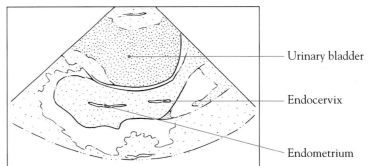

- Urinary bladder
- Endocervix
- Endometrium

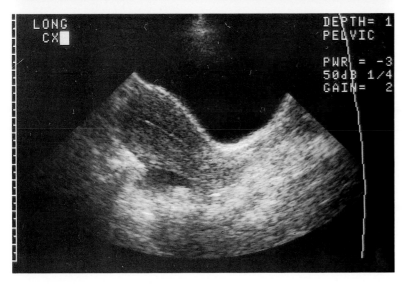

- Urinary bladder
- Endometrium
- Cervix
- Cul-de-sac fluid

figure 4.10

Two slides display logitudinal transabdominal ultrasounds of a normal uterus. The logitudinal axis of the uterus (top) is directed in a cephalocaudad plane because of marked distension of the urinary bladder. The endocervical and endometrial echoes are thin in this early proliferative phase of the menstrual cycle. The uterus (bottom) is mildly anteverted. The thin endometrium is characteristic of the early proliferative phase. The cervical canal is not as well visualized because of its oblique orientation relative to the ultrasound beam. There is minimal fluid in the cul-de-sac, which may be seen in normal patients.

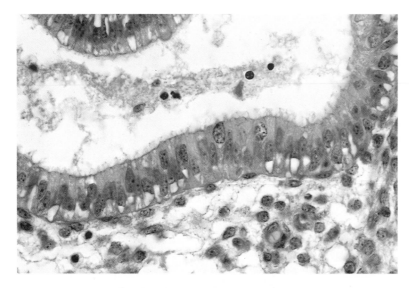

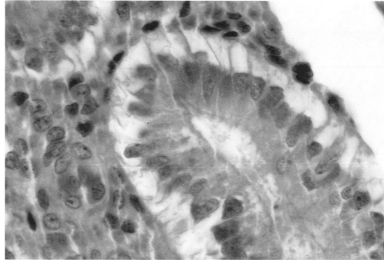

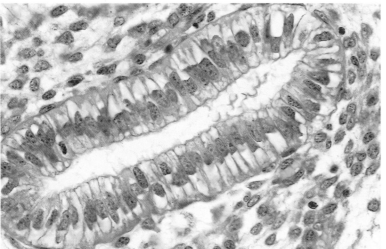

figure 4.11

The earliest subnuclear vacuoles (top left) are beginning to appear beneath the nuclei in this epithelium. At a later stage (top right) subnuclear vacuoles are generalized in this endometrial gland. The epithelial vacuoles (left) are largely subnuclear, but some slipped past the nucleus toward the lumen of this gland.

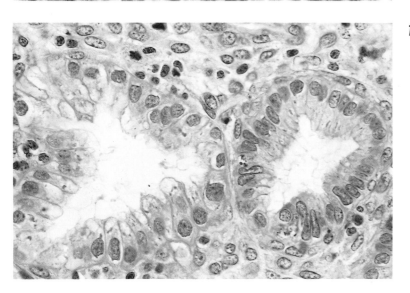

figure 4.12

The vacuoles seen here are being extruded from the luminal edge of the cell.

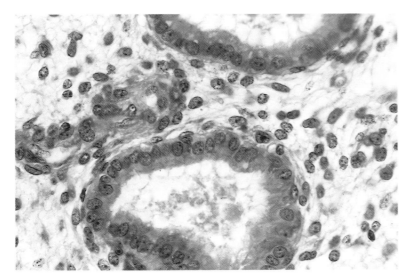

figure 4.13

Secretion within the lumen of this gland appears associated with shorter epithelial cells, but secretory vacuoles persist along their luminal edge. In addition, there is stromal edema.

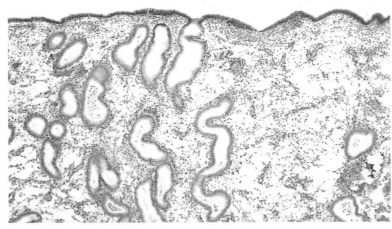

figure 4.14

Marked stromal edema (top) is present with maximal fluffy secretion in dilated glands. The brightly eosinophilic secretion in the lumen of this gland (bottom) is inspissated.

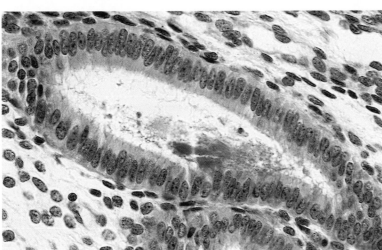

endometrium

IMPLANTATION

When implantation does occur, the result is the conversion of the endometrium to decidua, and the development of trophoblastic invasion at the implantation site (Fig. 4.15). The conversion to decidua is seen first around the spiral arterioles, where stromal cells with increasing amounts of cytoplasm begin to appear. By day 24, well-developed cuffs of predecidual cells have organized around the coiled links of the spiral arterioles (Fig. 4.16). In addition, a significant second wave of secretion has occurred within the glands, so that they begin to expand as fresh secretion is seen within their lumina, around the inspissated cores of the earlier wave of secretion (Fig. 4.17). With the production of additional glycogen, the epithelium of the glands begins to enlarge and become clear or hypersecretory in appearance (Fig. 4.18). By the 25th day, predecidual cells have developed extensively around the spiral arterioles and are extending beneath the surface capsule of the functional portions of the endometrium. On day 26, these predecidual changes have resulted in the formation of solid columns that extend up and down the course of the spiral arterioles and spread out underneath the capsule of the surface to form the zona compacta of the functionalis (Fig. 4.19). And on the 27th day, the endometrial granulocytes are becoming prominently differentiated (Fig. 4.20).

Subsequently, the epithelium of the glands becomes more fully hypersecretory in appearance and some of the epithelial cells develop the so-called Arias-Stella reaction, which is marked by the presence of an enlarged atypical nucleus produced by the 4N DNA associated with the hormonal changes of pregnancy (Fig. 4.21). The predecidual cells then mature into true decidual cells (only a matter of degree) and it is the combination of hypersecretory epithelium and enlarged stromal cells that is termed decidua. As the pregnancy advances and the decidua becomes fully established, the apocrine secretory mechanism of the epithelial cells results in their gradual shortening and atrophy; consequently, by term, many of these cells are flattened or mesothelial in appearance (Fig. 4.22). Simultaneously, dramatic decidual and granulocytic stromal differentiation continues to occur, such that the decidual cells become large and polygonal, producing an apparent mosaic that fills the stromal tissue of the endometrium with granulocytic cells scattered throughout (Fig. 4.23).

Additional differentiation may take place in the decidua. For unknown reasons, decidua occasionally is replaced by a process that initially looks inflammatory and fibroblastic but later results in the formation of smooth muscle (Fig. 4.24). During pregnancy the production of muscle nodules in the placenta or membranes as well as the formation of endometrial polyps suggestive of prolapsed submucous fibroids may result (Fig. 4.25). As this is an active

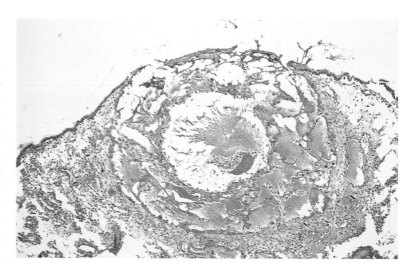

figure 4.15

A bilaminar disc and early amniotic sac are present in this early implantation. The expanded chorionic membrane forms a labyrinth around them. Maternal blood passively circulates in these interconnecting spaces.

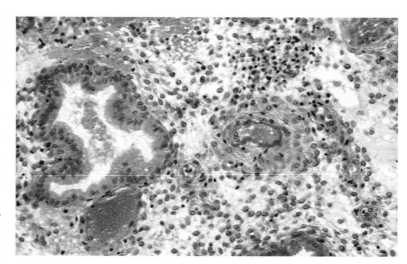

figure 4.16

Photomicrograph of a spiral arteriole that is surrounded by a collection of decidualized stromal cells that form a so-called periarteriolar cuff.

4.8

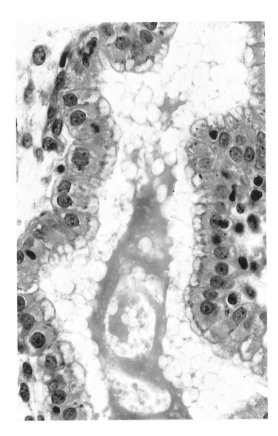

figure 4.17

Inspissated secretion lies in the lumen of this gland, but the epithelium has formed a new generation of secretory vacuoles that are about to be extruded into the glandular lumen.

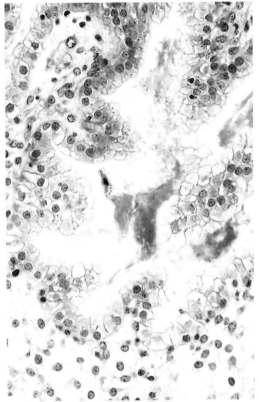

figure 4.18

Inspissated secretion lies in the lower portion of the gland's lumen, with fresher secretion above. The epithelium consists of enlarged, clear or hypersecretory cells. Stromal edema is present.

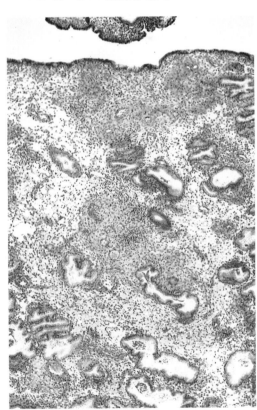

figure 4.19

An apparent "blush" in the center of this piece of endometrium (top left) indicates that the column of cells around a spiral arteriole are beginning to accumulate cytoplasm. This is an early stage of decidualization. The blush of decidualization (right) is seen not only around a spiral arteriole in the spongiosa, but beneath the surface epithelium as well. The blush of decidualization (bottom left) is becoming generalized beneath the surface epithelium and is developing into a zona compacta.

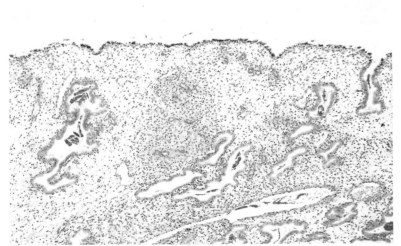

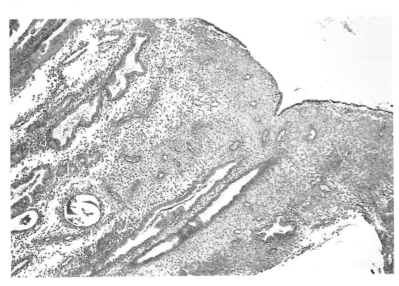

endometrium

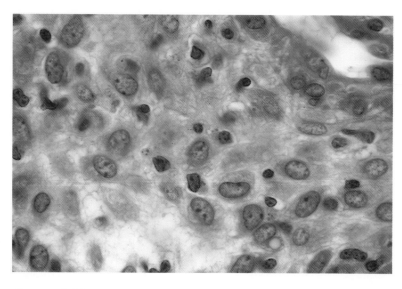

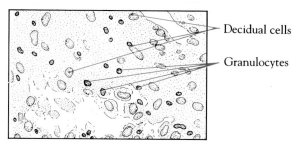

Decidual cells

Granulocytes

figure 4.20

The decidual cells possess enlarged vesicular nuclei and ample eosinophilic cytoplasm. The granulocytes possess small dark nuclei and clear to reddish cytoplasm.

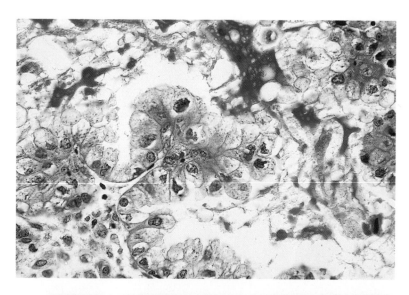

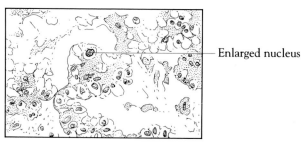

Enlarged nucleus

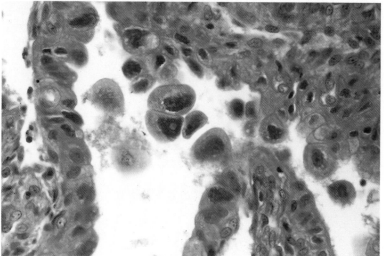

figure 4.21

One of the hypersecretory cells in this epithelium (top) contains an enlarged atypical nucleus. This is the Arias-Stella reaction. In these post-abortal curettings (bottom) the presence of atypical nuclei (in the center of the field) is the most dramatic feature as the epithelium is degenerating.

atlas of gynecologic pathology

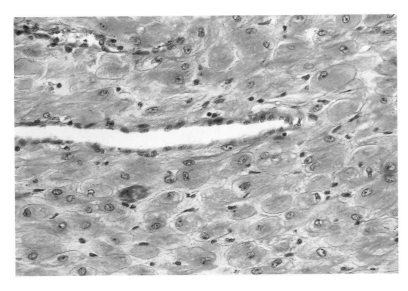

figure 4.22

The gland in this mature decidua is lined by low flat epithelium.

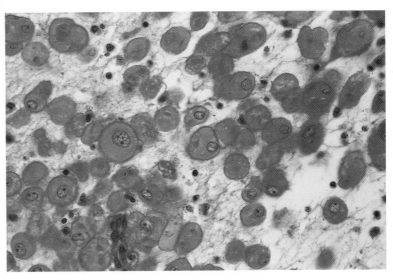

figure 4.23

Both endometrial granulocytes and decidual cells are seen clearly in this edematous decidua. The decidual cells have eccentric vesicular nuclei and large amounts of eosinophilic cytoplasm within clear-cut cell membranes.

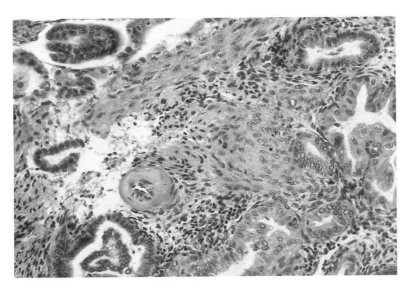

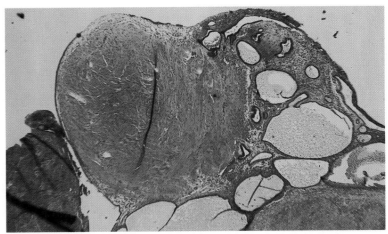

figure 4.25

A focus of smooth muscle without a pushing border (top) is located in the most distal portion of this endometrial polyp. Endometrial tissue (bottom) merges with a similar structure in this polyp, with the myometrium below.

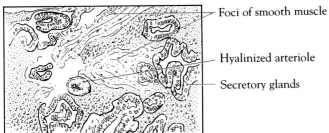

Foci of smooth muscle

Hyalinized arteriole

Secretory glands

figure 4.24

The hyalinized spiral arteriole in the lower left and the secretory glands below and to the right indicate a recent pregnancy. In the center and above, small foci of smooth muscle are developing.

endometrium

process, mitoses may be present, and leiomyosarcoma occasionally has been diagnosed mistakenly. The same process may also occur in pelvic lymph nodes (Fig. 4.26).

Following trophoblastic invasion, the endometrium at the implantation site is altered in several ways. Those glands that are most lateral to the implantation are pushed laterally, such that they deviate from a straight course to swing around the implantation. Both glands and vessels within the path of the invading trophoblast are entered, and they discharge their contents directly into the labyrinthine space of the early syncytiotrophoblast (Fig. 4.27). In addition, isolated trophoblastic cells infiltrate the maternal tissue and differentiate into large mononuclear and multinuclear intermediate trophoblastic cells, many of which are capable of producing human placental lactogen. These cells infiltrate the endometrium and myometrium, producing a pattern known as syncytial endomyometritis (Fig. 4.28). Exaggerated forms of this infiltration result in the placental site tumor (Fig. 4.29). Most of these tumors are benign, but some examples have malignant potential (Fig. 4.30). The vessels that serve the implantation site become nonreactive vascular channels, because trophoblastic cells invade and destroy their walls (Fig. 4.31). In addition, trophoblastic cells invade the walls of the spiral arterioles that serve the implantation site (Fig. 4.32). Postpartum, they are additionally converted into hyaline masses that are apparent weeks and months after pregnancy ends (Fig. 4.33).

PUERPERIUM

After the end of a normal pregnancy the drop in chorionic gonadotropin and progesterone levels, together with placental removal, results in endometrial slough. With the onset of estrogen secretion, regrowth of the endometrium occurs over the placental implantation site as well as elsewhere; complete reepithelialization of the implantation site may take as long as six weeks. This information, ascertained by Dr. J. Whitridge Williams (*Am J Obstet Gynecol* 1931; 22:664–696), is the basis for the common but misleading assumption that women are physiologically recovered from their pregnancy by approximately six weeks postpartum.

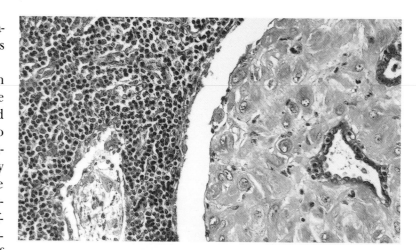

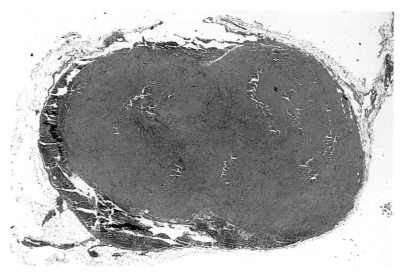

figure 4.26

A large focus of decidua in a pelvic lymph node (top) is seen in a woman undergoing a radical hysterectomy for invasive carcinoma of the cervix, complicating her pregnancy. A smooth muscle nodule (bottom) has replaced a focus of decidua in a pelvic lymph node similar to the one seen in the top slide. It does not destroy the node. It occupies the hilum of the node, where decidual deposits are seen; it does not involve the peripheral sinuses, where metastases occur.

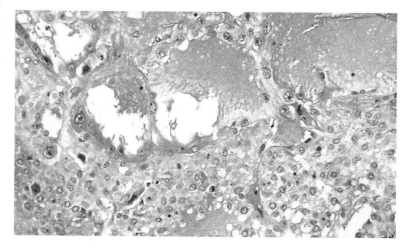

figure 4.27

The syncytiotrophoblast located above created a labyrinthine space that contains maternal blood. When the trophoblast invaded the maternal tissue, it opened a maternal capillary to the right.

NONIMPLANTATION

In cycles where implantation does not occur, the histologic sequence described above develops only abortively, and the histologic appearance of such endometria may be distinguished from that characterizing the implantation cycle by approximately day 24 (Fig. 4.34). In the absence of implantation, the secondary wave of secretion mentioned previously does not begin, and the glandular epithelium remains low and cuboidal. In addition, the edema that developed on the 21st day disappears from the endometrium by the 24th day, and consequently that endometrium, while possessing the predecidual changes described above for the implantation cycle, is more compact and dense (Fig. 4.35). On the 25th day, predecidual change develops beneath the surface epithelium. By the 26th day, it has formed columns around the spiral arterioles (Fig. 4.36). By day 27, granulocytes are prominent in the endometrial stroma (Fig. 4.37). Thus, the immediate premenstrual endometrium possesses a superficial zona compacta composed of predecidua with periarteriolar columns of predecidua extending into the middle zone, or zona spongiosa. The basalis, which does not respond to progesterone, does not participate in any of these changes (Fig. 4.38). Furthermore, ultrasonograms reveal that the endometrium becomes much thicker in the secretory phase of the cycle (Fig. 4.39).

MENSTRUATION

Menstruation is still not well understood although it is known to consist of the patchy loss of varying portions of the zonae compacta and spongiosa from the most functional areas of the endometrium, namely, the anterior and posterior walls. Histologically, the first change noticed is the presence of small collections of darkened clumped stromal cells, with perhaps some associated extravasated blood or fluid and an inflammatory infiltrate (Fig. 4.40). Subsequently, larger areas will show necrosis (Fig. 4.41). Fibrin thrombi may be present, and in many cases, some metaplastic epithelial repair is apparent from even the earliest examples of menstruation (Fig. 4.42). After several days of bleeding, epithelial repair is a routine observation in curettings that are very extensive (Fig. 4.43). The immediately postmenstrual endometrium is low, with a repairing epithelium on its surface (Fig. 4.44). Just beneath the surface is an inflammatory infiltrate with some necrotic tissue that has not yet been resolved. The topmost portion of the remaining glands may

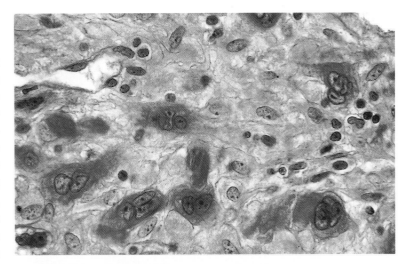

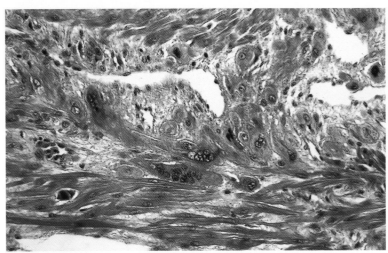

figure 4.28

The darker cells (top), some of which appear multinucleated, are trophoblastic cells invading the decidua. Large multinucleated trophoblastic cells (bottom) are invading the myometrium.

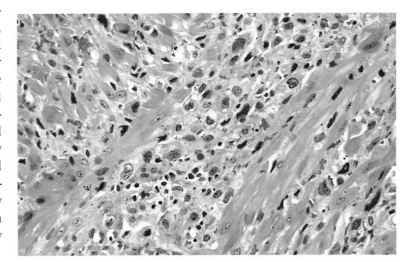

figure 4.29

This sheet of intermediate-type trophoblast invading but not destroying the adjacent muscle bundles constitutes the placental site tumor. Note the absence of syncytial-type trophoblast.

endometrium

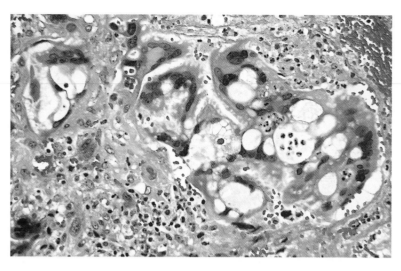

figure 4.30

A focus of developing syncytial-type trophoblast in this placental site tumor may represent an early choriocarcinoma.

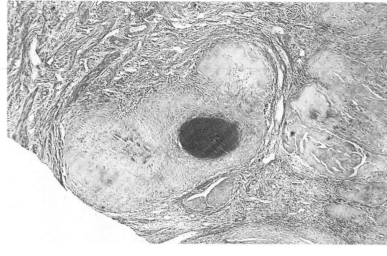

figure 4.31

At term, the walls of the spiral arterioles consist of large masses of scar containing pipelike vascular channels.

4.14

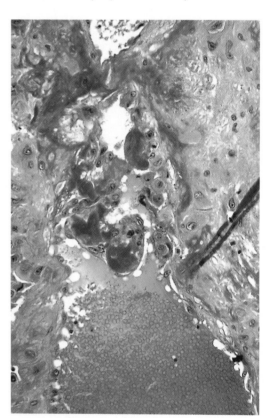

figure 4.32

Above, trophoblast lines the vascular channel. Below, it is lined by endothelium.

Trophoblast

Endothelium

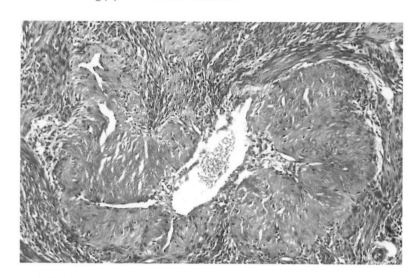

figure 4.33

Postpartum, the wall of the spiral arterioles becomes collagenized. Some reendothelialization is suggested here.

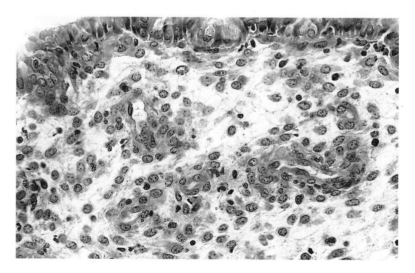

figure 4.34

The very earliest development of a periarteriolar blush is suggested here, as very early decidualization is occurring.

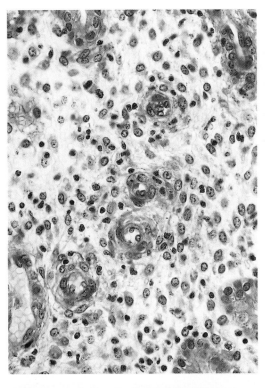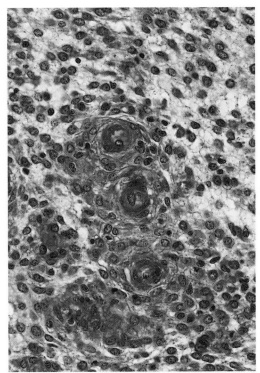

figure 4.35

A more clear-cut periarteriolar blush (left) is seen in this photomicrograph. A clear-cut collection of predecidual cells (right) outlines the spiral arteriole.

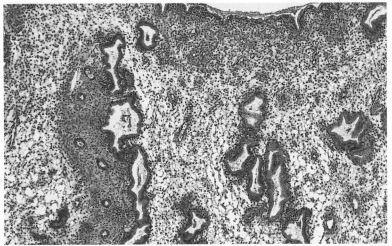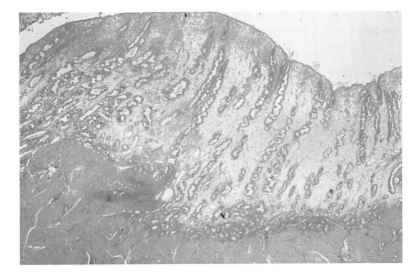

figure 4.36

Both a column of periarteriolar decidualization and a subepithelial surface blush are present. Edema is not a prominent feature.

figure 4.37

The decidual cells seen in this photomicrograph are distinguishable from the granulocytes, but they are not well developed.

figure 4.38

This fully developed premenstrual endometrium possesses the three-layered structure of classic endometrial histology. The basalis is the dense layer below. The spongiosa is loose and edematous and occupies the middle zone. The compacta, formed by subepithelial decidualization, occupies the topmost portion.

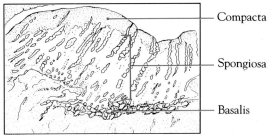

Compacta

Spongiosa

Basalis

endometrium

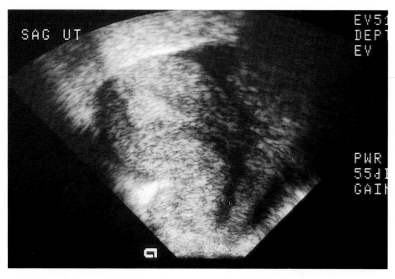

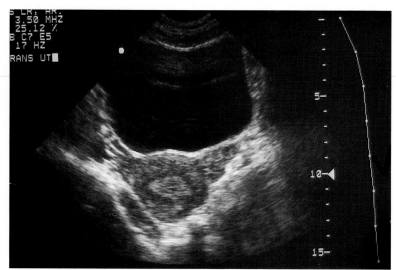

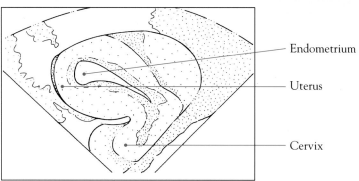

Endometrium

Uterus

Cervix

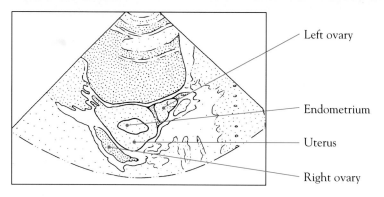

Left ovary

Endometrium

Uterus

Right ovary

4.16

figure 4.39

Sagittal endovaginal ultrasound of a normal uterus taken with the ultrasound probe (left) placed in the vagina for better delineation of the endometrium. The endomertrium is slightly thickened, compatible with a late secretory phase. Transverse transabdominal ultrasound of a normal uterus (right) depicts the uterus as triangular in cross-section. The endometrium is markedly thickened, compatible with a late secretory phase. The left ovary is seen just lateral to the uterus. The right ovary is partialy imaged in the cul-de-sac.

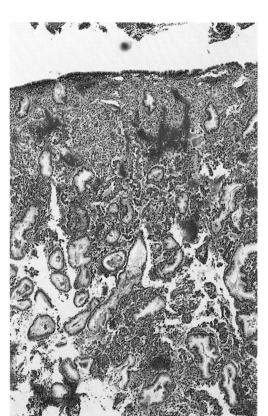

figure 4.40

This endometrial fragment appears to have separated at the level of the spongiosa. The glands are tortuous and fragmented. The stroma consists of dark necrotic fragments. Free hemorrhage is present in the tissue.

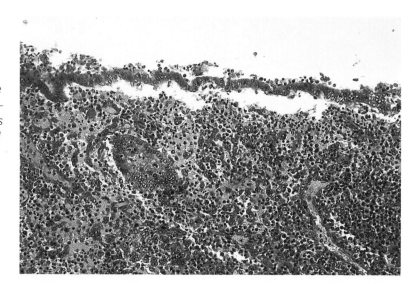

figure 4.41

Photomicrograph of total necrosis with only ghosts of glands present.

atlas of gynecologic pathology

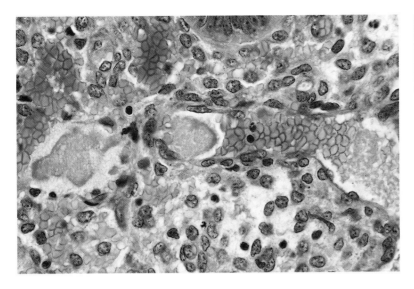

figure 4.42

In this case of abnormal bleeding, fibrin thrombi (left) occupy the left side of the capillary. Obstructed blood occupies the right side. The apparent clumping and darkening of the endometrial stromal cells (right) are the first signs of this tissue's impending slough. The brightly eosinophilic metaplastic epithelium on the surface represents an attempt at repair that in this case obviously failed.

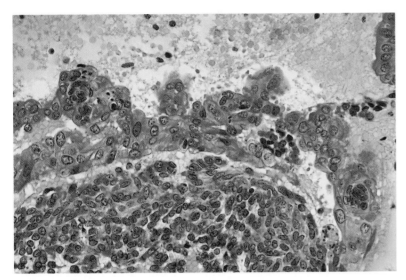

figure 4.43

This focus of metaplastic repairing epithelium both contains and overlies dark clumps of necrotic stroma.

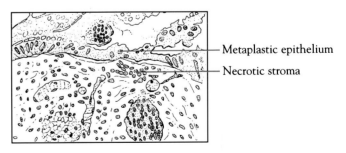

Metaplastic epithelium
Necrotic stroma

figure 4.44

Immediately postmenstrual, a small focus of necrotic stroma remains beneath the metaplastic epithelial repair.

4.17

endometrium

still appear secretory, although within a day or two they have been converted to a proliferative appearance (Fig. 4.45). Necrotic menstruating endometrium often is mistaken for malignancy (Fig. 4.46).

The changes described above typically occur in the middle portion of the anterior and posterior walls. The cornual areas, the lower uterine segment, as well as the sides and top of the fundus show lesser degrees of change and cannot be evaluated as easily.

benign Pathologic Conditions

EXOGENOUS HORMONE THERAPIES

Perhaps the most common changes seen in endometrium in clinical practice are those induced by exogenous hormone therapies. The changes induced by exogenous estrogen are the same as those induced by endogenous estrogen and are discussed below. Exogenous progestational agents produce decidualization, some edema, and stromal dominance; oral contraceptives act as progestational drugs in this context. Most exogenous agents produce more extensive decidualization than is produced during the normal luteal phase, and this may result in the complete decidualization of the endometrial cavity except for the basalis, which does not respond to the progestational drug (Fig. 4.47). The differentiating and growth-inhibiting influence of the progestational drug has several histologic effects. The glands become sparse relative to their number in the physiologic endometrium and are lined by low cuboidal or flattened epithelial cells. In addition, the total amount of endometrial tissue becomes smaller. Sometimes, muscle metaplasia occurs.

ENDOMETRITIS

Endometritis is a nonspecific diagnosis in the endometrium and implies a need to search for an etiology. Isolated lymphoid aggregates, some with germinal centers, are seen in the endometrium physiologically, most often just above the basalis (Fig. 4.48). The more widespread presence of inflammatory cells constitutes the diagnosis of endometritis, although this finding may be difficult to establish as both round cells and polymorphonuclear leukocytes may be confused with stromal cells of the routine or granulocytic type. Invasion of the epithelium of the glands by inflammatory cells, destruction of the epithelium, and accumulation of pus in endometrial glands are signs of true endometrial inflammation (Fig. 4.49).

4.18

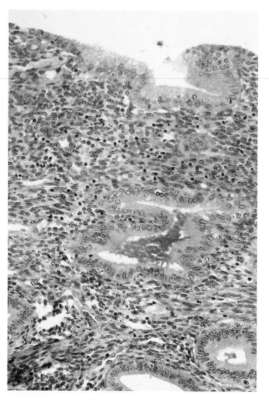

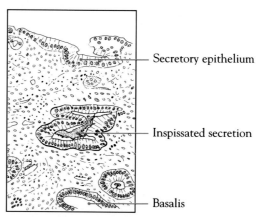

— Secretory epithelium

— Inspissated secretion

— Basalis

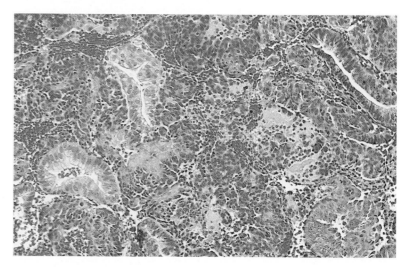

figure 4.46

This collection of fragmenting necrotic glands and stroma (probably representing the stage illustrated in Fig. 4.40) is a typical example of the type of curettings frequently misinterpreted as adenocarcinoma.

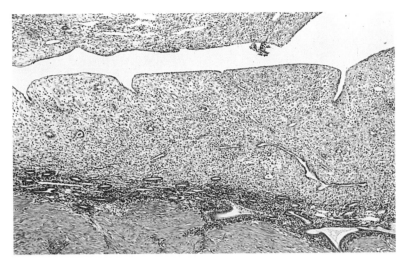

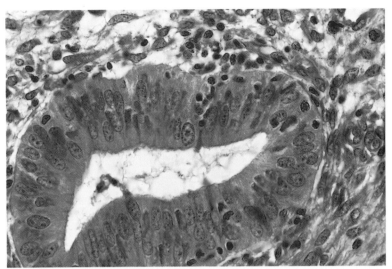

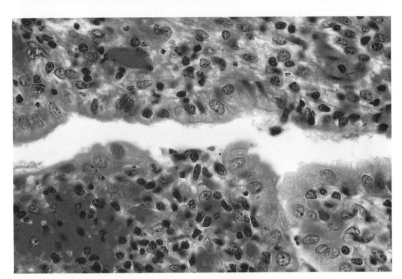

figure 4.47

Rather than the three layers of classic histology, this endometrium (top) has been converted to two by megestrol acetate therapy. The basalis does not respond even to pharmacologic doses of progestogen. At higher power (bottom), note the relative absence of glands and the stromal edema.

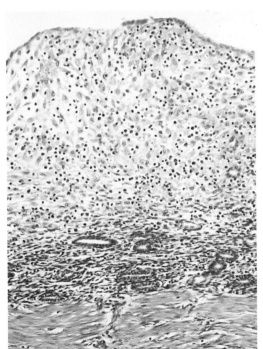

figure 4.48

The lymphoid nodule seen in this photomicrograph is immediately above the basalis in an otherwise normal proliferative endometrium.

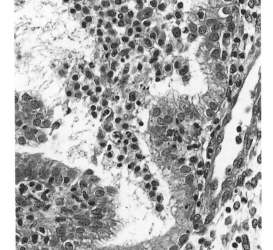

figure 4.49

Inflammatory cells (top) invade the epithelium of this gland. Focally, the epithelium (center) has been destroyed and replaced with a collection of inflammatory cells. Pus (bottom) fills the lumen of this gland.

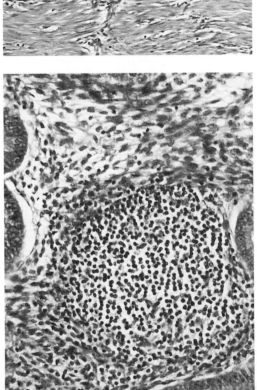

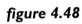

endometrium

The most common cause of endometrial inflammation is the termination of pregnancy. The endometrium under these circumstances will usually show at least some degree of secretory change. More complete decidualization, or even the Arias-Stella reaction, may be present. Old decidua in the endometrium results in hyalinized plaques, which are characteristic (Fig. 4.50); spiral arterioles may be particularly hyalinized (see Fig. 4.24). Degeneration in the decidua may result in enlarged atypical nuclei, some of which appear multiple. This appearance suggests trophoblast and can be mistakenly diagnosed as such (Fig. 4.51). Occasionally, gestational products may be found, including placental polyps. Bony fetal parts have been retained in the uterus for years and may be a significant inflammatory stimulus. The second most common cause of endometritis is a foreign body, of which the IUD is most ubiquitous (Fig. 4.52). IUDs produce an acute, but most importantly a chronic, response that is most likely to be intense only locally. The endometrium in contact with the device may be depressed and so inflamed as to consist of granulation. Squamous metaplasia may occur as a repair phenomenon. IUDs also fragment and become infested with large quantities of bacteria. Some of these organisms, like Actinomyces, are unusual in the absence of foreign bodies. Both IUD fragments and bacteria may be seen in curettings or hysterectomy specimens (Fig. 4.53).

An acute endometritis may exist in the acute phase of ascending pelvic inflammatory disease. The glands are filled with pus, and both epithelium and stroma are infiltrated with polymorphonuclear leukocytes and may be necrotic. This portion of the disease usually subsides spontaneously if drainage is adequate. Thinned endometrium caused by submucous fibroids or to postmenopausal atrophy is frequently irritated (Fig. 4.54). If this is combined with stenosis or with obstruction of the cervix, then pyometra may result.

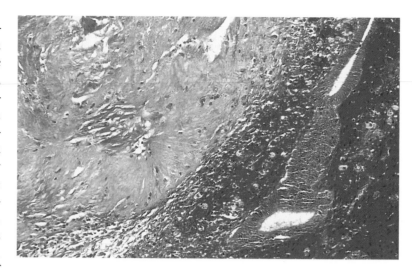

figure 4.50

A focus of hyalinized decidua occupies the top left portion of this photomicrograph. Below, the endometrium is proliferating.

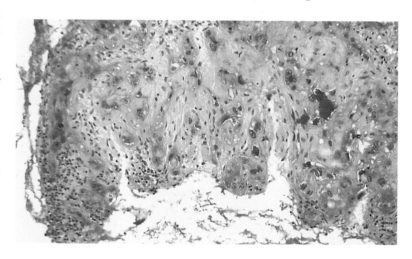

figure 4.51

While the darker cells in this necrotic decidua resemble the trophoblastic infiltration seen in Figure 4.28, they are the result of degeneration of single decidual cells. This patient had an ectopic implantation.

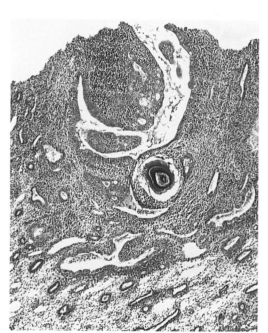

figure 4.52

The focus of inflammation developed around a calcified foreign body of unknown etiology.

4.20

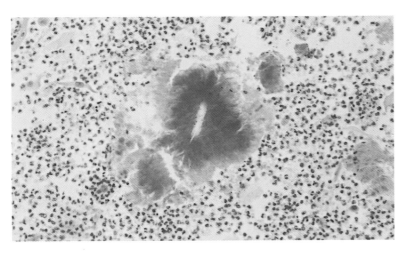 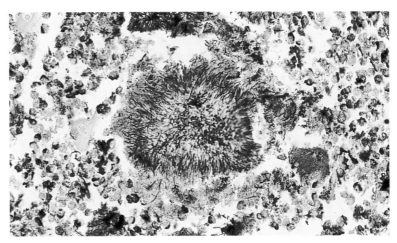

figure 4.53

This "sulfur granule" (left) was found in the curettings from a uterus that also contained an IUD. A methenamine silver stain of the same specimen (right) reveals the fibrillar appearance of Actinomyces.

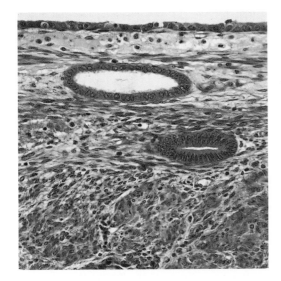 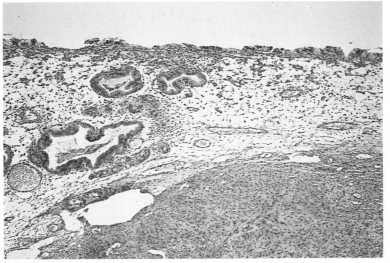

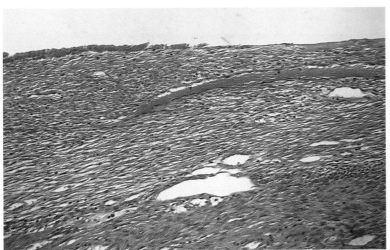 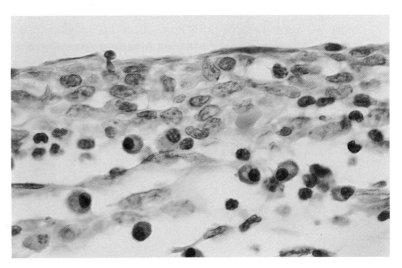

figure 4.54

This thinned postmenopausal endometrium (top left) possesses a subepithelial inflammatory infiltrate. The submucous myoma below (top right) causes thinning of the secretory endometrium, which is seen as one moves from left to right. In the same case but farther to the right, the thinned endometrium over the submucous myoma (bottom left) is inflamed and becomes ulcerated as epithelium is lost. A thin, metaplastic, repairing epithelium (bottom right) barely covers the inflamed surface of this submucous myoma. Plasma cells, not normal constituents of the endometrium, are numerous.

endometrium

Pyometra is frequently associated with tumor or with radiation of previous cervical tumor (Fig. 4.55). A specific bacterial infection that today is seen most commonly in endometrial biopsies taken in the course of infertility evaluations is tuberculosis. Endometrial tuberculosis is usually secondary to tubal disease (Fig. 4.56).

HYPERPLASIA

Attention has already been called to the fact that the endometrium is not uniformly responsive to hormone stimulation and that even the progesterone-responsive portion of the endometrium is focally heterogeneous in its capacity to respond to progesterone. Consequently, foci are routinely present within the endometrium that do not respond to the progesterone levels achieved during the normal cycle (Fig. 4.57). These foci do not differentiate and may not slough with each cycle; instead, they grow continuously in response to estrogen. Their continuous growth results in hyperplasia and in the development of thick-walled vascular stalks, which eventually become polypoid (Fig. 4.58). These foci may be recognized before they are grossly polypoid, however, on the basis of focal hyperplasia and the vascular stalks. Adenomyosis, which appears to be a response of the basalis to the same continuing estrogenic stimulation, also develops in some individuals (Fig. 4.59). If decidualization is subsequently achieved in either of these overgrowths and the muscle metaplasia mentioned above does take place, then an adenomyoma develops either within the myometrium or in the form of a polyp.

Hyperplasia, whether it occurs in adolescents with anovulatory cycles, in foci of decreased responsiveness to progesterone, or in anovulatory or postmenopausal women, is likely to have the same histologic characteristics. Initially, there is overgrowth of both epithelium and stroma (Fig. 4.60; see also Fig. 4.58). As the epithelium is more sensitive to estrogen than is the stroma, continuous growth results in the gradual overgrowth of the epithelium vis-à-vis the stroma. In the early stages, endometrial glands tend to become obstructed at their necks by epithelial growth and adjacent stromal pressure. Resulting intraluminal pressure produces varying degrees of cystic dilatation of the glands, and the histology thus consists of a combination of large and small

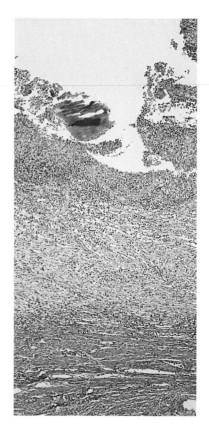

figure 4.55

This pyometra (top) was associated with a uterine tumor. A "sulfur granule" lies on the surface of the endometrium, which has been replaced by granulation tissue and pus. Squamous metaplasia, an attempt at repair (bottom), is occurring on the surface of the inflamed endometrium in this example of pyometra.

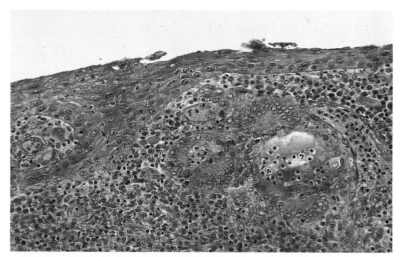

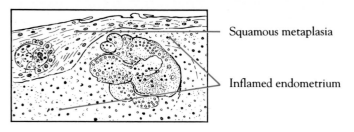

Squamous metaplasia

Inflamed endometrium

atlas of gynecologic pathology

epithelial cysts embedded in a dense stroma (Fig. 4.61). This is benign cystic hyperplasia. Subsequently, continued growth and glandular crowding tend to produce intraluminal papillary folding and glandular tortuosity, known by a variety of terms of which adenomatous hyperplasia is one of the common ones (Fig. 4.62).

Premenopausal hyperplasia, arising as it does in nonresponsive foci, often is itself only a focal process (Fig. 4.63).

When adenomatous hyperplasia has progressed to such a degree that the glands are back to back and the stroma has been completely crowded out, then adenocarcinoma is thought to exist (Fig. 4.64). Individual cell atypicality suggesting this diagnosis may occur in some hyperplastic epithelia prior to the complete development of back to back crowding (Fig. 4.65). When it does, malignancy is suggested (Fig. 4.66). For unknown reasons, stromal hyperplasia occasionally occurs (Fig. 4.67), in which case the stromal proliferation crowds out the epithelium. The factors controlling this development are unknown. In this type of hyperplasia a sequence is difficult to define, as endometrial stromal histology does not differ over a wide spectrum of clinical entities, from mild stromal hyperplasia to low-grade sarcomas.

METAPLASIA

Metaplasia of a variety of types may be seen in early or late hyperplastic endometria. Perhaps the most common form is that of so-called tubal metaplasia (Fig. 4.68). While the presence of ciliated cells in endometrium has been mentioned previously, with estrogen production large portions of endometrial epithelium may be converted to ciliated cells and may produce a brightly eosinophilic epithelium more typical of the fallopian tube. On occasion this epithelium is quite papillary, similar to the tube. However, this type of papillary pattern is not as ominous as is the papillary folding associated with adenomatous hyperplasia. Of course, the two may be combined. Furthermore, squamous metaplasia is commonly seen in hyperplastic endometria and is histologically benign and similar to that seen in the cervix (Fig. 4.69). However, it may produce quite dramatic foci. Other rare forms of metaplasia are occasionally seen (Fig. 4.70).

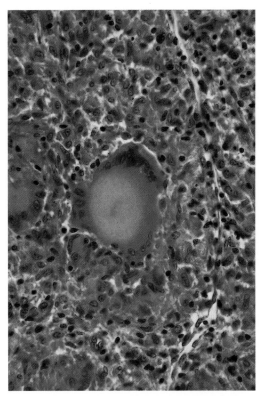

figure 4.56

This photomicrograph of tubercubus endometritis is characterized by a typical Langhans'-type giant cell and associated nonspecific inflammation.

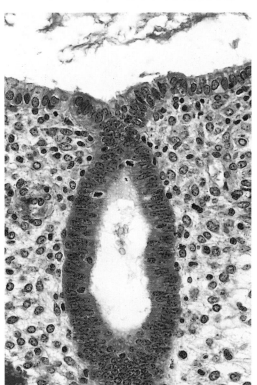

figure 4.57

This photomicrograph shows a secretory endometrium, but an isolated focus of unresponsive epithelium extends all the way to the surface. It contains mitoses and is sharply demarcated from the secretory epithelium on both sides of its surface extent.

4.23

endometrium

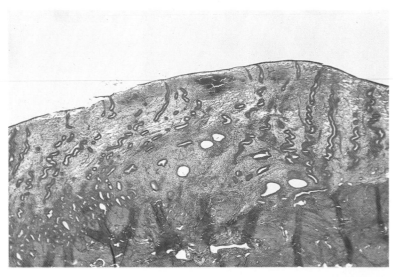

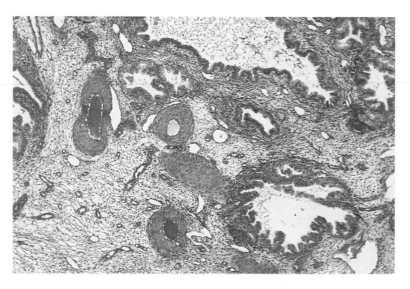

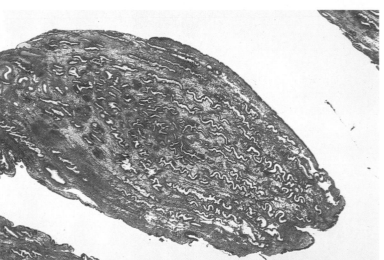

figure 4.58

A focus of basal-type endometrium (top left) is enlarging into the functional portion of the endometrium. The thick-walled vessels (top right) indicate the long-term existence of this focus of endometrial tissue removed when a pregnancy terminated. Although there is some secretory change in the glands, the rest of the endometrium was fully decidualized. The core of this endometrial polyp (left) contains denser proliferating endometrium, whereas the surface has undergone secretory change.

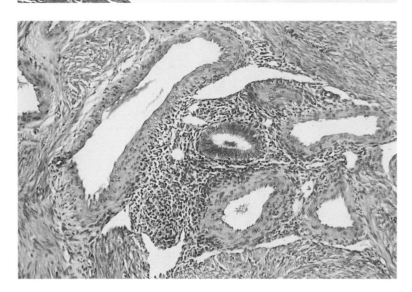

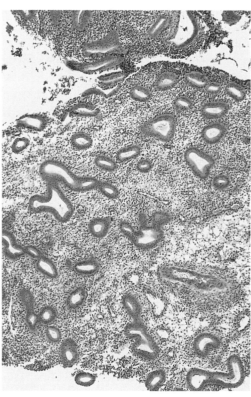

figure 4.60

A band of mild hyperplasia extends from the lower left to the upper right. The stroma is denser than the surrounding endometrium and the glands are slightly dilated.

figure 4.59

In this photomicrograph depicting adenomyosis, a small focus of endometrial stroma and glands has penetrated deep within the myometrium.

atlas of gynecologic pathology

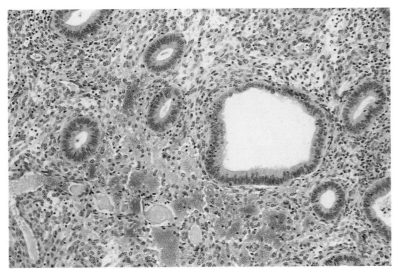

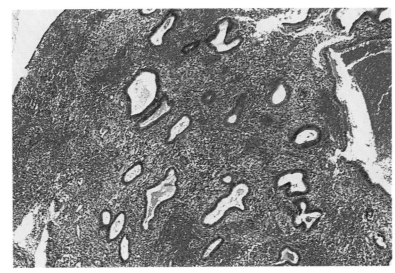

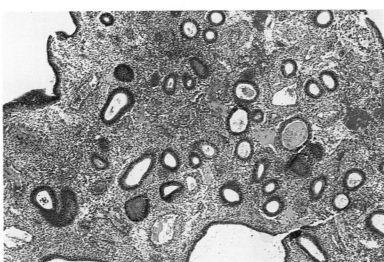

4.25

figure 4.61

This cystically dilated gland (top left) shows some epithelial atrophy with associated bleeding. It comes from a case of abnormal vaginal bleeding, in which most of the endometrium was proliferative but focal areas like this one also were present. The hyperplasia here (top right) is mild but more generalized. The stroma is dense, but some glandular crowding is just beginning. Glandular crowding (left) is more apparent here than in the previous view, but the stroma is still dense. The glands are mostly round.

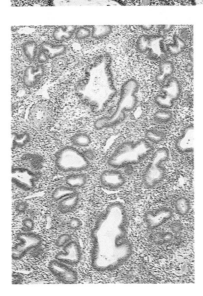

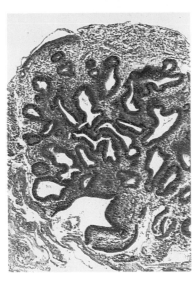

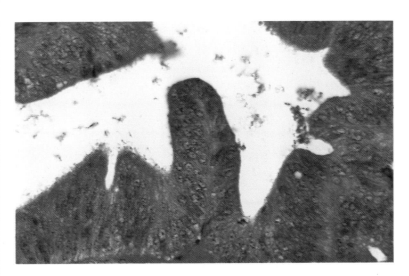

figure 4.62

The glands in this endometrium (left) are crowded and beginning to look irregular in shape as well as in size and number. Glandular budding and crowding (center) are prominent in this endometrium. True

piling up of epithelium (right) has occurred in this example. Epithelial papillae have developed.

endometrium

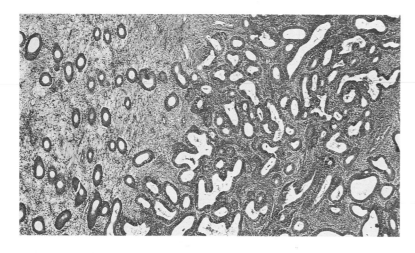

figure 4.63

Significant hyperplasia occupies the right side of the field and is separated clearly from the normal proliferative endometrium to the left.

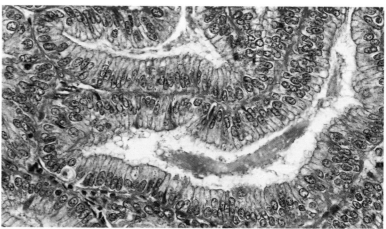

figure 4.64

Photomicrograph showing a focus of well-differentiated adenocarcinoma, characterized by atypical epithelium, lining glands that have completely crowded out all but the most minimal supporting stroma. The nuclei are similar to those seen in rapidly proliferating endometrium.

4.26

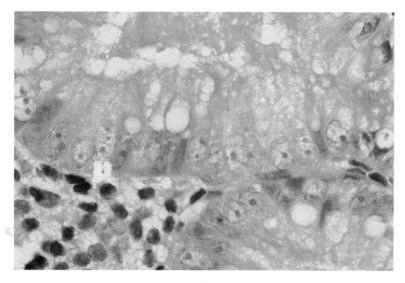

figure 4.65

Enlarged nuclei with prominent, and in some cases, multiple nucleoli represent nuclear atypicality and suggest the premalignant nature of a hyperplasia.

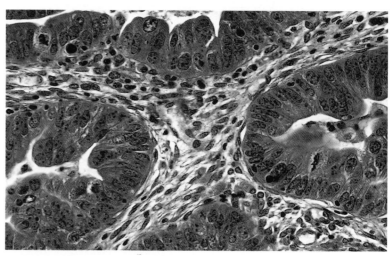

Abnormal mitotic figures

figure 4.66

Although some stroma remains, cytologic atypicality in this case is inconsistent with a benign process. Two and possibly more clearly abnormal mitotic figures are seen.

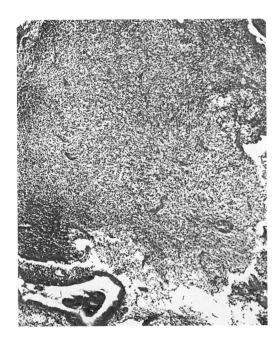

figure 4.67

In this case, proliferating stroma has crowded out the glands. Although only an isolated focus, its malignant potential is hard to assess.

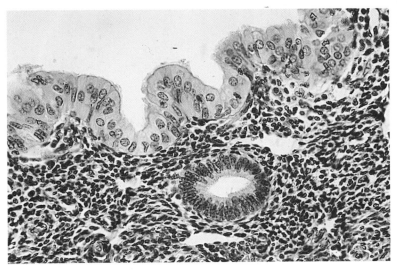

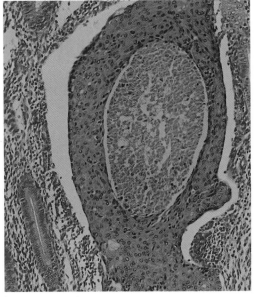

figure 4.69

A focus of squamous metaplasia in an otherwise routine curetting.

figure 4.68

A strip of eosinophilic ciliated cells tending to form papillae characterizes this example of tubal metaplasia.

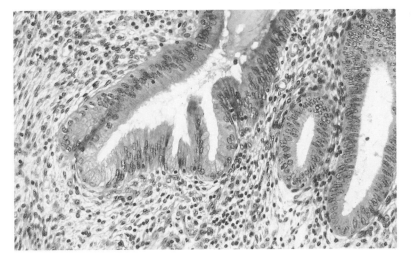

figure 4.70

This isolated focus of mucinous epithelium was an incidental finding in a hysterectomy specimen.

endometrium

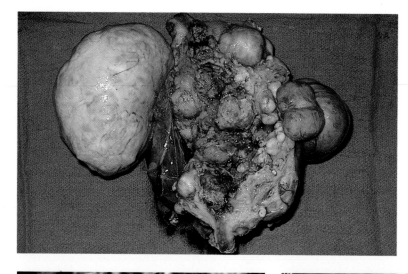

figure 4.71

Multiple leiomyomata, including a large pedunculated one, involved the uterus of this patient with endometrial carcimona.

4.28

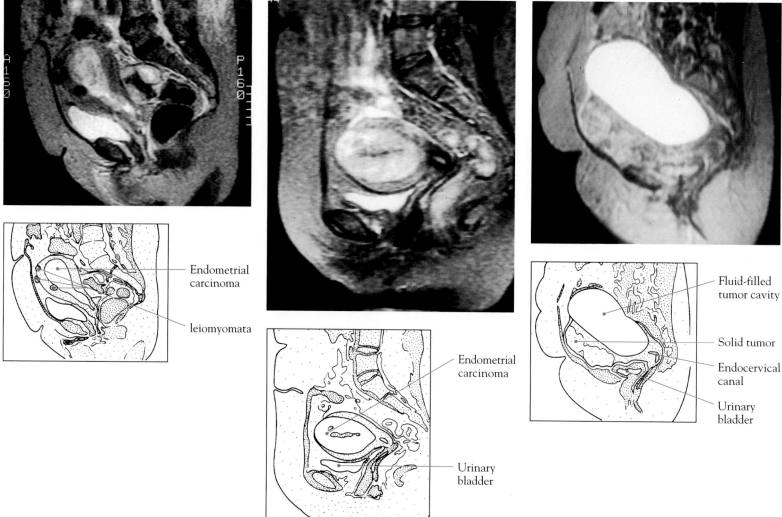

Endometrial carcinoma

leiomyomata

Endometrial carcinoma

Urinary bladder

Fluid-filled tumor cavity

Solid tumor

Endocervical canal

Urinary bladder

figure 4.72

These three slides illustrate sagittal T2-weighted MRIs of endometrial carcinoma. The endometrial cavity (left) is expanded by a bright signal mass that has penetrated into the deep myometrium, obliterating the junctional zone. Several low signal, small leiomyomata are seen within the anterior myometrium. The endometrial mass (center) has penetrated deep into the myometrium, extending anteriorly to the serosal sur-

face. The junctional zone is again obliterated and the urinary badder is displaced inferiorly. Only the endocervical canal (right) is identifiable. The uterine body is replaced by a heterogeneous mass, with a fluid-filled posterior half and a solid anterior half. The plane between the uterus and the contracted urinary bladder is obliterated, suggesting tumor extension into the vesico-uterine space.

Endometrial Cancer

TYPICAL ADENOCARCINOMAS

Most endometrial adenocarcinoma develop in the immediate postmenopausal years as a continuation of the hyperplastic process just described and in association with estrogen secretion. In the absence of ovarian estrogen, gonadotropins rise and ovarian androgen production is stimulated. Obese women convert this androgen in peripheral lipid tissue to estrone, and thus continue to experience estrogen stimulation. Therefore, such women are at a higher than average risk for the development of endometrial cancer. Exogenous estrogen administration has also been associated with an increased risk of the development of endometrial cancer as well as other estrogen related disorders (Fig. 4.71). As a result of these factors, most endometrial cancers are adenocarcinomas, histologically similar to hyperplasia; most are low grade (see Fig. 4.64). This is important, as grade is an important prognostic variable for endometrial cancer and is correlated with other prognostic factors such as depth of myometrial invasion and extent of nodal metastases. MRI sometimes allows for striking preoperative visualization of the depth of myometrial invasion (Fig. 4.72). An exception to the case of depth is the lesion that arises in preexisting adenomyosis (Fig. 4.73). Grade is determined histologically by the degree to which the glandular pattern of the endometrium is preserved. If this pattern is fully preserved, the tumor is grade I (Fig. 4.74); if glandular bridging has occurred and there is partial loss of the original pattern,

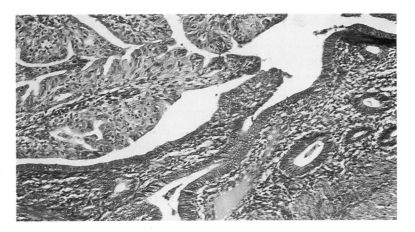

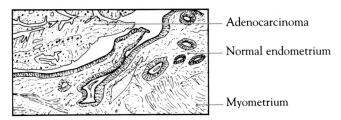

Adenocarcinoma

Normal endometrium

Myometrium

figure 4.73

In this focus of adenomyosis, adenocarcinoma (above) is present with normal endometrium (below). This does not constitute myometrial invasion.

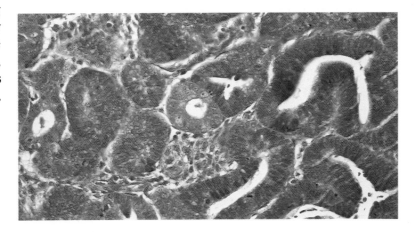

figure 4.74

The glands are well preserved in this grade I adenocarcinoma, indicating continuing differentiation.

endometrium

then grade II is the proper diagnosis (Fig. 4.75); a solid tumor is grade III disease (Fig. 4.76). The gross appearance is variable (Fig. 4.77). Moreover, pyometra is sometimes associated with endometrial cancer (Fig. 4.78).

Histiocytes are common accompaniments of both endometrial cancer and hyperplasia, and they may produce a striking appearance (Fig. 4.79). Endometrial cancer is complicated by the fact that it can drain to either the pelvic or the para-aortic lymph nodes, with fundal lesions being more likely to drain to the para-aortic nodes, and lower segment tumors or those involving the cervix are more likely to involve the pelvic nodes. In clinical experience, each set of nodes is involved in about half of the cases in which any nodes are involved.

OTHER EPITHELIAL TYPES

A variety of other types of histologies are seen in endometrial cancer. But except in those cases in which variation is an indication of grade, it is not necessarily significant. Mucinous epithelium frequently is present in endometrial adenocarcinomas and usually has no bearing on grade (Fig. 4.80). Squamous epithelium is also common. If the squamous epithelium is well differentiated and is seen in association with very low-grade adenocarcinomas, then the tumor is termed an adenoacanthoma and has a good prognosis. If the squamous epithelium is poorly differentiated and is seen with more aggressive adenocarcinomas, then the tumor is termed adenoepidermoid or adenosquamous, depending upon the maturity of the epithelium (Fig. 4.81). Such tumors are more likely to involve the myometrium deeply and thus are associated with less favorable outcomes. Rarely, pure squamous cell cancer occurs in the endometrium (Fig. 4.82). Clear cell adenocarcinoma of the endometrium is a high-grade tumor and has a poor prognosis. Its histology is similar to that of the clear cell tumor seen elsewhere in the genital canal (Fig. 4.83). Both solid sheets of clear cells and tubulopapillary patterns are found. Hobnail cells are characteristic in the latter. Papillary adenocarcinomas occur in the endometrium. They illustrate histologies more typical of those tumors seen in the ovary; most are high grade (Fig. 4.84). Rarely, foci of hyperplasia develop that are secretory in character and may be sufficiently exuberant as to suggest secretory carcinoma (Fig. 4.85). This lesion is very low grade, however, and its significance is questionable.

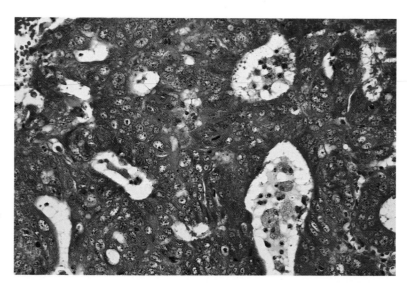

figure 4.75

In this example of grade II adenocarcinoma a cribriform pattern has resulted from the piling up and bridging of malignant epithelium within gland spaces.

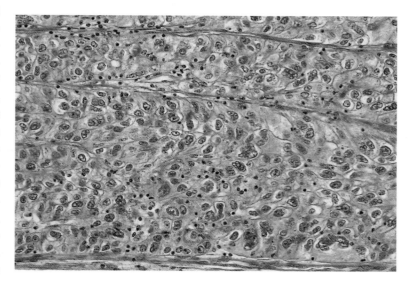

figure 4.76

This example of grade III adenocarcinoma shows solid sheets of cancer that have lost all glandular organization.

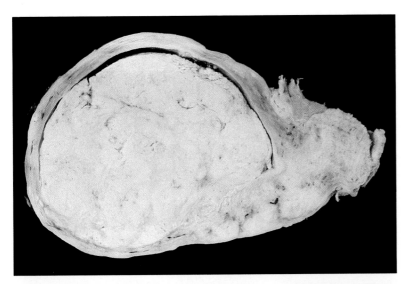

figure 4.77

The cut surface of this endometrial tumor involves the cervix and invades the posterior wall of the myometrium, particularly in the lower uterine segment. The anterior myometrial wall is free of disease (from Tuuk and Fletcher, 1985).

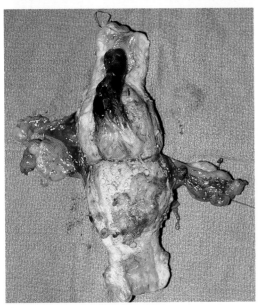 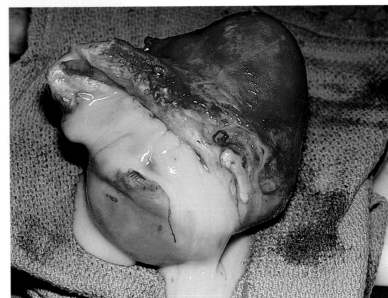

figure 4.78

Polypoid and more endophytic components (left) characterize the gross behavior of this endometrial cancer. This fluid-filled uterus (right) of a patient with endometrial cancer contained a large quantity of pus. (Courtesy of Dr. D. Bard.)

4.31

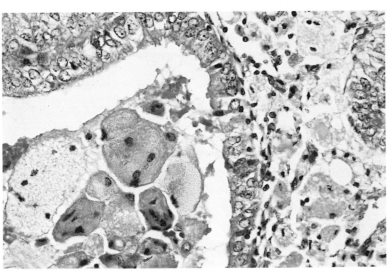 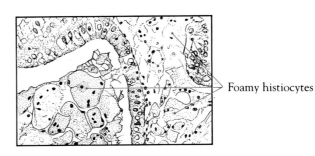

Foamy histiocytes

figure 4.79

Large foamy histiocytes occupy both the glandular lumen and the stroma of this tumor.

endometrium

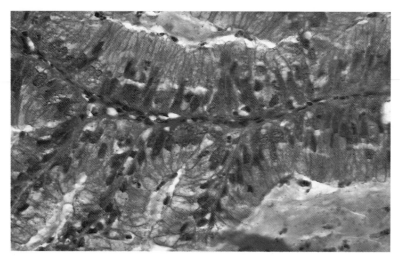

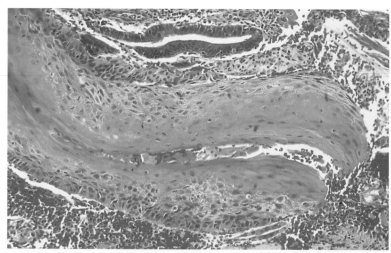

figure 4.80

Mucinous epithelium, albeit atypical, is seen in this endometrial adeno-carcinoma.

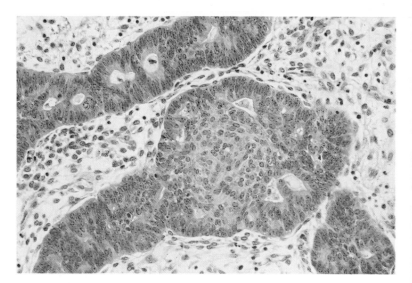

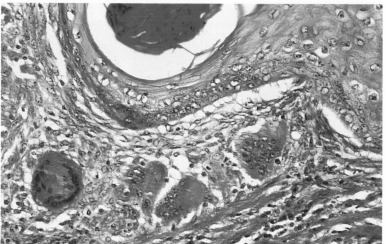

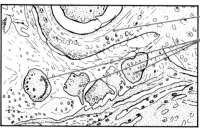

Squamous cancer

Giant cell reaction

figure 4.81

This moderately differentiated adenocarcinoma (top) possesses both glands and foci of immature squamous epithelium. In this endometrial tumor (bottom) the squamous epithelium is more mature, almost achieving keratinization.

figure 4.82

This strip of malignant squamous epithelium (top) was seen in other-wise normal proliferative curettings and misinterpreted as cervical. This hysterectomy specimen from the same case (bottom) showed pure squamous cell cancer deeply invading the myometrium and not involv-ing the cervix. A giant cell inflammatory reaction is part of the host response.

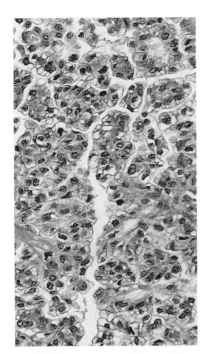

figure 4.83

Photomicrograph shows an example of a clear cell carcinoma in endometrial curettings.

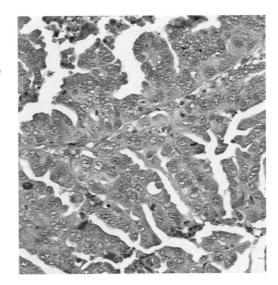

figure 4.84

This papillary carcinoma contained a variety of cell types, all poorly differentiated.

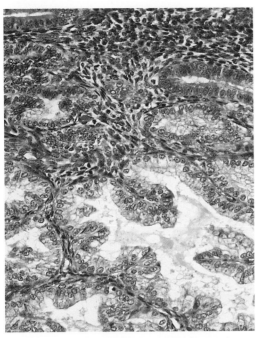

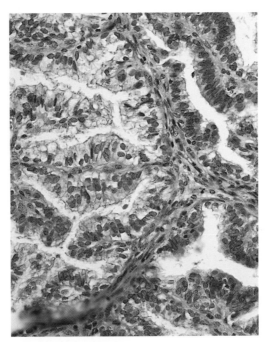

figure 4.85

The proliferative endometrium in the top portion of this photograph (top left) is on the surface of the endometrium. It is not basal. The papillary secretory-appearing glands were in the basalis and appeared to constitute an enlarging focus of atypical secretory growth. This well-differentiated focal adenocarcinoma in a premenopausal woman (top right) contained both secretory and nonsecretory epithelium. This well-developed secretory endometrium (bottom) characterized the uninvolved portion of the endometrial cavity that contained the tumor seen in the top right photograph.

4.33

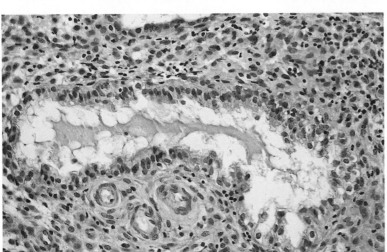

endometrium

If a woman is not obese when she becomes menopausal and if there is absence of exogenous estrogen, the endometrium will become atrophic or at least inactive (Fig. 4.86). The epithelium becomes low, and mitoses are absent. The stroma is sparse and equally nonproliferative. A preexisting pattern of hyperplasia may be preserved but this is misleading (Fig. 4.87). Alternatively, endometrial flattening results in shortening and simplification of the glands. If irritation occurs in this thinned tissue, squamous metaplasia may occur. After age 65, on average, the endometrium becomes atrophic even in obese women (Fig. 4.88).

When malignancies arise in atrophic endometrium, unassociated with estrogen, they are more likely to be of higher grade and to demonstrate the papillary and undifferentiated histologies described above (Fig. 4.89). In addition, they are more likely to be widespread when diagnosed.

Endometriosis

Endometrial tissue develops spontaneously, apparently as a result of biologic variability at all levels of the genital canal and at various other more distant mesodermal sites (Fig. 4.90). The factors that determine the development of clinical endometriosis remain a matter of debate, but in the form of

4.34

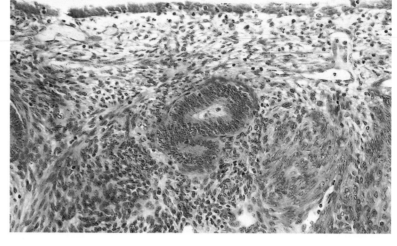

figure 4.86

Photomicrograph of a very thin atrophic postmenopausal endometrium.

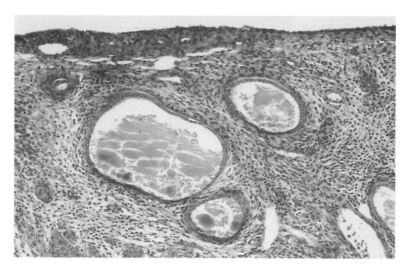

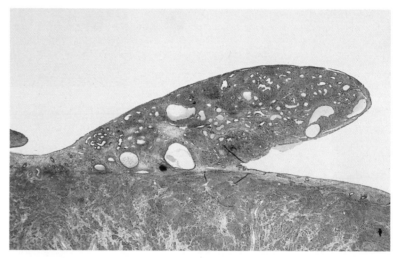

figure 4.87

Although the glands look cystically dilated in this postmenopausal endometrium (top), their epithelium is low and flat and the stroma is sparse. This endometrial polyp (bottom) in a postmenopausal woman no longer displays histologic evidence of active growth. The cystically dilated glands may represent preexisting hyperplasia that is no longer present.

microscopic foci endometriosis is ubiquitous throughout the genital canal and into the peritoneal cavity. At whatever site, its histology is likely to be similar to that of endometrium as described above, and as such, it is subject to the same disease processes, including tumor formation. When decidualization takes place in foci of endometriosis, the concomitant cell death results in its replacement (Fig. 4.91). Muscle metaplasia in such sites may result in a variety of unusual histologies (Fig. 4.92). Perhaps the most dramatic of these histologies is that of leiomyomatosis peritonealis disseminata, in which the presence of widespread subperitoneal decidua and its subsequent conversion to smooth muscle result in the development of smooth muscle nodules all over the peritoneal cavity.

When in the absence of complete differentiation repeated cyclic function takes place in foci of endometriosis, the histology is likely to be that of the associated inflammation and scarring (Fig. 4.93). Initially the stroma is obliterated, leaving epithelial remnants embedded in apparent scar (Fig. 4.94). The epithelium is then lost, but the copious capillary vasculature of the preexisting disease is likely to persist (Fig. 4.95). Inclusion cysts may occur if the epithelium is not eradicated. In the ovary, endometriosis tends to result in cysts that function and produce painful internal bleeding. The stroma in the wall of such a cyst may be unidentifiable, either because it has been replaced by scar as described above or because it is filled with hemosiderin-laden macrophages (Fig. 4.96).

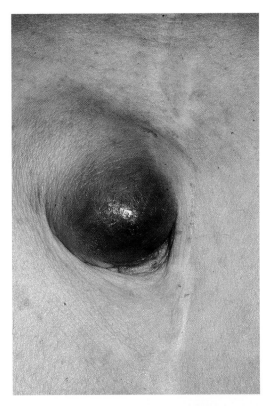

figure 4.88
A Sister Mary Joseph's nodule presents in the umbilicus of a patient with high grade, disseminated endometrial cancer. (Courtesy of Dr. D. Bard.)

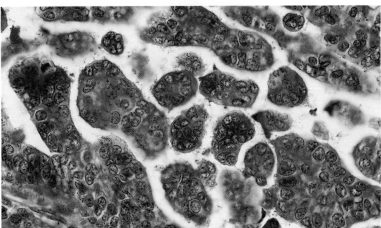

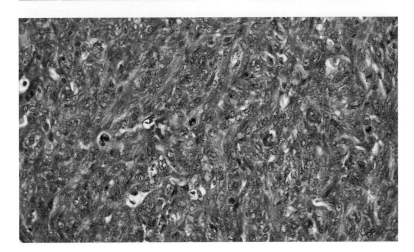

figure 4.89
This highly undifferentiated papillary adenocarcinoma (top) is typical of the malignancies that arise in the endometrial cavity of very elderly women. This solid tumor (bottom) is so undifferentiated that its nature is debatable.

endometrium

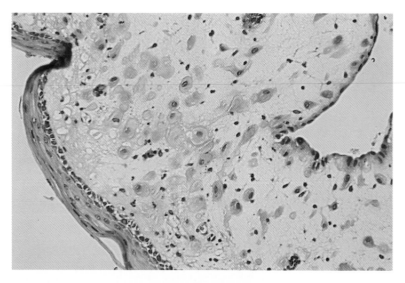

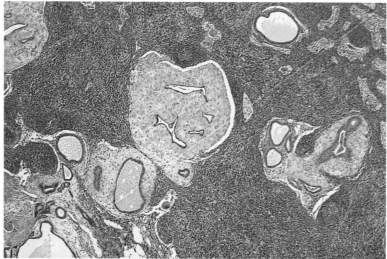

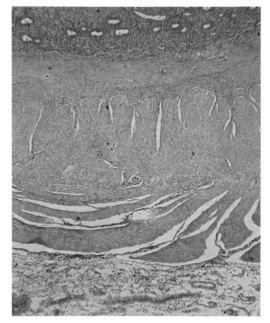

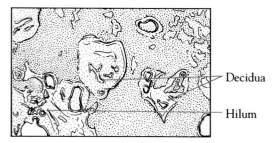

figure 4.90

Photomicrograph (top left) of a focus of decidualized glands and stroma removed from beneath the vaginal mucous membrane in pregnancy. Decidua in this pregnant woman's pelvic lymph node (top right) has a central rather than peripheral distribution. Proliferative endometrium on the surface of the bowel wall (left) is not invading the muscle.

figure 4.91

A focus of decidua immediately beneath the peritoneal surface of a peritubal adhesion removed at the time of postpartum tubal ligation.

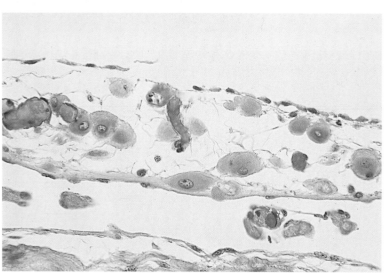

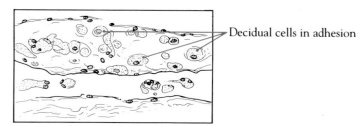

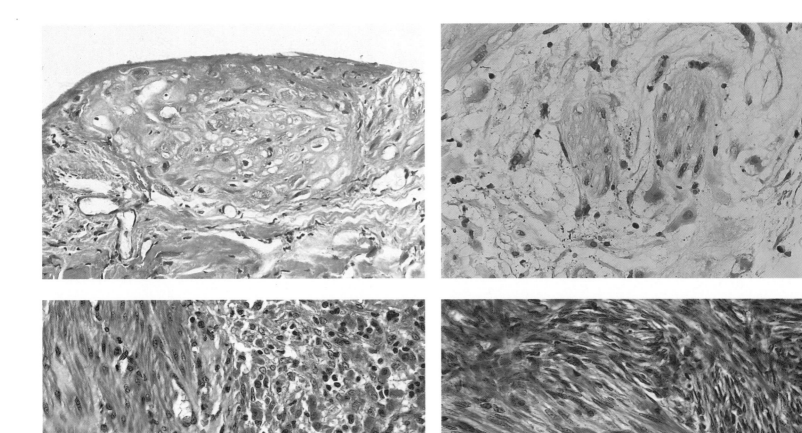

figure 4.92

A focus of subperitoneal decidua in the omentum (top left) is beginning to degenerate. In this focus of subperitoneal omental decidua (top
right) most of the cells look fibroblastic, but two foci of muscle are
developing. Clear-cut muscle (bottom left) is present to the left in this
omental nodule. Persisting inflammation from the preexisting process
remains to the right. A small focus of smooth muscle (bottom right)
has developed in the ovarian cortex.

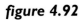

endometrium

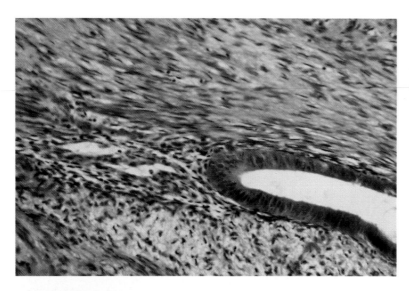 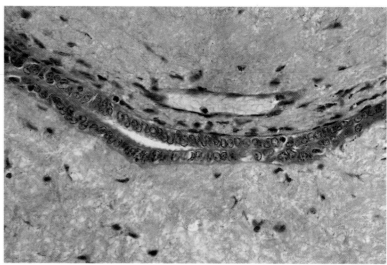

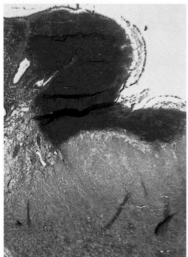

figure 4.93

A gland and a thin strip of remaining stroma (top left) are embedded in developing scar from this case of endometriosis. The stroma in this site (top right) has been eliminated entirely and only an epithelial inclusion remains. Clear-cut endometriosis (left) is present on the ovarian surface to the left. To the right only inflammation and scar are present.

4.38

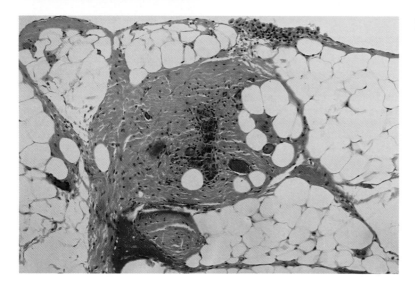

figure 4.94

An epithelial inclusion surrounded by scar containing capillaries is seen in this piece of omentum from a case of endometriosis. The diagnosis is obviously not apparent from this tissue in isolation.

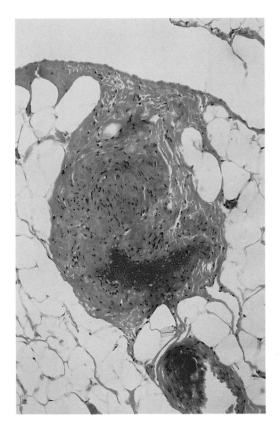

figure 4.95

Immediately adjacent to the site seen in Figure 4.94 is this tiny scar containing only capillaries.

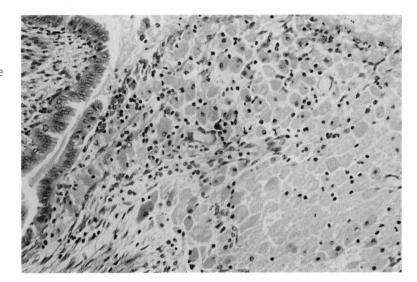

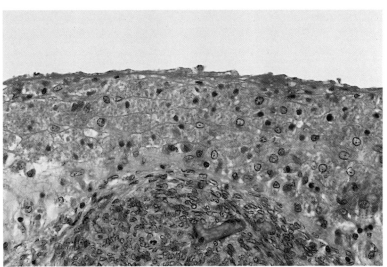

figure 4.96

The wall of this ovarian "chocolate" cyst (top) is lined by epithelium and stroma on the left but only hemosiderin-laden macrophages on the right. Large foamy histiocytes (bottom) are all that is left of the preexisting endometriosis in this ovary.

endometrium

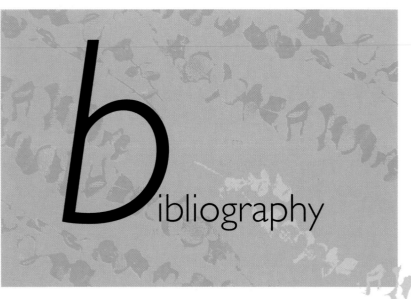

bibliography

Abell MR, Ramirez JA: Sarcomas and carcinosarcomas of the uterine cervix. *Cancer* 31:1176, 1973.

Coppleson M, Reid B: *Preclinical Carcinoma of the Cervix Uteri,* ed 1. Oxford, Pergamon Press, 1967.

Crum CP, Ikenberg H, Richart RM, Gissman L: Human papillomavirus type 16 and early cervical neoplasia. *New Engl J Med* 310:880, 1984.

Fluhmann CF: *The Cervix Uteri and its Diseases.* Philadelphia, WB Saunders Co., 1961.

Fujii T, Crum C, Winkler B, et al: Human papillomavirus infection and cervical intraepithelial neoplasia: Histopathology and DNA content. *Obstet Gynecol* 63:99, 1984.

Gardner HL: Cervical and vaginal endometriosis. *Clin Obstet Gynecol* 9:358, 1966.

Glucksmann A, Cherry CP: Incidence, histology, and response to radiation of mixed carcinomas (adenoacanthomas) of the uterine cervix. *Cancer* 9:971, 1956.

Kurman RJ, Jenson AB, Lancaster WD: Papillomavirus infection of the cervix II. *Am J Surg Pathol* 7:39, 1983.

Lawrence WD, Shingleton HM: Early physiologic squamous metaplasia of the cervix: Light and electron microscopic observations. *Am J Obstet Gynecol* 137:661, 1980.

Meisels A, Roy M, Fortier M, Morrin C: Condylomatous lesions of the cervix, morphologic and colposcopic diagnosis. *Am J Diagn Gynecol Obstet* 1:109, 1979.

Ostor AG, Pagano R, Davoren RAM, et al: Adenocarcinoma in situ of the cervix. *Int J Gynecol Pathol* 3:179, 1984.

Papanicolaou GN, Traut HF: The diagnostic value of vaginal smears in carcinomas of the uterus. *Am J Obstet Gynecol* 42:193, 1941.

Richart RM: Cervical intraepithelial neoplasia. In Sommers SC (ed.): *Pathology Annual.* New York, Appleton-Century-Crofts, 1973.

Shingleton HM, Orr JW: Cancer of the cervix. *Current Reviews Obstetrics & Gynecology.* New York, Churchill Livingstone, 1983.

Singer A: The uterine cervix from adolescence to the menopause. *Br J Obstet Gynecol* 82:81, 1975.

Terruhn V: A study of impression moulds of the genital tract of female fetuses. *Arch Gynecol* 229:207, 1980.

Tuck JL, Fletcher CDM: *Royal College of Surgeons of England Slide Atlas of Pathology.* Reproductive System, London, Gower Medical Publishing, 1985.

Van Nagell JR, Greenwell N, Powell DF, et al: Hanson MB, Gay EC: Microinvasive carcinoma of the cervix. *Am J Obstet Gynecol* 145:981, 1983.

Woodruff JD, Braun L, Cavalieri R, et al: Immunologic identification of papillomavirus antigen in condyloma tissue from the female genital tract. *Obstet Gynecol* 56:727, 1980.

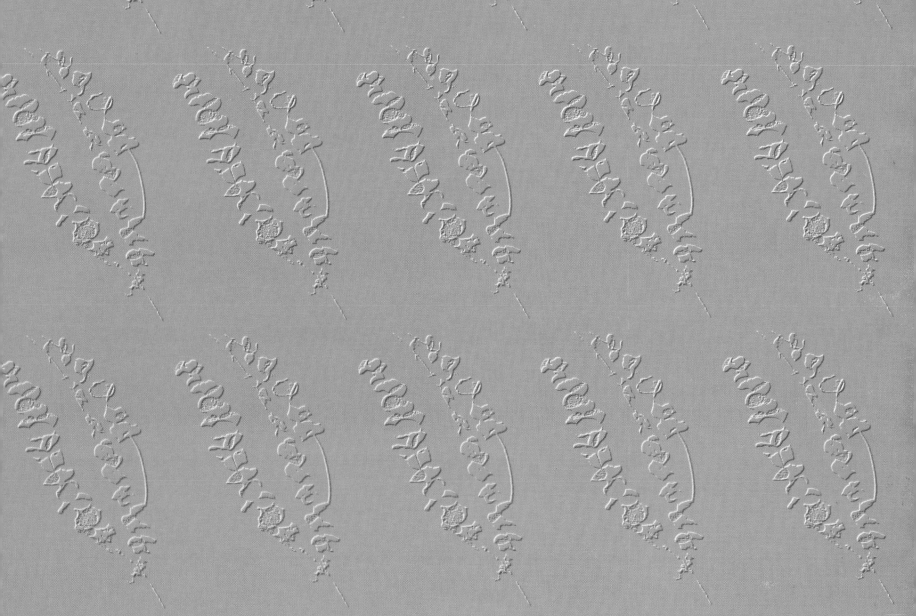

mesenchymal tumors

tumors

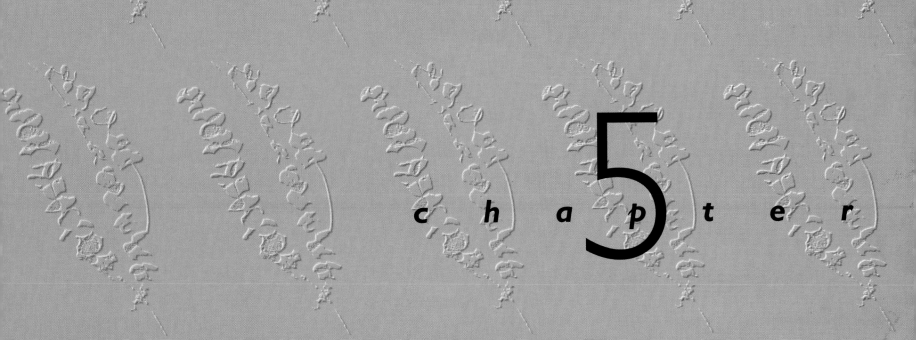

chapter 5

Origin of Mesenchymal tumors

The mesenchymal lesions of the uterus arise in the myometrium and in the endometrial stroma. As the myometrium develops from the lateral portion of the mesodermal wall of the müllerian duct and the endometrial stroma develops from the medial portion of the same structure, the two tissues are closely related (Fig. 5.1). Consequently, proliferative disorders in either tissue may resemble those in the other; in fact, because all of the mesenchyme of the genital canal are closely related, the description that follows is applicable to mesenchymal lesions at all levels.

A fully differentiated myometrium consists largely of smooth muscle cells arranged in interlacing bundles (Fig. 5.2) and is roughly organized in two layers (Fig. 5.3). The hormones of pregnancy produce additional differentiation in the myometrium, which is manifest as tremendous hypertrophy of the smooth muscle cells, with an apparent increase in ground substance (Fig. 5.4). Additional myometrial changes attributable to pregnancy are the infiltration by intermediate-type trophoblasts (Fig. 5.5) and the conversion of the spiral arterioles of the myometrium to hyaline masses that persist as evidence of a previous implantation (Fig. 5.6). After the menopause, the myometrial muscle cells atrophy. The myometrial tissue tends to consist of acellular areas containing mostly collagen, alternating with areas that appear to be highly cellular, in which the muscle cell cytoplasm has shrunk to the point that only small, crowded nuclei remain (Fig. 5.7). Failure of the müllerian ducts to fuse can result in varying degrees of uterine reduplication (Fig. 5.8).

The endometrial stroma is a loose reticulum in which small fibroblastic-type cells are suspended. Its border with the myometrium is not only anatomically irregular, but

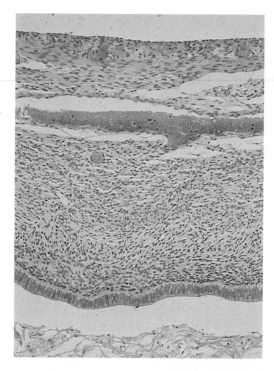

figure 5.1

The entire wall of the embryonic uterus is seen in this photomicrograph. The epithelium of the müllerian duct is evident below. Above, the myometrium and the endometrial stroma are not yet sufficiently differentiable as to be distinguishable from one another.

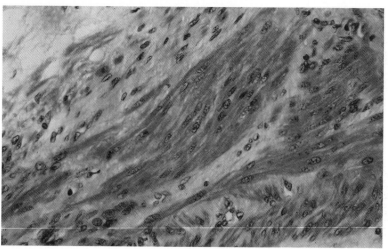

figure 5.2

Photomicrograph of a nonpregnant uterus from a normal cycling woman. Smooth muscle bundles appear almost parallel, oblique, and perpendicular to the plane of the section as one moves from the upper left center to the lower right.

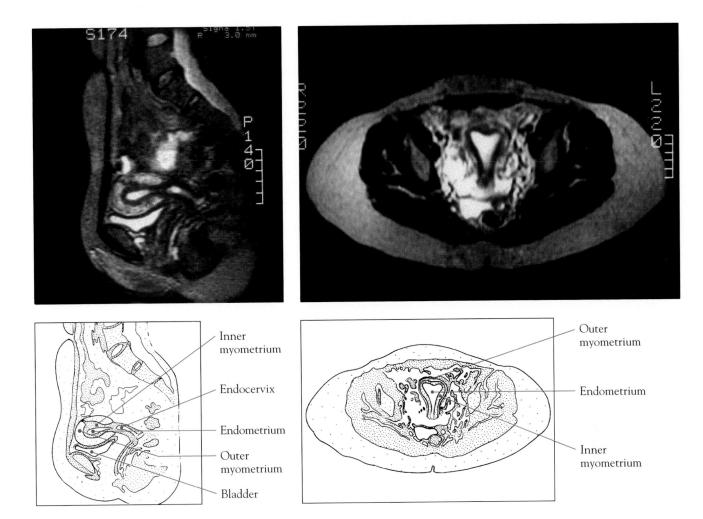

figure 5.3

Sagittal T2-weighted MRI (left) shows a normal uterus anteverted with the fundus indenting the superior aspect of the bladder. Three distinct layers are identified: a bright central signal representing the endometrium, a low intensity rim representing the superficial myometrium, and a medium intensity rim representing a deep myometrium. The cervix

shows two layers: the bright endocervix and the low signal cervical stroma. Axial T2-weighted MRI (right) displays a coronal view of a normal uterus. Three distinct layers are equally appreciated in this view as in the sagittal view. A normal bright signal arising from the parametria and fluid containing bowel can be seen around the uterus.

figure 5.4

This photomicrograph, taken at the same magnification as Figure 5.2, reveals the tremendous hypertrophy of the myometrial smooth muscle cells that results from pregnancy.

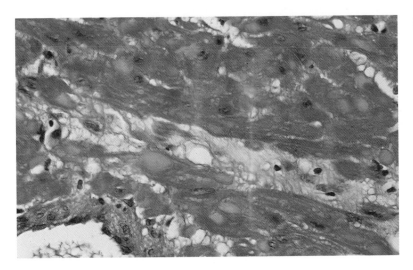

mesenchymal tumors

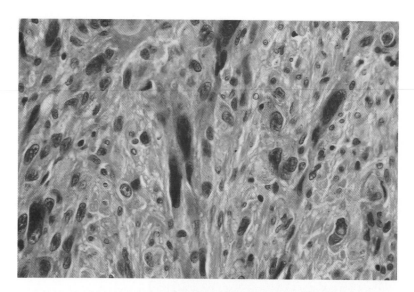

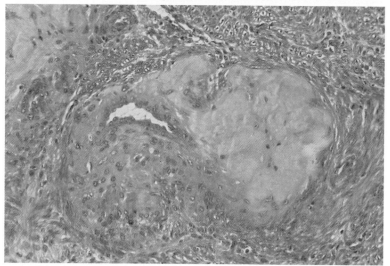

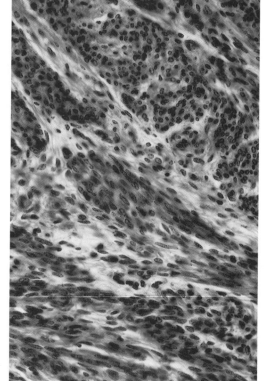

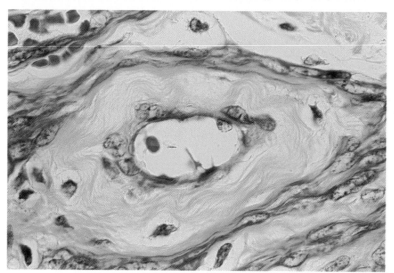

figure 5.5

Large mononuclear and multinuclear intermediate trophoblastic cells infiltrate the myometrium in this section from the uterine wall immediately beneath the implantation site.

figure 5.7

This photomicrograph, taken at the same magnification as Figures 5.2 and 5.4, illustrates the shrunken myometrial cells of the postmenopausal atrophic uterus. Areas of cellularity alternate with acellular ones.

figure 5.6

Trophoblastic invasion during a prior pregnancy (top) has converted the wall of this spiral arteriole into an acellular scar. Even years later this myometrial vessel (bottom) beneath an old implantation site possesses a hyalinized wall.

atlas of gynecologic pathology

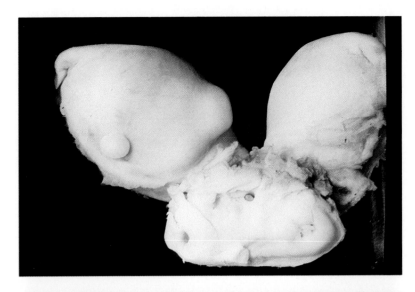

figure 5.8

The didelphic uterus (top) consists of completely separate tracts (from Tuck and Fletcher, 1985). The uterus (center) possesses a fundal indentation indicating the site of the septum that divides the cavity into two compartments. (Courtesy of Dr. D. Bard.) Transverse transabdominal ultrasound of a septate uterus (bottom) exhibits a section taken through two uterine cavities with artifactual acoustic enhancement, posteriorly. The septum separating the uterine cavities appears hypoechoic because of its parallel orientation to the ultrasound beam. The endometrial echoes are bright due to the presence of decidual reaction in this pregnant patient.

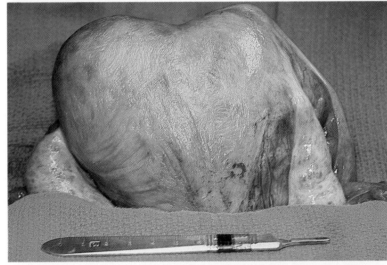

5.5

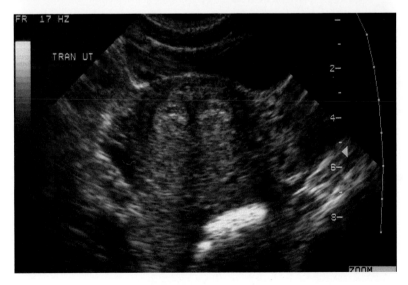

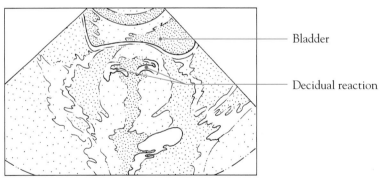

Bladder

Decidual reaction

mesenchymal tumors

physiologically unstable as well (Fig. 5.9). There is evidence that myometrial cells differentiate from undifferentiated stroma along this border, at least until the menopause. In an estrogenic environment, the basal endometrium (both glands and stroma) may grow deeply into the myometrium, resulting in adenomyosis (Fig. 5.10). Function in such sequestered foci may produce pain (Fig. 5.11). In addition, all of the pathologic processes known to occur in endometrium may occur in these foci (Fig. 5.12). Perhaps the two most significant of these processes are:

1. The development of adenocarcinoma in adenomyosis, which gives the false impression of myometrial invasion (Fig. 5.13).
2. The development of muscle hypertrophy, possibly by metaplasia, around the focus of adenomyosis.

This second process produces an adenomyoma (Fig. 5.14).

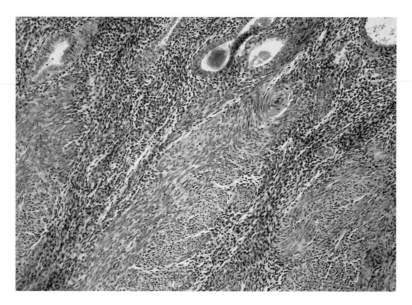

Smooth Muscle tumors

LEIOMYOMAS

The most common mesenchymal tumor is the leiomyoma, which is found in up to 40% of women, depending upon how the figure is ascertained. Leiomyomas resemble hyperplasia in that they are estrogen-dependent and grow only in its presence. Developing at any location within the myometrium, their clinical manifestations depend upon their site and size, and are highly variable (Fig. 5.15). Leiomyomas may also occur at other levels in the genital canal. Microscopically, they consist of whorled bands of interlacing smooth muscle, alternating with more cellular foci (Fig. 5.16). This picture results from a planar section that is both parallel and tangential to the long axis of muscle bundles. Occasional examples show remarkable palisading of nuclei (Fig. 5.17). This pattern has no known significance, although it has been interpreted by some to be evidence of a neural origin. Consistent with their benignity, leiomyomas have only a pushing border (Fig. 5.18).

Leiomyomas are often multiple, although each is a unique clone of cells arising from a single progenitor cell. Characteristically, they possess less arterial blood supply than the surrounding myometrium, and the truly large ones have usually achieved a parasitic blood supply from the omentum (Fig. 5.19). Because of their decreased blood flow, leiomyomas are extremely susceptible to infarction and to histologic degen-

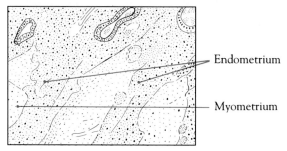

figure 5.9

The endometrium above extends deeply between muscle bundles into the myometrium below. This results in an irregular endomyometrial border.

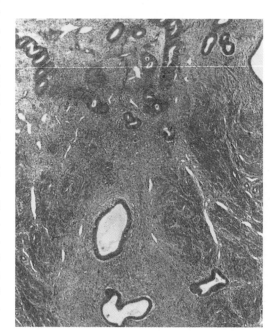

figure 5.10

The normal endometrium above is extending into the myometrium below. The endometrium within the myometrium is slightly hyperplastic in contrast to that above.

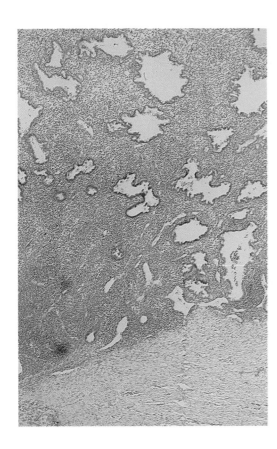

figure 5.11

In this focus of adenomyosis the endometrial tissue immediately adjacent to the myometrium resembles basalis; however, further removed from the myometrium it is displaying secretory function.

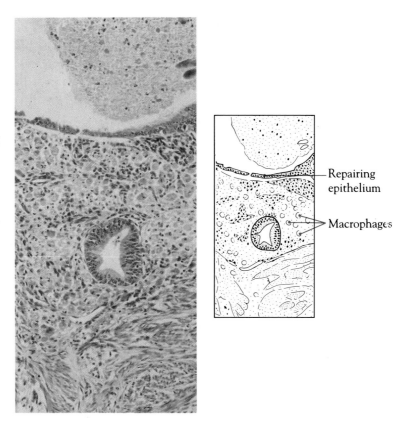

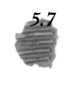

Repairing epithelium

Macrophages

figure 5.12

Hemosiderin-laden macrophages in the stroma, in this focus of adenomyosis, indicate recent bleeding. The epithelium is repairing.

5.7

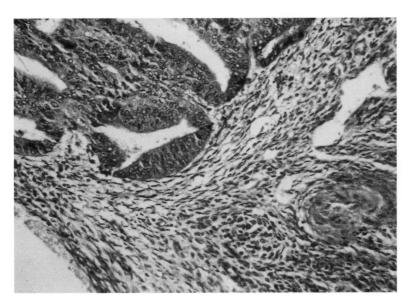

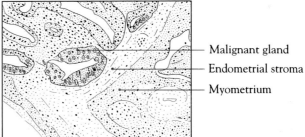

Malignant gland
Endometrial stroma
Myometrium

figure 5.13

Malignant glands are seen deep within the myometrium, but they are embedded in normal endometrial stroma, suggesting that they are located in a preexisting site of adenomyosis.

mesenchymal tumors

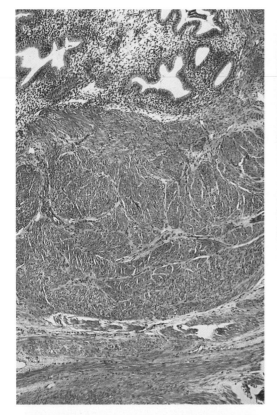

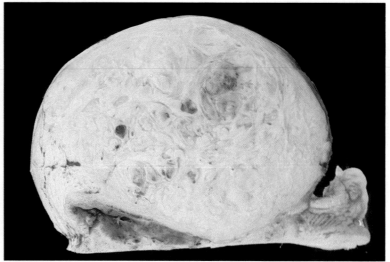

figure 5.14

A focus of adenomyosis seen above (left) appears to be supported by and embedded in a band of hypertrophic muscle that completely encircled the endometrial-type tissue. This example of an adenomyoma (above) shows the characteristic alteration of yellowish muscle tissue with darker hemorrhagic areas of functioning endometrial tissue (from Tuck and Fletcher, 1985).

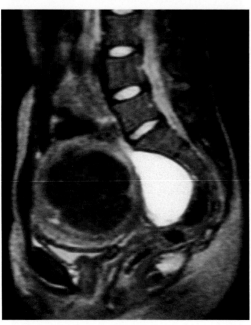

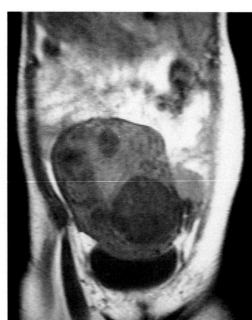

figure 5.15

Sagittal T2-weighted MRI of a leiomyoma (left) shows the endometrial echo displaced anteriorly by a low signal mass and surrounded by a circumferential rim of myometrium. The pulse sequence defines the intramural location of this myoma accurately due to its ability to discriminate between normal myometrium and endometrium. A moderate fluid collection is seen in the cul-de-sac with a typical bright signal. Coronal T1-weighted MRI of a uterine leiomyomata (right) shows the uterus markedly enlarged with several leiomyomata distorting the uterine contour. On this pulse sequence, the masses are of medium signal intensity. The low signal urinary bladder is seen inferiorly.

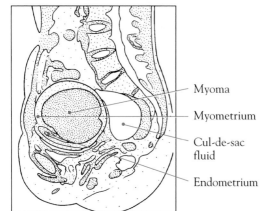

Myoma

Myometrium

Cul-de-sac
fluid

Endometrium

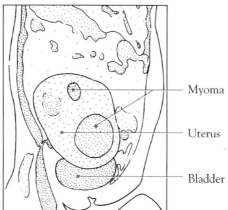

Myoma

Uterus

Bladder

atlas of gynecologic pathology

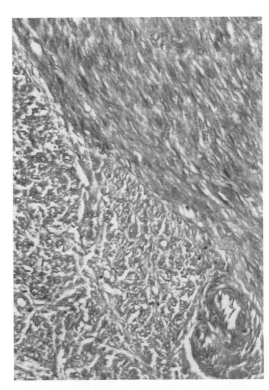

figure 5.16

Above and to the right in this photomicrograph, the muscle bundles run parallel to the plane of the section. Below and to the left, the plane of the section cuts across the muscle bundle.

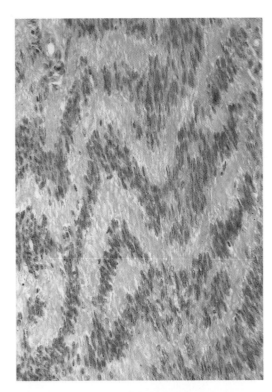

figure 5.17

The nuclei of these muscle cells are arranged in wavy palisades. This pattern was focal in this myoma.

5.9

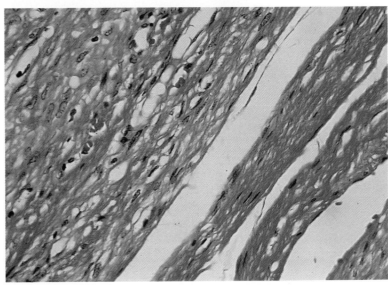

figure 5.18

The myoma above and to the left is a solid cellular mass. It has pushed the surrounding myometrium into linear strands, from which it has retracted during the course of fixation.

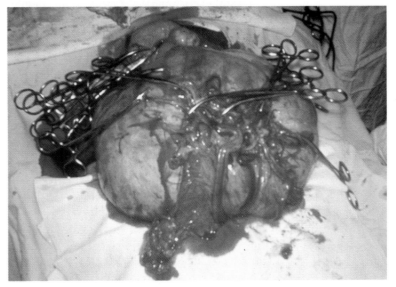

figure 5.19

This large myoma filled the abdominal cavity. Large vessels in the attached omentum represent the additional blood supply.

mesenchymal tumors

eration. The most common change is focal or generalized hyalinization, which may be very extensive (Fig. 5.20). Secondary calcification routinely takes place in hyalinized leiomyomas, particularly after the menopause (Fig. 5.21). If liquefaction occurs, large or small cystic spaces result (Fig. 5.22).

When mesenchymal cells begin to degenerate, they may become enlarged with huge vacuolated nuclei that falsely suggest malignancy. If this change is generalized, the result is a bizarre leiomyoma (Fig. 5.23). When mitoses are present in this context, malignancy is closely simulated. However, atypicality due to degeneration is usually distinguishable from true sarcoma (Fig. 5.24). Focal cell death, with necrosis and secondary inflammation, may result from progestational hormone administration. So-called *carneous degeneration* of a myoma is a hemorrhagic infarct resulting from venous obstruction (Fig. 5.25). Since the venous supply of myomas is usually quite large, carneous degeneration occurs most commonly during pregnancy, when significant architectural rearrangements take place between the myoma and the surrounding muscle. If a myoma is acutely infarcted, systemic symptoms may result, including pain, fever, leukocytosis, and disseminated intravascular coagulation. Occasionally, degenerating myomas are infiltrated by lipid-absorbing macrophages, resulting in fatty degeneration; true uterine lipomas have been reported but are rare (Fig. 5.26).

If routine myomas are only foci of hyperplasia in muscle, there exist other entities that are more likely to be true neoplasms. *Cellular myomas* are defined as myomas that are more cellular than the surrounding myometrium (Fig. 5.27). Small ones, however, may only be developing myomas, which lacking any degeneration appear more cellular (Fig. 5.28). Some cellular myomas, however, appear to consist of immature muscle cells that lack cytoplasmic differentiation (Fig. 5.29). Most are solitary nodules with pushing borders. Since myomas may contain foci of stromal differentiation (Fig. 5.30), in some cases the distinction between a cellular

5.10

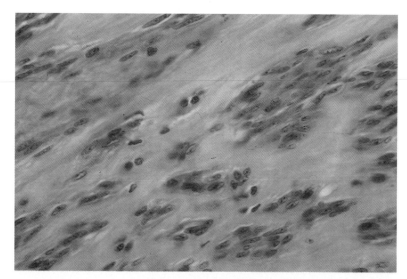

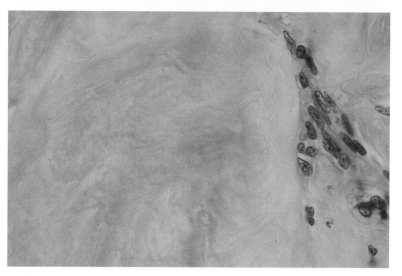

figure 5.20

Early hyalinization in this myoma (top) separates collections of muscle cells, producing a pattern of alternating cellularity and acellularity. In this myoma (bottom), extensive hyalinization has converted almost the entire nodule into an acellular mass with only a few muscle cells remaining.

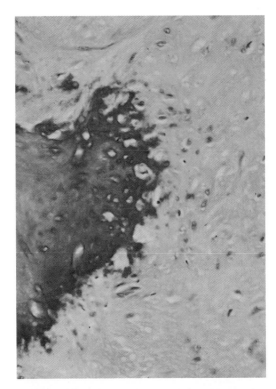

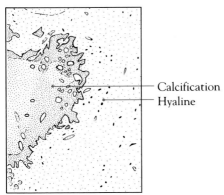

Calcification
Hyaline

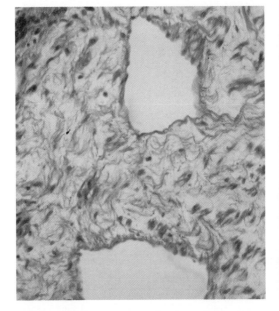

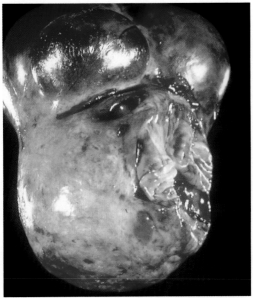

figure 5.22

Cystic spaces (left) have developed in the edematous acellular center of the myoma where most of the tissue substance has been liquefied. The myoma's multiple large cysts (right) result from a more dramatic example of the process seen at left.

5.11

figure 5.23

The nuclei in this degenerating myoma are multiple, enlarged, and atypical in appearance. In addition, they are smudged and in some cases vacuolated, showing the characteristic signs of degeneration. They were generalized over a large portion of the mass.

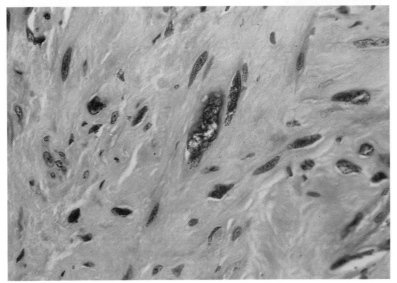

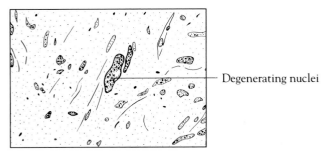

Degenerating nuclei

mesenchymal tumors

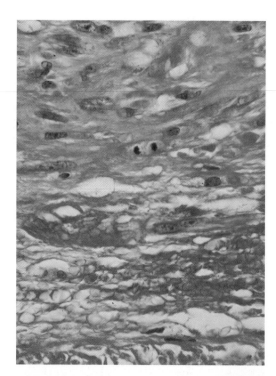

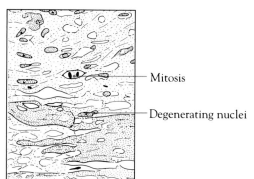

Mitosis

Degenerating nuclei

figure 5.24

Mitosis seen in a myoma, in the still living tissue at the edge of the central area of infarction, is only reactive. Some of the adjacent nuclei are degenerating and show minor atypicality.

5.12

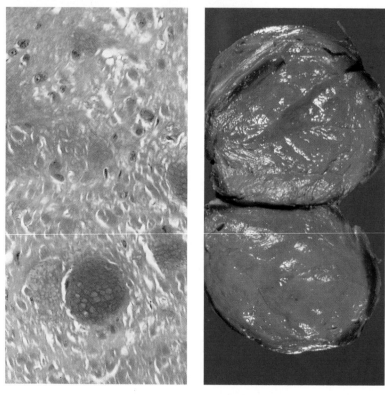

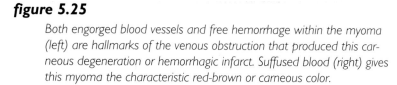

figure 5.25

Both engorged blood vessels and free hemorrhage within the myoma (left) are hallmarks of the venous obstruction that produced this carneous degeneration or hemorrhagic infarct. Suffused blood (right) gives this myoma the characteristic red-brown or carneous color.

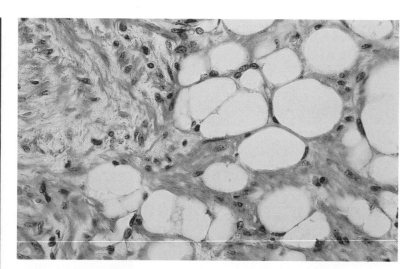

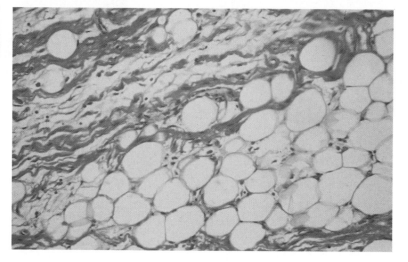

figure 5.26

Fat cells (top) infiltrate the muscle of the myoma in this example of fatty degeneration. Fat cells (bottom) compose this lipoleiomyoma from the broad ligament. (Courtesy of Dr. Ibrahim Ramzy.)

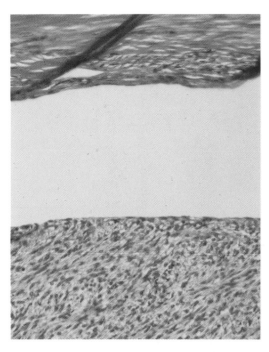

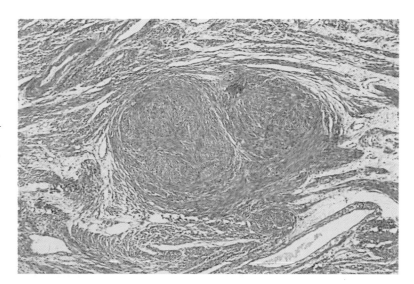

figure 5.27

The normal myometrium seen above contrasts with the increased cellularity of the cellular myoma seen below. The latter has retracted from the surrounding myometrium, causing an artifactual separation of the two.

figure 5.28

This small, relatively young myoma appears superficially more cellular than the surrounding myometrium.

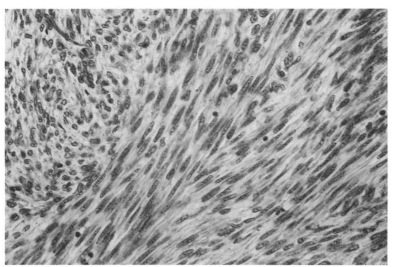

figure 5.29

The cells of this cellular myoma, seen at a lower power in Figure 5.27, lack the cytoplasmic differentiation of fully mature smooth muscle cells.

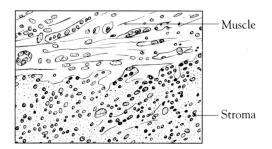

Muscle

Stroma

figure 5.30

Normal muscle seen above contrasts with a focus of endometrial stromal differentiation seen below. This focus represented only a small portion of an otherwise routine myoma.

mesenchymal tumors

myoma and a solitary stromal nodule is not clear-cut (Fig. 5.31). Neither cellular myomas nor isolated stromal nodules have malignant potential.

Smooth muscle tumors, composed of cells with distinctive cytoplasmic differentiation suggesting epithelial cells, may occur. These epithelioid myomas are found in two forms:

1. Cells that have a small amount of relatively dense eosinophilic cytoplasm (Fig. 5.32).
2. Cells that have larger amounts of clear cytoplasm (Fig. 5.33). Small epitheloid myomas have been called *plexiform tumorlets* (Fig. 5.34). Although in general they are not malignant, most observers require only five mitoses per ten high-power fields to label them as such, in contrast to the ten mitoses per ten high-power fields required to label a cellular leiomyoma as sarcoma.

LEIOMYOMATOSIS

Intravenous leiomyomatosis is a rare condition consisting of the infiltration of the pelvic veins by benign smooth muscle (Fig. 5.35). The epithelioid type of leiomyoma is significantly represented among these cases. The tumor produces worm-like masses that fill the pelvic veins. Rarely, they progress via the vena cava to the tricuspid valve in the right atrium, where they may be lethal (Fig. 5.36). Intravenous leiomyomatosis does not metastasize outside of the veins, but occasionally has been either multicentric or metastatic within them. Multiple attachment sites to vein walls may be seen (Fig. 5.37). Surgical excision, perhaps with the assistance of vascular surgical techniques, is the preferred therapy.

Leiomyomatosis peritonealis disseminata is an unusual condition that in most cases consists of muscle metaplasia in preexisting, decidualized, endometrial-type stroma. Examples are found, however, in which subperitoneal muscle nodules seem to arise under conditions that suggest little hormone stimulation or support. Such cases should possibly be viewed as autonomous neoplasms, although only rarely have they been reported to pursue a malignant clinical course. Muscle metaplasia is an important process, which, as mentioned above, probably occurs physiologically in the endometrial cavity, but sporadically it occurs throughout the pelvis. Although it may occur by several mechanisms, it commonly begins with fibrosis in decidual tissue (Fig. 5.38). Subsequently, the tissue is converted to muscle, and may result in nodules at a variety of unusual sites (Fig. 5.39). This condition requires no treatment.

5.14

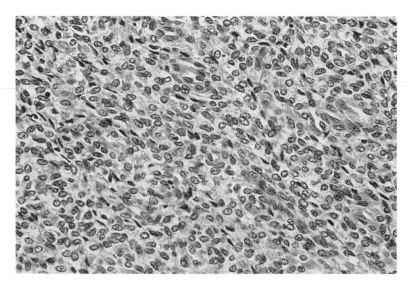

figure 5.31

This nodule in the myometrium is composed of hypercellular tissue that resembles both stroma and muscle.

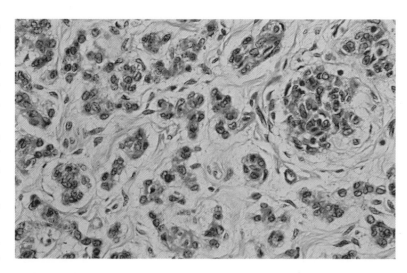

figure 5.32

In this myometrial nodule, the individual cells are epithelioid with dense eosinophilic cytoplasm. They are arranged in nests, further contributing to their epithelial appearance.

LEIOMYOSARCOMA

Leiomyosarcomas arise in myomas or in the myometrium. Rarely found before age 40, they tend to be low grade and confined to the uterus in premenopausal women, and high grade and more extensive in postmenopausal women (Fig. 5.40). Most leiomyosarcomas are associated with characteristic malignant cellular atypicality (Fig. 5.41). However, since degeneration in smooth muscle tumors can simulate this atypicality, it is widely accepted that mitoses are the appropriate criteria for the diagnosis and grading of leiomyosarcomas (Fig. 5.42). In general, if the muscle tumor has one mitosis per high-power field in ten high-power fields, it qualifies as leiomyosarcoma; if it has less than five mitoses per ten high-power fields, it is benign. Between these two limits are rare cases that are viewed with suspicion but without certainty. Such cases usually look like cellular myomas, but a few have pursued progressive and lethal courses. If the muscle tumor is of an epithelioid variety, then many observers accept five mitoses per ten high-power fields as the diagnostic level of malignancy. In recent years, the question of mitoses has become more complicated as it has been shown that some benign forms possess mitoses, particularly in the luteal phase of the cycle. Most leiomyosarcomas are not subtle, however, and in addition to large numbers of atypical mitoses per high-power field, they possess many atypical cellular features. Poor prognostic indicators are high mitotic counts, infiltrative borders, vascular invasion, and advanced stage or advanced age, but all of these are correlated with one another (Fig. 5.43). At present, if surgical removal is not curative, there is no truly effective therapy.

Stromal tumors

Occasionally, foci of tissue resembling other types of mesenchyme develop within the myometrium. These may be foci of apparent metaplasia, or they may take the form of tumors. The tissue type may be truly unusual, such as adipose tissue or fibrous tissue, but most often the anomalous focus resembles endometrial stroma (Fig. 5.44). Tumors with stromal differentiation occur in a spectrum (Fig. 5.45). Solitary nodules of histologically normal stroma occurring in the myometrium are referred to as isolated stromal nodules, and these nodules possess a pushing border. They pursue a benign clinical course with only local enlargement. Grossly, they are indistinguishable from myomas. Hemangiopericytomas have been described in the uterus. These consist of lesions that in

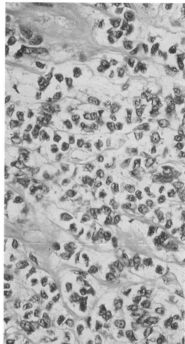
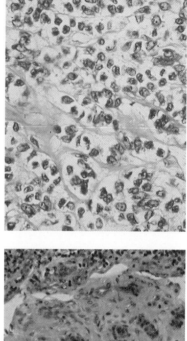

figure 5.33

The cells in this example have an abundant clear cytoplasm. The nests are separated by relatively acellular ground substance.

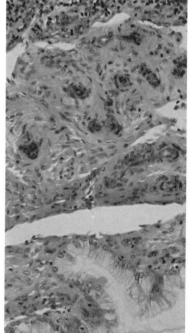

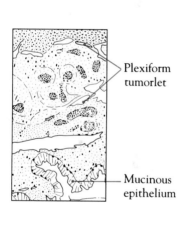

Plexiform tumorlet

Mucinous epithelium

figure 5.34

The tiny epithelioid leiomyoma above was located in the basal endometrium. This plexiform tumorlet is associated with epithelial metaplasia in the adjacent endometrium, where a focus of mucinous epithelium is seen.

5.15

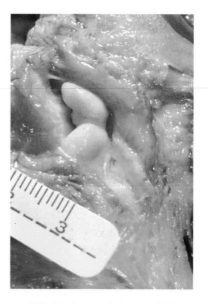 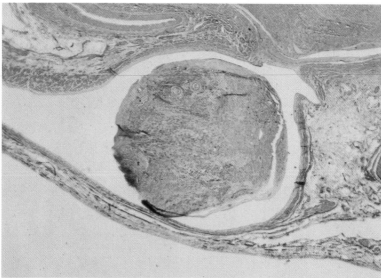

figure 5.35

Multiple fingerlike extensions of muscle (left) extend into the broad ligament in this intravenous leiomyomatosis. A large dilated pelvic vein (right) contains a smooth muscle mass that is histologically benign. This is a trichrome stain. (Courtesy of Dr. Belur Bhagavan.)

5.16

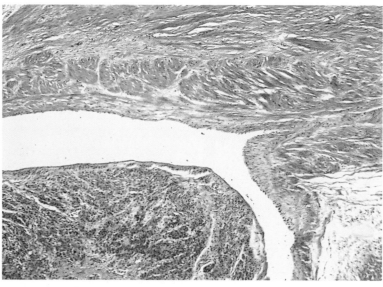 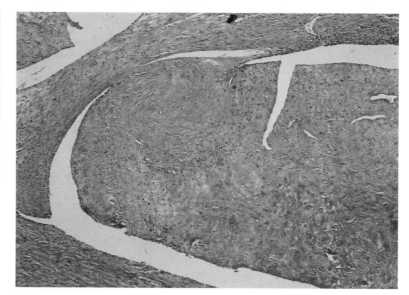

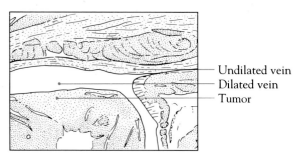

Undilated vein
Dilated vein
Tumor

Venous wall
Tumor

figure 5.36

A mass of benign smooth muscle has dilated the vein on the left side of the picture. That portion of the vein which lies to the right has not yet been entered or dilated. (Courtesy of Dr. Belur Bhagavan.)

figure 5.37

The mass of muscle in the vein is attached to the venous wall in the upper left portion of the photomicrograph.

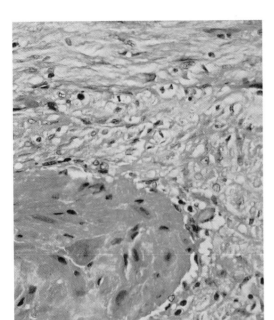

figure 5.38

A focus of decidua with degenerating decidual cells (top) is seen below and to the left in this nodule of apparent fibrosis immediately beneath the peritoneum. This microscopic focus of muscle immediately beneath the peritoneum (bottom) has the nodular shape and distribution of the focus of decidua that preceded it.

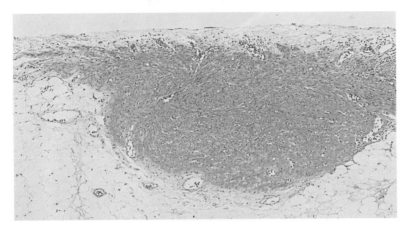

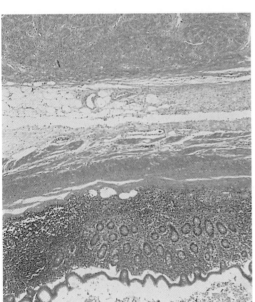

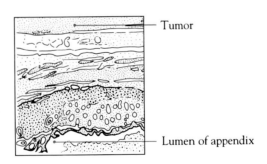

Tumor

Lumen of appendix

figure 5.39

This nodule of muscle is subperitoneal in the mesoappendix. The appendiceal epithelium is seen below. (Courtesy of Dr. Shingo Fujii.)

mesenchymal tumors

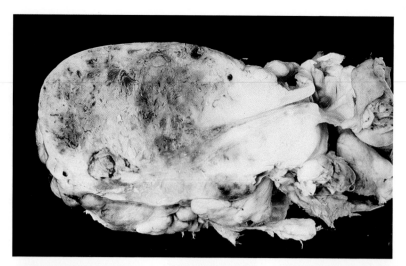

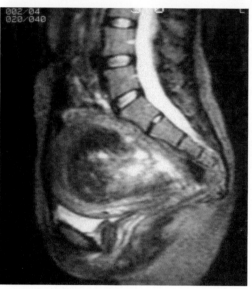

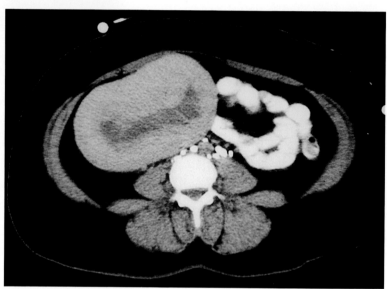

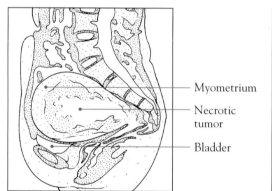

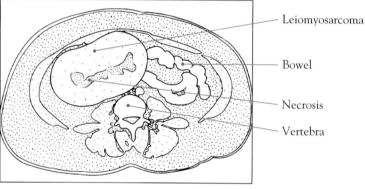

figure 5.40

The cut surface of this leiomyosarcoma (top left) indicates that it massively involves the surrounding myometrium and has penetrated to the serosal surface at several sites. This gross appearance is highly associated with a high grade lesion (from Tuck and Fletcher, 1985). Sagittal T2-weighted MRI of a uterine leiomyosarcoma (bottom left) shows the uterus markedly enlarged by a posterior uterine mass. This mass is predominantly low in signal intensity but has multiple areas of bright signal, suggesting marked necrosis and degeneration. Axial CT of a uterine leiomyosarcoma (bottom right) shows a section of the abdomen above the iliac crest. On lower sections, the large mass to the right of the midline appeared to be arising from the uterus. The low density center designates areas of necrosis within this leiomyosarcoma.

Myometrium

Necrotic tumor

Bladder

Leiomyosarcoma

Bowel

Necrosis

Vertebra

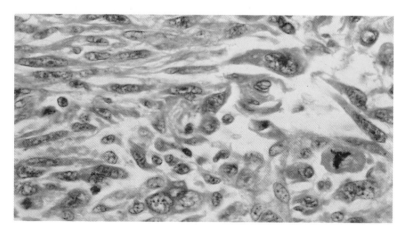

figure 5.41

Atypical nuclei and bizarre mitotic figures clearly identify the malignant nature of this leiomyosarcoma.

5.18

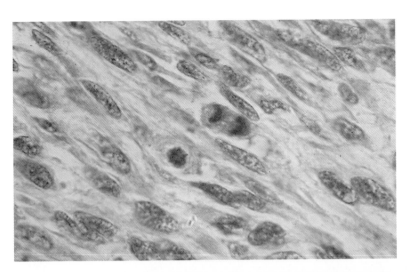

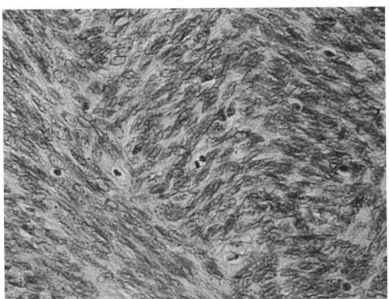

figure 5.43
The organization of this tissue (left) is not too atypical for a myoma, but the nuclei are enlarged and multiple mitotic figures are present. A poorly differentiated leiomyosarcoma (right) is seen invading the vascular channels at the edge of an infiltrating tumor.

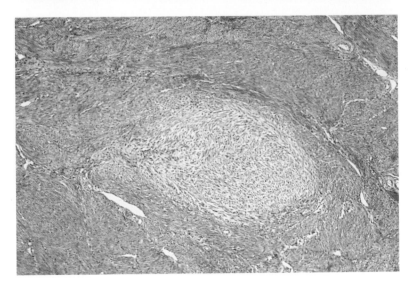

figure 5.44
This focus of stromal differentiation deep within the myometrium does not appear to be expanding. It may represent only a focus of aberrant differentiation rather than a tumor.

figure 5.45
Above, stromal tissue forms a nodule within the myometrium. Mitoses are rare, but the border is not truly a pushing one. Elsewhere in this tumor, infiltration was present.

mesenchymal tumors

some areas appear stromal and in other areas appear to be composed of cells specifically organized around small blood vessels (Fig. 5.46). Moreover, they are likely to be isolated nodules with no malignant potential.

STROMATOSIS

When histologically benign stroma does not possess a pushing border but instead infiltrates the surrounding myometrium and separates muscle bundles without tissue destruction, then it constitutes stromatosis or low-grade stromal sarcoma (Fig. 5.47). Stromatosis probably arises more frequently in the endometrium than in the myometrium. This entity has been evaluated on the basis of both mitotic counts and degree of differentiation, and certainly some examples with very high mitotic counts or with less than maximal differentiation are more aggressive than others (Fig. 5.48). Routinely, stromatosis infiltrates locally throughout the pelvis and may recur in the upper abdomen after surgical removal; it does not usually metastasize to distant extraperitoneal sites. Surgical removal is the primary therapy. Stromatosis may respond to progesterone, and, when it does, indefinite treatment is indicated. Relatively low-grade stromal tumors with epithelial components have been described as sex-cord stromal tumors (Fig. 5.49). Their behavior is assessed by evaluating the grade of the stromal component, as the epithelial cell clone imparts no additional clinical significance.

Less differentiated sarcomas composed of endometrial stromal-like tissue occur in the uterine mesenchyme or elsewhere in the genital canal. They are difficult to distinguish from mixed mesodermal tumors to which they are undoubtedly closely related (Fig. 5.50). If enough sections are taken, most seemingly pure stromal sarcomas will display some type of variation in cell type, so that, depending on the pathologist's philosophy, they may be labeled as mixed. Probably the most frequent example of this phenomenon is the combined appearance of leiomyosarcoma at some sites and what appears to be more typical of endometrial stroma at other sites. When more sophisticated levels of analysis are used, such as electron-microscopic searches for rhabdomyoblasts, most seemingly pure stromal sarcomas will turn out to be impure (Fig. 5.51). Stromal sarcomas are treated by surgery.

5.20

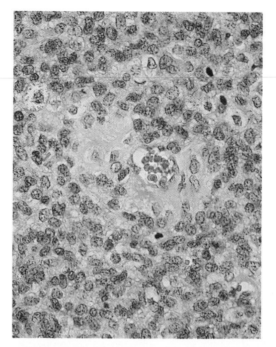

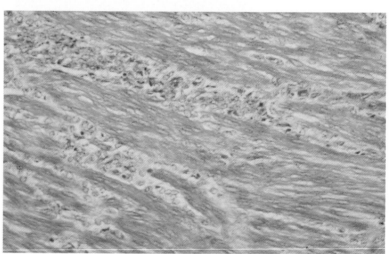

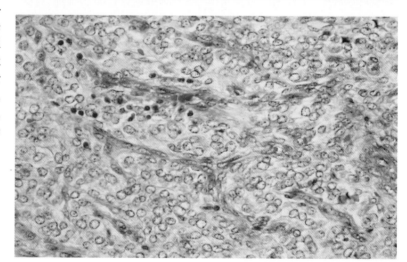

figure 5.47

This example of stromatosis (top) illustrates the infiltrative behavior of this lesion. There is no tissue destruction, however, only separation of the muscle bundles. The mass of this tumor (bottom) is hypercellular but not atypical, and mitoses are infrequent.

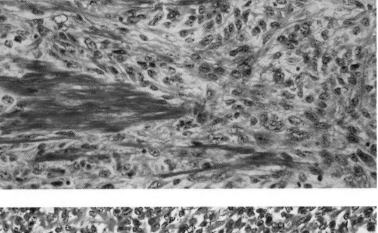

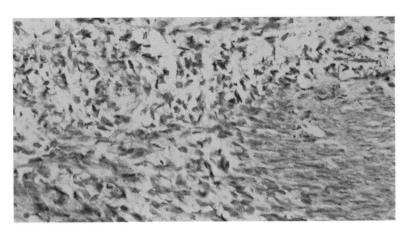

figure 5.48

Mitoses are infrequent in this stromal lesion, which is infiltrating without tissue destruction, but the differentiation is poor.

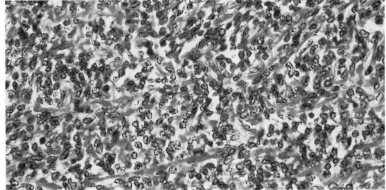

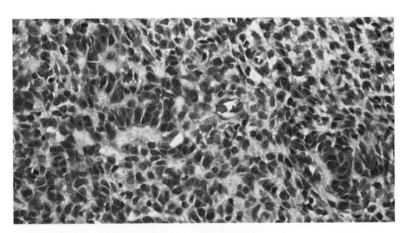

figure 5.49

In this stromal nodule (top) a few of the cells are organized in cordlike arrangements and have a tendency to look epithelial. In this stromal nodule (bottom), clear-cut epithelial-type cells have formed a gland in the stroma.

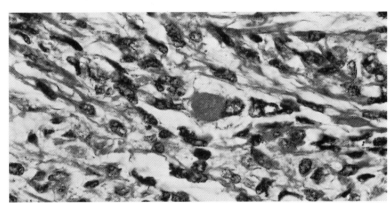

figure 5.50

Highly atypical stromal cells (top) infiltrate the surrounding myometrium. Mitoses were frequent and atypical. This stromal tumor (bottom) consists of smaller cells, but the atypicality is marked.

Gland

Stroma

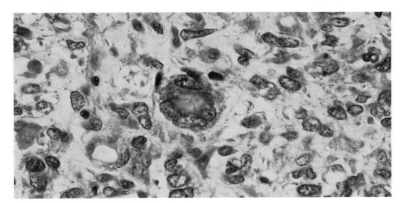

figure 5.51

An isolated cell (top) resembling a rhabdomyoblast is seen in this field, in which most of the cells appear stromal. In this apparent stromal tumor (bottom), a small focus of epithelium results in an apparent gland.

mesenchymal tumors

mixed tumors

Mesenchymal mixed tumors may occur at any level in the genital canal, although the myometrium and endometrium are most common, with the latter site as the more common of the two. The tumors may contain different types of stroma, or both epithelium and stroma (Fig. 5.52). The mesenchymal tissues may be heterologous or homologous, but these variations are important clinically only when they reflect grade. Histologically, however, they are dramatic and fascinating, as their wide spectrum illustrates the many different types of mesenchymal differentiation. Cartilage, bone, muscle, fibrous tissue, and epithelium in varying states of differentiation are the most common tissue types seen (Fig. 5.53). Familiarity with embryonic mesenchyme aids in the interpretation of these tumors (Fig. 5.54). Characteristi-

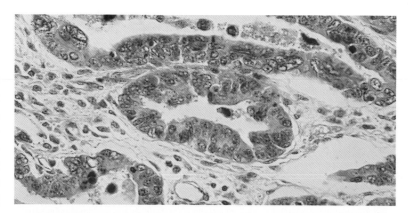
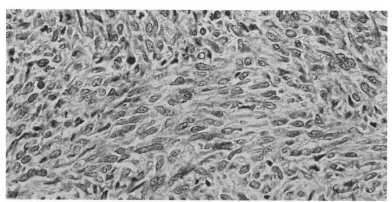
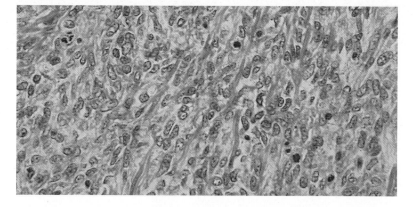
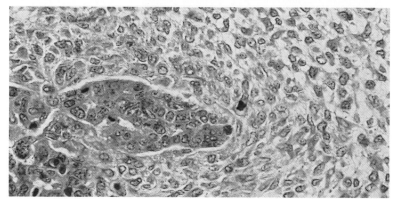

figure 5.52

These four photomicrographs are all from the same tumor. In the portion seen in the topmost photograph, the apparent diagnosis is adenocarcinoma. In the portion of the tumor seen below that, the tissue organization suggests the whorls of a muscle tumor; the impression is that of a leiomyosarcoma. In the third photomicrograph, the tissue organization seen is more consistent with a stromal sarcoma. In the fourth photomicrograph, both epithelium and stroma are malignant and carcinosarcoma is present.

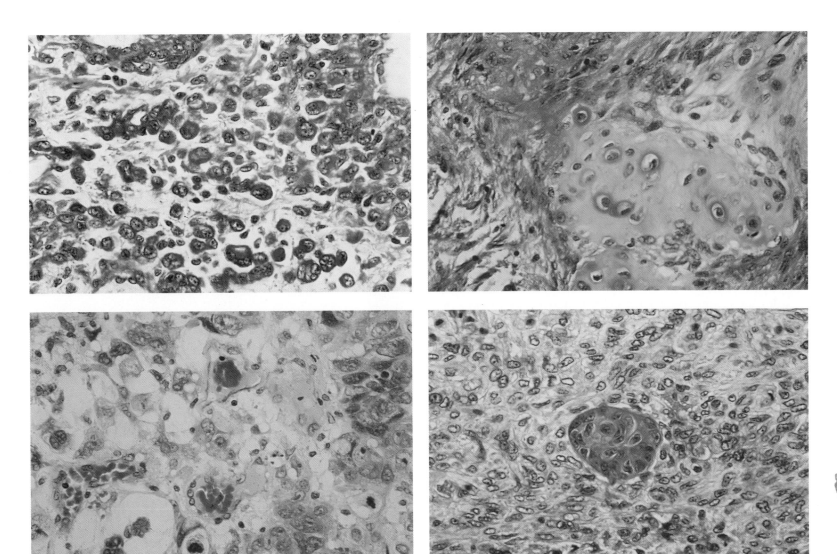

figure 5.53

Tissue organization and undifferentiated malignant cells, not clearly stromal or epithelial (top left), characterize most of this tumor. Heterologous atypical cartilage (top right) is differentiating in the middle of this malignant mixed tumor. Elsewhere this tumor (bottom left) was more obviously composed of both epithelium and stroma; here, only undifferentiated large cells are arranged in an amorphous pattern. An island of squamous epithelium (bottom right) is differentiating in the midst of malignant stroma of this mixed tumor.

figure 5.54

In the upper left portion of the photomicrograph, this normal embryonic mesenchyme contains a focus of immature cartilage. Immature striated muscle is present in the upper right, and nonspecific soft tissue is below.

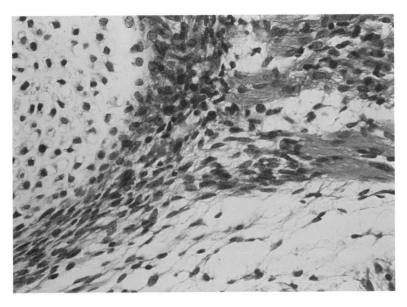

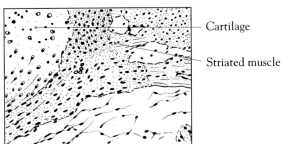

mesenchymal tumors

cally, the most aggressive malignant mixed tumors produce polypoid masses that result in bleeding or discharge. They may protrude through the cervix into the vagina (Fig. 5.55).

Malignant mixed mesodermal tumors are very aggressive and have only a 60% salvage rate when they are confined to the uterus at the time of surgical extirpation. They metastasize early, both to nodes and to distant extraperitoneal body sites, and if not surgically curable, they do not usually respond to other therapies.

Exceptionally low grade or benign mixed tumors may contain all of these tissue types in well differentiated form. Those containing both epithelium and stroma are *adenofibromas* (Fig. 5.56). Here, as well as in the most malignant types, an aggressive search will reveal a variety of tissue types. Mixed tumors with intermediate degrees of malignancy may be seen, and these have been called *adenosarcomas* (Fig. 5.57). Adenosarcomas possess a clear-cut malignant stromal component, where the epithelium is not atypical in that it does not look malignant. However, the epithelium in the glands of adenosarcomas does not usually resemble any of the mature types of epithelium seen in the genital canal, and, in this sense, it is atypical. When locally confined, adenosarcomas are cured by surgical removal. However, they do have malignant potential, and may extend or spread in the abdominal cavity.

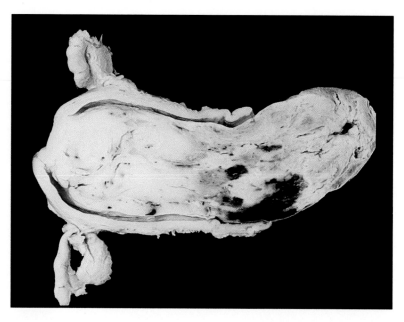

figure 5.55

This malignant mixed tumor has the characteristic gross appearance. Although arising in the fundus, it produces a large polypoid mass that protrudes through the cervix.

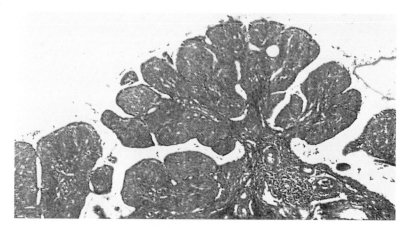

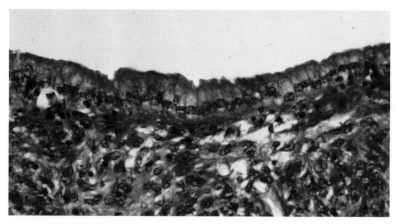

figure 5.56

This papillary fibroepithelial polyp, confined to the endometrium within the endometrial cavity (top), consists of benign tissue. Well differentiated mucinous epithelium and benign stroma (bottom) are seen in this higher power view.

atlas of gynecologic pathology

Other Uterine tumors

Adenomatoid tumors are benign mesotheliomas that occur most often on the epithelial or mesothelial surfaces of the pelvis, although they may arise anywhere, including the myometrium (Fig. 5.58). Usually, they are small and detected incidentally when the myometrium is sectioned; however, they may be large and discrete enough to suggest a myoma, grossly. Histologically, they are characterized by a minimal fibrous stromal reaction around cleftlike spaces lined by mesothelial or cuboidal epithelium (Fig. 5.59). This cuboidal epithelium is most often mucinous. While locally infiltrative, adenomatoid tumors are clinically insignificant. Rarely, adenocarcinomas display similar histologic patterns (Fig. 5.60). Vascular tumors arise in the myometrium and may be purely vascular or have significant components of uterine mesenchyme (Fig. 5.61). Whether these tumors are primarily vascular tumors or are highly vascular mesenchymal tumors is debatable. While benign, they can be responsible for clinically significant hemorrhage. Metastatic cancer in the myometrium commonly originates in the cervix or ovary (Fig. 5.62).

While the preceding description implies a series of clearly defined entities in the myometrium, there are in fact many variations and mixtures, with different philosophies about how these tumors should be classified. If multiple sections are taken, it is not uncommon to find a tumor having patterns that place it in more than one of the diagnostic categories described. If different levels of analysis are used, such as electron microscopy or immunoperoxidase staining for specific proteins, additional heterogeneities are detected. Accordingly, what is most important clinically is the grade of the neoplasm, regardless of its cell type or types. Poorly differentiated muscle tumors, stromal tumors, or mixed tumors behave badly, and at the moment have only insignificant clinical differences. On the other hand, well differentiated lesions of any histologic type tend to remain confined to their site of origin and respond to local surgery.

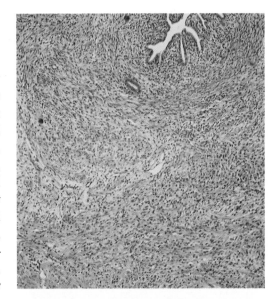

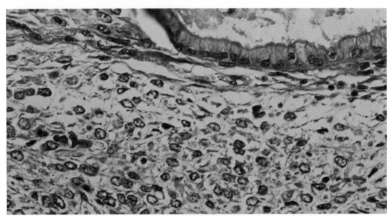

figure 5.57

Epithelium (top) that is not obviously atypical forms glands in a stroma that is atypical. The lesion is infiltrating the myometrium below. A higher power view of the lesion seen above (bottom) portrays the epithelium as typical. The stroma, however, is atypical.

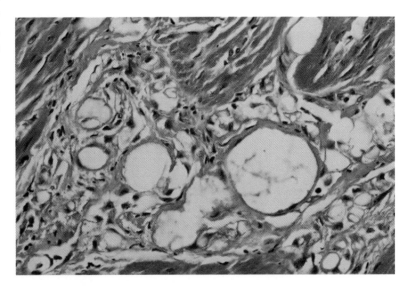

figure 5.58

The adenomatoid tumor seen here is infiltrating the muscle bundles of the myometrium, but it will not metastasize.

mesenchymal tumors

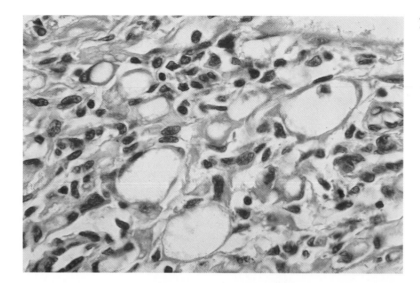

figure 5.59

Cleftlike spaces are lined by flattened mesothelial cells. There is a stromal component.

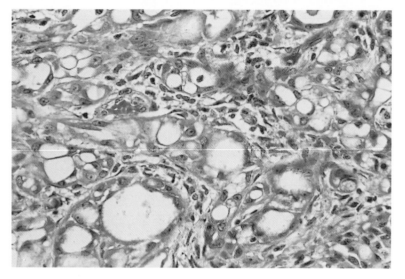

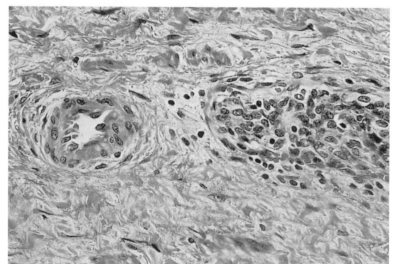

figure 5.60

This very rare tumor (left) has the general histology of an adenomatoid tumor, but the individual cells are atypical. Elsewhere in the same tumor (right) the pattern is more like those papillary mesothelial lesions seen higher in the genital canal and usually labeled ovarian.

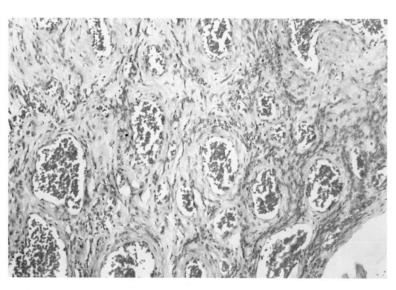

figure 5.61

This apparent myoma consisted of engorged blood vessels supported by a stroma composed of smooth muscle.

figure 5.62

A plug of epidermoid carcinoma from the cervix is infiltrating a myometrial tissue space near an arteriole.

atlas of gynecologic pathology

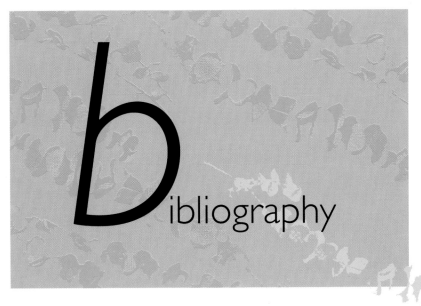

bibliography

Clement PB, Scully RE: Müllerian adenosarcoma of the uterus: A clinicopathologic analysis of 10 cases of distinctive type of müllerian mixed tumor. *Cancer* 34:1138, 1974.

Clement PB, Scully RE: Uterine tumors resembling ovarian sex-cord tumors. *Am J Clin Pathol* 66:512, 1976.

Cramer SF, Robertson AL Jr., Ziats NP, Pearson OH: Growth potential of human uterine leiomyomas: Some in vitro observations and their implications. *Obstet Gynecol* 66:36, 1985.

Ferenczy A, Fenoglio J, Richart RM: Observations on benign mesothelioma of the genital tract (adenomatoid tumor). A comparative ultrastructural study. *Cancer* 30:244, 1972.

Fleming WP, Peters WA, Neelan KB, Morley GW: Autopsy findings in patients with uterine sarcoma. *Gynecol Oncol* 19:168, 1984.

George M, Pejovic MH, Kramer A, Gynecologic Cooperating Group of French Oncology Centers: Uterine sarcomas; prognostic factors and treatment modalities. Study on 209 patients. *Gynecol Oncol* 24:51, 1986.

Goldfarb S, Richart RM, Okagaki T: Nuclear DNA content in endolymphatic stromal myosis. *Am J Obstet Gynecol* 106:525, 1970.

Hendrickson MR, Kempson RL: *Surgical Pathology of the Uterine Corpus.* Major problems in Pathology, Philadelphia, WB Saunders Co., 1980, vol 12.

Kahanpaa KV, Wahlstrom T, Grohn P, Heinonen E, Nieminen U, Widholm O: Sarcomas of the Uterus: A clinicopathologic study of 119 patients. *Obstet Gynecol* 67:417, 1986.

Kempson RJ, Bari W: Uterine sarcomas. *Hum Pathol* 1:331, 1970.

Kempson RL: Sarcomas and related neoplasms, in Hertig AT, Norris HJ, Abell MR (eds.): *The Uterus.* Baltimore, Williams and Wilkins, 1973.

Kurman RJ, Norris HJ: Mesenchymal tumors of the uterus VI: Epithelioid smooth muscle tumors including leiomyoblastoma and clear cell leiomyoma. *Cancer* 37:1853, 1976.

Norris HJ, Parmley TH: Mesenchymal tumors of the uterus V: Intravenous leiomyomatosis: A clinical and pathologic study of 14 cases. *Cancer* 36:2164, 1975.

Norris HJ, Roth E, Taylor HB: Mesenchymal tumors of the uterus II: A clinical and pathologic study of 31 mixed mesodermal tumors: *Obstet Gynecol* 28:57, 1966.

Norris HJ, Taylor HB: Mesenchymal tumors of the uterus III: A clinical and pathologic study of 31 carcinosarcomas. *Cancer* 19:1459, 1966.

Ober WB: Uterine Sarcomas: Histogenesis and taxonomy. *Ann NY Acad Sci* 75:568, 1959.

Piver MS, Rutledge FN, Copeland L, et al: Uterine endolymphatic stromal myosis: *Obstet Gynecol* 64:173, 1984.

Rubin SC, Wheeler JE, Mikuta JJ: Malignant leiomyomatosis peritonealis disseminata. *Obstet Gynecol* 68:126, 1986.

Sternberg WH, Clark WH, Smith RC: Malignant mixed müllerian tumor (mixed mesodermal tumor of the uterus). *Cancer* 7:704, 1954.

Sutton GP, Stehman FB, Michael H, et al: Estrogen and progesterone receptors in uterine sarcomas. *Obstet Gynecol* 68:709, 1986.

Taylor HB, Norris HJ: Mesenchymal tumors of the uterus IV:Diagnosis and prognosis of leiomyosarcomas. *Arch Pathol* 82:40, 1966.

Thatcher SS, Woodruff JD: Uterine stromatosis: A report of 33 cases. *Obstet Gynecol* 59:428, 1982.

Townsend DE, Sparkes RS, Baluda MC, et al: Unicellular histogenesis of uterine leiomyomas as determined by electrophoresis of glucose-6-phosphate dehydrogenase. *Am J Obstet Gynecol* 107:1168, 1970.

Tuck JL, Fletcher CDM: *Royal College of Surgeons of England Slide Atlas of Pathology.* Reproductive System, London, Gower Medical Publishing Ltd, 1985.

Vellios F, Ng ABP, Reagan JW: Papillary adenofibroma of the uterus. *Am J Clin Pathol* 60:543, 1973.

fallopian tube

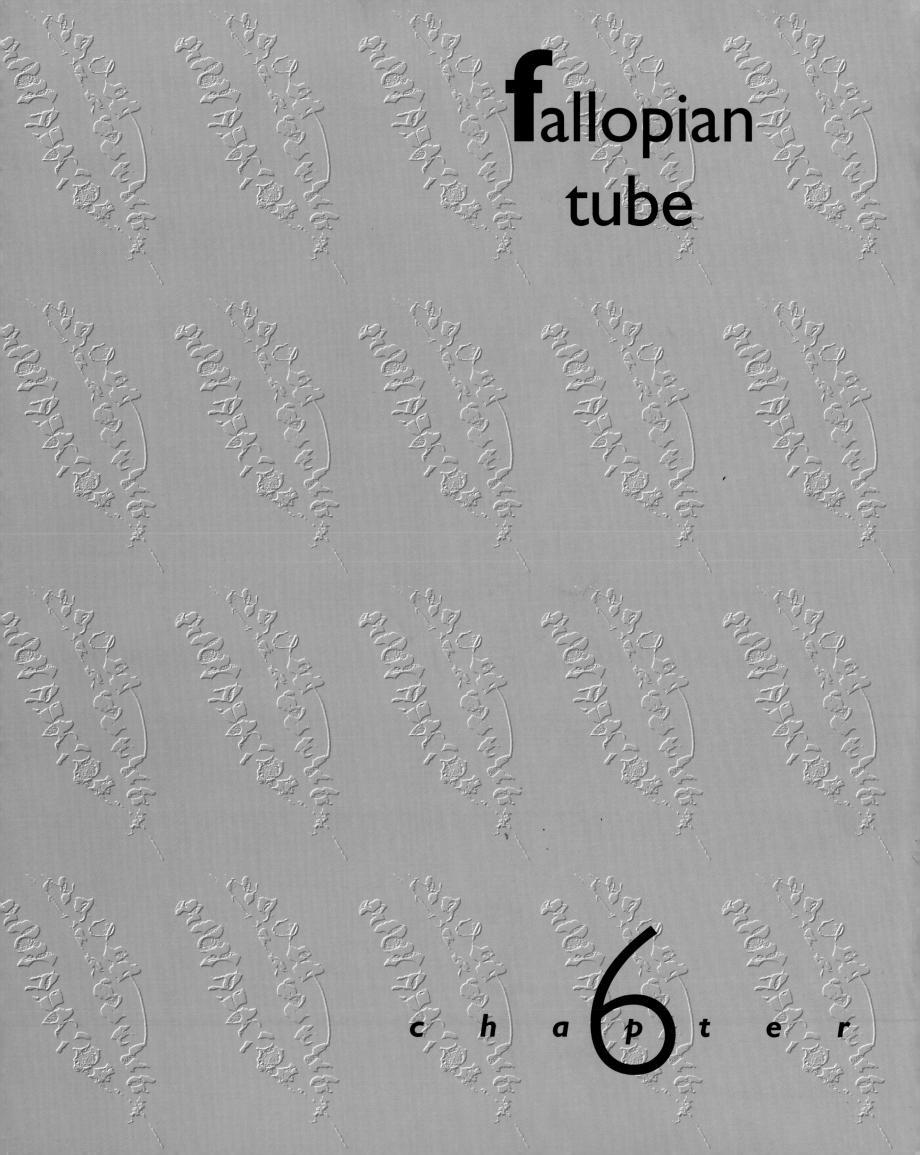

chapter 6

development and histology

During the fifth week of embryonic life, the fallopian tubes begin as multiple evaginations of the coelomic epithelium on the lateral surface of the urogenital ridge. During the sixth week, these multiple evaginations fuse into the müllerian duct, which migrates along the course of the wolffian duct into the underlying urogenital ridge (Fig. 6.1). The müllerian duct lies on the lateral surface of the wolffian duct until it reaches the pelvis. It then crosses the wolffian duct anteriorly, and lies on its medial surface. Here, during the seventh week of embryonic life, the bilateral müllerian ducts fuse and abut on the posterior wall of the urogenital sinus, between the orifices of the two wolffian ducts (Fig. 6.2). The most cranial portions of the müllerian duct remain unfused, however, and develop into the fallopian tubes. The embryologic relationship of the tubes to the wolffian duct is revealed in the persistence of wolffian duct remnants in the adult mesosalpinx (Fig. 6.3).

During the second and third trimesters of life, the mesoderm of the tubal wall develops into an internal lamina propria and an external muscular wall. The muscle is thick and clearly demarcated at the cornual end of the tube (Fig. 6.4), and becomes more attenuated as the fimbria are approached (Fig. 6.5). The peritoneal serosa of the surface of the broad ligament is firmly attached to the tube at the uterine end, but is less so more distally. Here the tube is separated from the serosa by loose connective tissue that is highly vascular (Fig. 6.6).

The lumen of the fallopian tube is simple in its cornual and isthmic portions and becomes more complex nearer the ampulla and fimbria. This complexity initially consists of more and more arborization of papillary fronds projecting into the lumen. Many of the papillary fronds seem to arise from only a few primary folds (Fig. 6.7). The primary folds themselves consist of a loose stromal extension of the lamina propria, and they contain a vascular supply. The arborization of the papillary fronds is maximal at the fimbriated end of the tube, where primary folds are less distinctive. Rare tubal polyps apparently consist of the exaggerated development of one of these folds and its papillary fronds (Fig. 6.8).

Tubal epithelium differentiates into ciliated and secretory cells during the second and third trimesters. The ciliated cells are more numerous near the fimbriated end of the tube. They are characterized by an eosinophilic brush border and a round nucleus with perinuclear clearing, which produces a halo appearance (Fig. 6.9). The secretory cells are tall and columnar, with oval nuclei arranged perpendicular to the basal lamina of the epithelium (Fig. 6.10). Their cytoplasm is more basophilic than that of the ciliated cells. So-called intercalary, or peg, cells are secretory cells; while prominent enough to project above the ciliated surface in the secretory phase, secretory cells are lower in the prolifera-

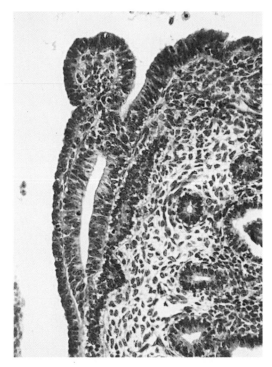

figure 6.1

The müllerian duct (top) seen in this photomicrograph is open to the coelomic cavity. It runs just beneath the coelomic epithelium, immediately adjacent to the wolffian duct. A day or two later (bottom), the müllerian duct is no longer so closely associated with the wolffian duct, but it is still just beneath the coelomic epithelium.

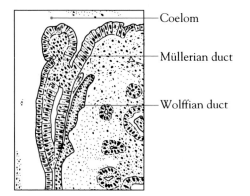

— Coelom

— Müllerian duct

— Wolffian duct

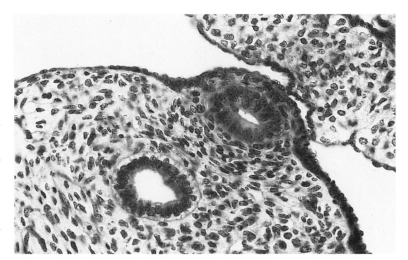

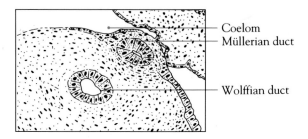

— Coelom
— Müllerian duct

— Wolffian duct

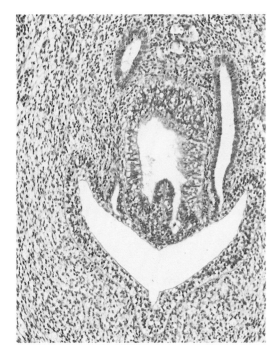

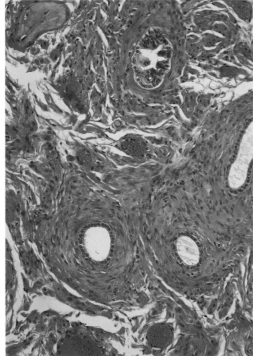

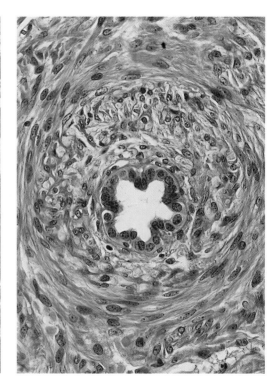

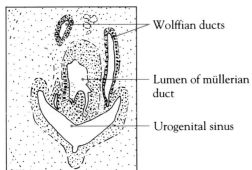

- Wolffian ducts
- Lumen of müllerian duct
- Urogenital sinus

figure 6.3

Multiple wolffian duct remnants (left) lie in the mesosalpinx. One has papillary epithelium, but the rest are flattened. The simple cuboidal epithelium of this wolffian duct remnant (right) contains a few ciliated cells.

The organization of the surrounding stroma reveals an inner longitudinal and outer circular layer, suggesting its homology with the vas deferens.

figure 6.2

The lumen of the tip of the müllerian duct is present between the two wolffian ducts and is abutting upon the wall of the urogenital sinus.

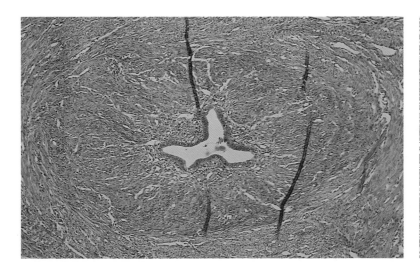

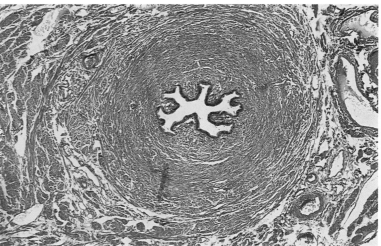

figure 6.4

The interstitial tube (left) has a simple lumen with three or four primary folds and a massive amount of surrounding musculature. Immediately external to the cornua (right), the isthmic tube has well-developed

musculature, and a few more primary folds supported by a slightly more conspicuous lamina propria.

fallopian tube

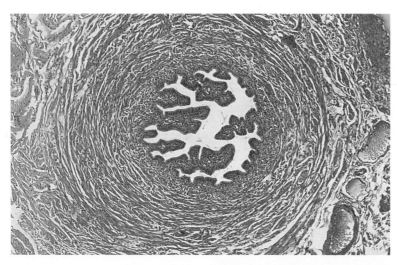
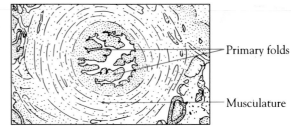

Primary folds

Musculature

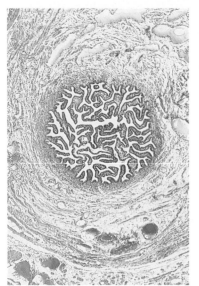
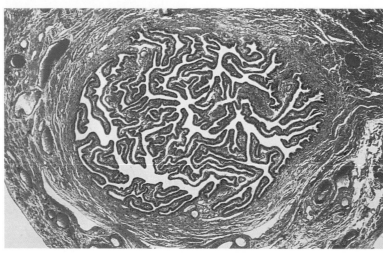

6.4

figure 6.5

In the more distal isthmus (top), primary folds are more complexly arborized and the tubal musculature is less discrete. In the ampulla (bottom left), the papillary fronds fill the tubal lumen, with primary folds being much less apparent. The tubal musculature is almost inapparent as a discrete layer. Nearer the infundibulum (bottom right), the complex papillary frond architecture of the tubal lumen is its most prominent feature. Tubal musculature is not apparent as a specific layer.

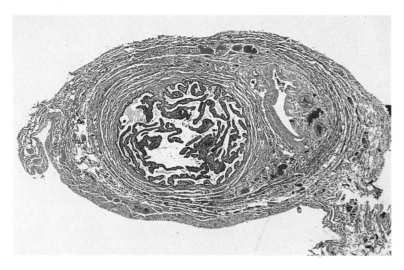
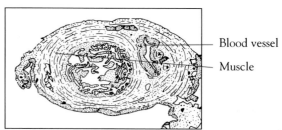

Blood vessel

Muscle

figure 6.6

The tubal lumen is surrounded by a relatively discrete muscle layer, external to which there is a looser vascular layer. Immediately beneath the peritoneal serosa, a dense layer also contains some muscle. A large vessel runs through the loose vascular layer.

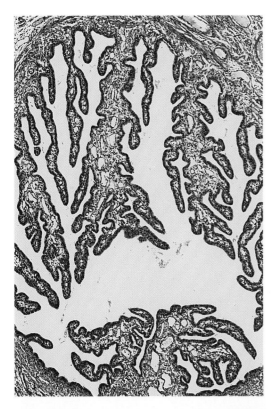

figure 6.7

Most, but not all, of the papillary fronds in this tubal lumen arise from a few large folds that arborize. The dilated vasculature in the lamina propria of these folds is particularly prominent.

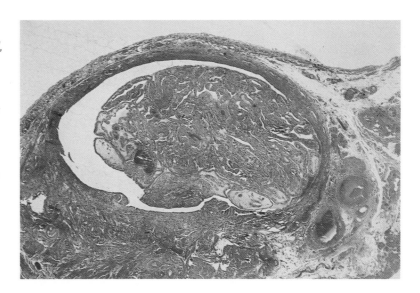

figure 6.8

A tubal polyp filling and dilating this tubal lumen appears to be the result of the excessively complex development of a primary fold.

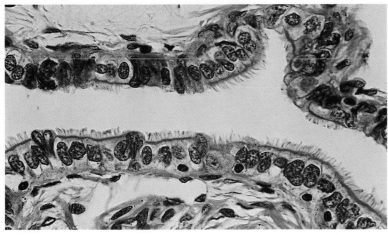

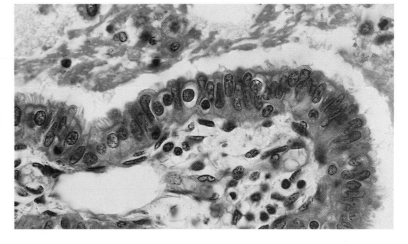

6.5

figure 6.9

Ciliated cells in this tubal epithelium produce extensive patches of cilia. The individual cells have prominent eosinophilic borders. Patches of ciliated cells are separated by protruding secretory cells and are underlain by undifferentiated cells isolated along the basement membrane.

figure 6.10

While fundamentally the same, this epithelium contains more secretory cells than those seen in the previous figure.

figure 6.11

In this proliferative-phase tubal epithelium, the secretory cells are not projecting above the level of the ciliated cells as they are in Figures 6.9 and 6.10.

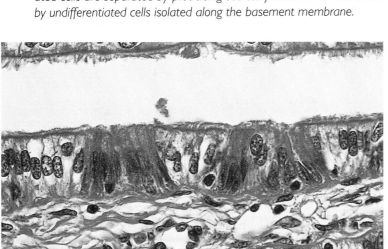

fallopian tube

tive phase (Fig. 6.11). The third cell type is the basal cell—a small undifferentiated cell with little cytoplasm, which lies along the basement membrane of the epithelium and serves as the cell of origin for the tubal epithelium (see Figs. 6.9 through 6.11). Mitoses are rare in normal tubal epithelium (Fig. 6.12).

Postmenopausally, in the face of estrogen deficiency, the tubal epithelium becomes low and flat (Fig. 6.13). Undifferentiated basal cells are uncommon. The papillary fronds are short and less arborized, with a more dense collagenous stroma than is seen premenopausally (Fig. 6.14). Estrogen replacement tends to restore premenopausal histology. Both atrophy and recovery may be present irregularly (Fig. 6.15).

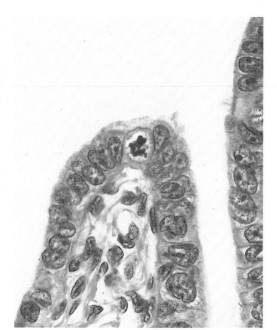

figure 6.12

This mitotic figure seen in tubal epithelium is very rare. Its significance is unknown.

tubal anomalies

STRUCTURAL ANOMALIES

Anomalies of tubal structure often consist of inappropriate or inadequate fusion of the multiple coelomic evaginations that give rise to the tube. The most common example of the failure of one of these multiple evaginations to coalesce is the so-called hydatid cyst of Morgagni. Usually less than a centimeter in diameter, this cystic structure is lined by tubal-like epithelium and suspended from the broad ligament by a fine stalk (Fig. 6.16). Very rarely, the epithelium within these cysts is proliferative, and gives rise to tumors (Fig. 6.17); this accounts for some of the epithelial neoplasms with typical tubal or ovarian histology that arise in paratubal locations. Paratubal cysts also may become clinically important simply by enlargement secondary to fluid accumulation (Fig. 6.18), and these cysts may become as large as true ovarian cysts (Fig. 6.19). Inappropriate or inadequate fusion of the multiple evaginations of coelomic epithelium also may give rise to multiple tubes or, more precisely, to one tube with multiple orifices (Fig. 6.20). Some of these accessory lumina may seal over to form diverticula; anomalous tubal structure occasionally is associated with ectopic pregnancy (Fig. 6.21).

ANOMALIES OF DIFFERENTIATION

Anomalies of differentiation are much more common than are anomalies of structure. An example of an anomaly of differentiation is the development of mucinous epithelium in the fallopian tube (Fig. 6.22). Mucinous epithelial differentiation is rare. Squamous metaplasia is uncommon within the

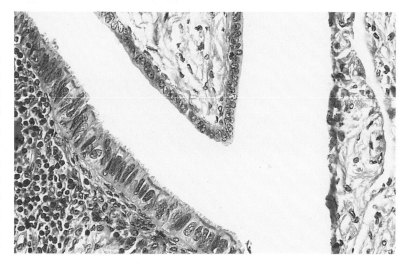

figure 6.13

The epithelium is totally flattened, cuboidal, or relatively normal at different sites in the postmenopausal tube seen in this photomicrograph.

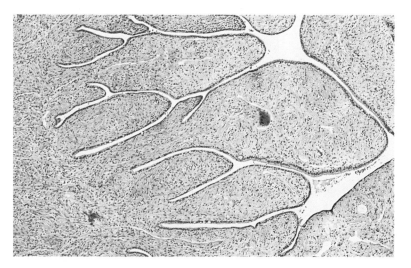

figure 6.14

Papillary fronds are blunted and the lamina propria is fibrotic and avascular, as is typical postmenopausally.

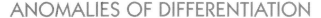

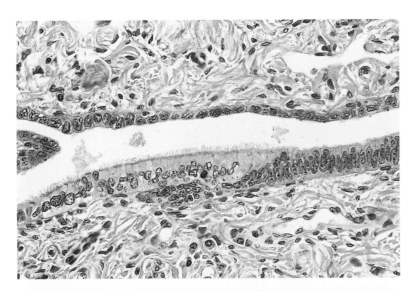

figure 6.15

Flattened atrophic epithelium above contrasts with alternating patches of well-developed ciliated cells and secretory cells below.

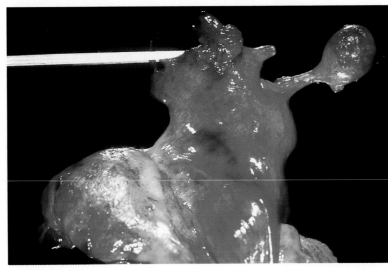

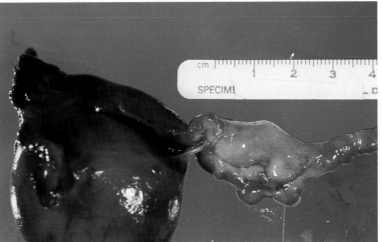

figure 6.16

A hydatid of Morgagni (left) is attached to the broad ligament near the fimbria by a thin, fibrous stalk. A rudimentary papillary frond (right) extends from the wall of this hydatid cyst. This is typical.

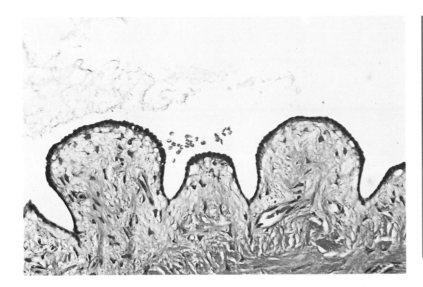

figure 6.17

In this paraovarian cyst, epithelial proliferation is associated with a significant stromal reaction. This is a papillary cystadenofibroma.

figure 6.18

This paraovarian cyst not only enlarged secondary to fluid accumulation, but also resulted in torsion and infarction of both itself and the adjacent tube.

fallopian tube

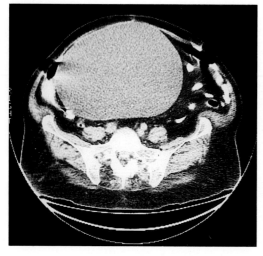

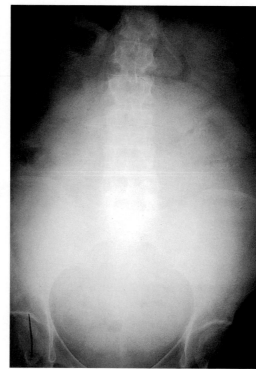

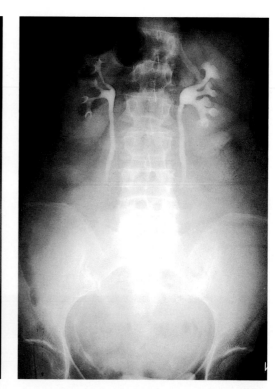

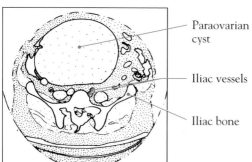

Paraovarian cyst

Iliac vessels

Iliac bone

6.8

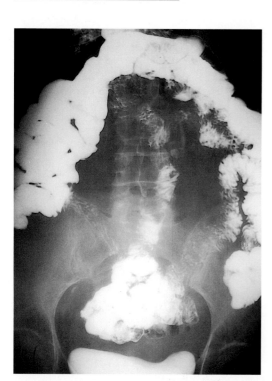

figure 6.19

CT scan (top left) presenting axial view of the pelvis. A large cystic mass occupies the right lower abdomen. On lower images the mass extended into the pelvis. Note the barium filled bowel displaced to the left side of the abdomen. X-ray film of the abdomen (top center) shows a soft tissue mass that creates an opacity which extends from the level of the umbilicus to the pelvis. Excretory urogram (top right) showing opacification of both kidneys with normal excretion into both ureters. The distal ureters are partially obstructed by the mass in the pelvis, causing mild hydronephrosis of the left kidney. Small bowel barium series (bottom), where loops of small bowel are opacified approximately one hour after barium ingestion. The bowel loops are draped around the mass and behind it. The urinary bladder is opacified from a prior excretory urogram.

atlas of gynecologic pathology

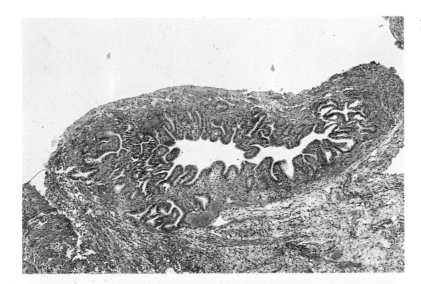

figure 6.20

The accessory tubal orifice seen here lacks a well-defined tubal wall.

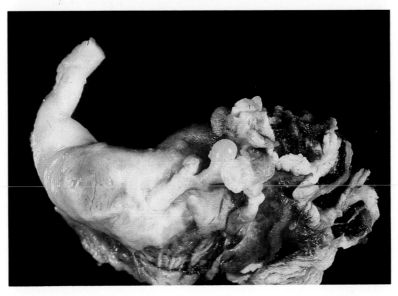

figure 6.21

Several accessory lumina and a diverticulum protrude from the surface of this tube, which contains an ectopic pregnancy.

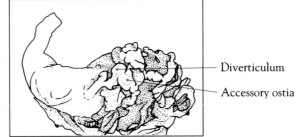

Diverticulum

Accessory ostia

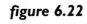

6.9

figure 6.22

Well-defined mucinous epithelium, normal for the endocervix, covers the papillary frond in this tubal lumen.

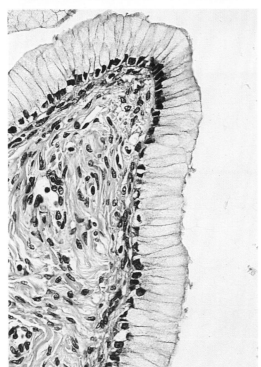

fallopian tube

lumen, but it is frequently seen on the tubal surface, where its presence in inclusion cysts is specifically termed a Walthard's rest (Fig. 6.23). Microscopic foci of endometrial-type tissue in the fallopian tube are ubiquitous (Fig. 6.24). The results are variable, depending on the site and extent of the abnormal differentiation. Repeated function in endometrial tissue within the isthmus of the tube results in dissection of the surrounding muscle, first by the breakdown of the endometrium, and then by its repair (Fig. 6.25). The result is the displacement of epithelium farther and farther out into the muscle. Early in the process, the endometrial nature of the tissue is apparent; but subsequently, only epithelial-lined spaces, and perhaps a little inflammation, are left. Ciliated cells are prominent in epithelial remnants of endometriosis. The result of this process is salpingitis isthmica nodosa (Fig. 6.26).

The appearance of endometriosis farther out in the isthmic, ampullary, or infundibular portions of the tube depends on its degree of development (Fig. 6.27). Extensive tubal endometriosis is one of the rare causes of hematosalpinx, when a tubal pregnancy is not present. In such a case, tubal obstruction may be present. If recent bleeding has occurred, the tubal wall will be only patchily lined by epithelium, and the stroma will be filled with siderophages, as in an endometrial cyst of the ovary (Fig. 6.28). If pregnancy has occurred or exogenous progesterone has been given, then the tube will be extensively decidualized (Fig. 6.29).

Less extensive foci of endometrial-type tissue are more common. They occur in the tips of the papillary fronds of the tube, where they are dramatically revealed by decidualization when pregnancy occurs (Fig. 6.30). If both epithelium and stroma participate, the epithelium will eventually become low and flat, and the stroma will contain characteristic decidual cells (Fig. 6.31). If the epithelium is not endometrial, then the stroma is decidualized underneath ciliated-type epithelium. The epithelium may react in the absence of a stromal response, and can produce an Arias-Stella-like picture (Fig. 6.32).

Endometriosis may develop within an obstructed tube—most often in the case of the short proximal segments that result from tubal ligation. Sampson (1930) described a case of this phenomenon. Laparoscopic tubal ligations, because they produce the shortest proximal stumps, are particularly likely to result in the development of intraluminal endometriosis (Fig. 6.33). This endometriosis with repeated function, as in the case of salpingitis isthmica nodosa, dissects into the muscular wall of the tube (Fig. 6.34). This may result in the development of tuboperitoneal fistulae; these are associated with the occurrence of laparoscopic sterilization failures, many of which are ectopic implantations. Before the fistula develops, the obstructed tube is dilated,

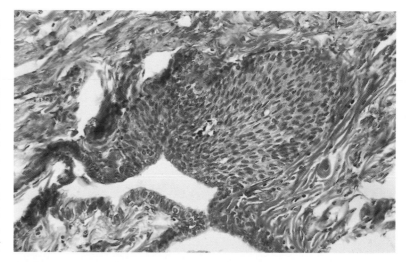

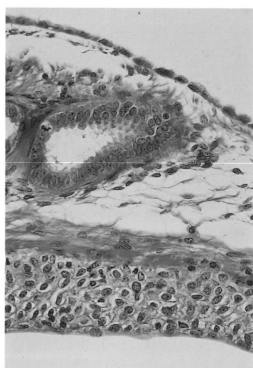

figure 6.23

Squamous metaplasia in the tubal epithelium (top) has resulted in the replacement of tubal epithelium with a squamous epithelium. Immediately beneath the peritoneum (bottom), there are two inclusion cysts. The small one is lined by tubal-type epithelium, while the large one is lined by immature squamous epithelium.

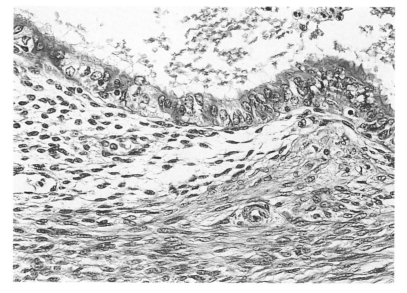

figure 6.24

Endometrial-type stroma supports the tubal epithelium in this tube.

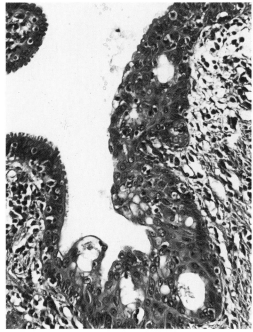

figure 6.25

After menstrual slough, the repairing meta-plastic epithelium looks squamous in this focus of tubal endometriosis.

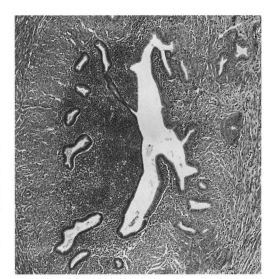

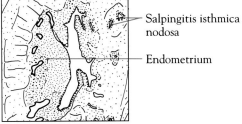

Salpingitis isthmica nodosa

Endometrium

figure 6.26

To the left, the lining of the tube (top) is typical endometrium; to the right are the isolated epithelial inclusions that result from repeated function and/or invasive prolifera-tion of the tissue seen to the left. This is salpingitis isthmica nodosa. In this example (bottom) from somewhat farther out in the isthmus, both near and far epithelial inclu-sions are apparent.

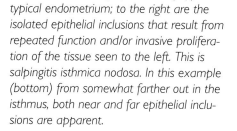

6.11

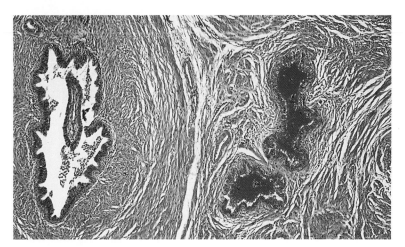

figure 6.27

Normal proliferative endometrium appears to occupy a portion of this tubal wall.

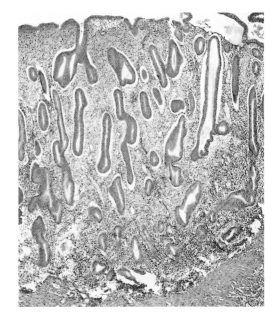

fallopian tube

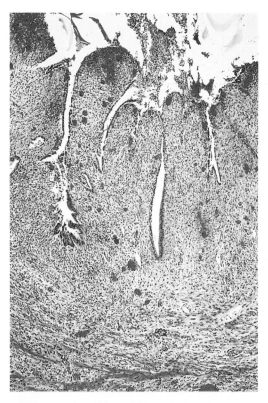

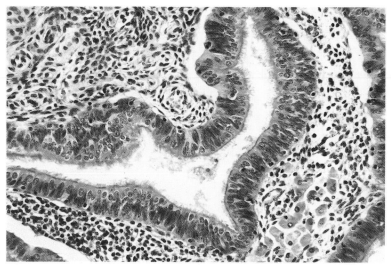

figure 6.28

The endometrial tissue seen in this photomicrograph (left) has cycled and sloughed; the result consists of repairing epithelium and stroma with inflammation. This focus of endometrium in the tubal wall (right) is laden with macrophages containing hemosiderin from previous bleeding.

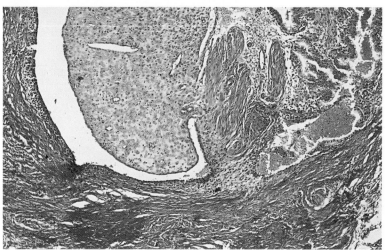

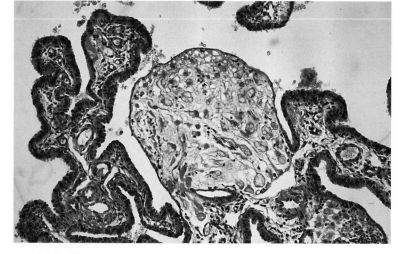

figure 6.29

This tubal lumen is filled with papillary fronds that have been decidualized.

figure 6.30

A focus of decidua occupies the tip of this papillary frond. This is typical.

figure 6.31

This focus of decidua is characterized by its location in the tip of a papillary frond, the decidualized nature of the stromal cells, and the flattened mesothelial nature of the epithelial cells.

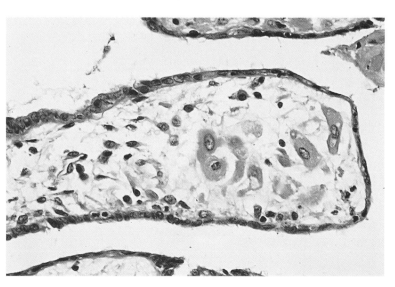

atlas of gynecologic pathology

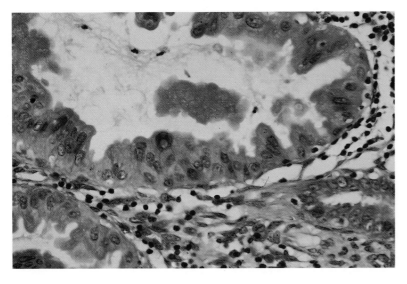

figure 6.32

Below and to the right, relatively normal tubal epithelium exists, but the rest of the epithelium is eosinophilic, with significant nuclear atypicality characteristic of the Arias-Stella reaction.

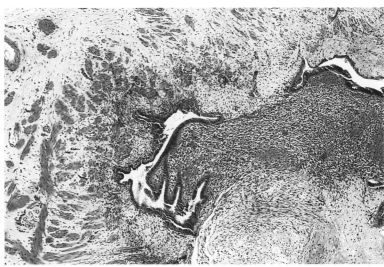

figure 6.33

Endometrial tissue occupies a lumen that is surrounded by muscle on the left but is unenclosed on the right.

figure 6.34

An apparent tubal lumen with expanded decidualized papillary fronds exists to the left, while epithelial extension of the tubal lumen perforates the muscle to the right.

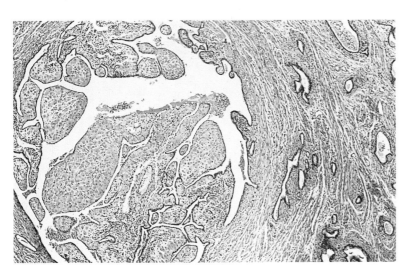

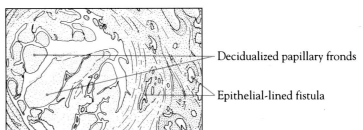

Decidualized papillary fronds

Epithelial-lined fistula

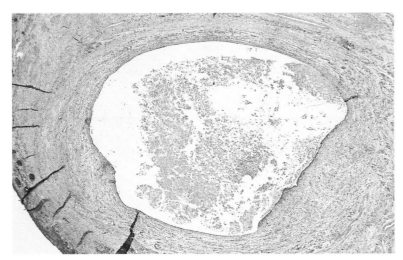

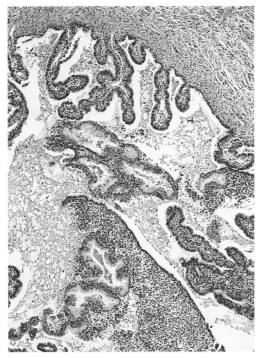

figure 6.35

This photomicrograph (left) shows a grossly dilated interstitial tube. This isthmic tube (right) contains fragments of secretory endometrium.

fallopian tube

presumably secondary to regurgitant flow (Fig. 6.35).

Foci of tubal endometriosis, when decidualized, also may go through the process of muscle metaplasia. This results first in an inflammatory fibrotic appearance (Fig. 6.36) and then in a tubal "myoma" (Fig. 6.37).

tubal Pregnancy

When tubal pregnancy occurs, the initial implantation may be at the tip of a papillary frond, where decidual foci are likely to be present. This is only a presumption however, as the implantation site routinely is destroyed by an invading trophoblast. This trophoblast soon expands the frond, and then extends through its base and through the muscular wall of the tube into the soft tissues between the tube and the peritoneal serosa (Fig. 6.38). In some cases, the trophoblast destroys the tube as it advances, but it also may grow in the peritubal soft tissue, sparing the tube, at least relatively (Fig. 6.39). In the peritubal soft tissue, the developing pregnancy enters maternal blood vessels resulting in hematoma formation, which expands the broad ligament (Fig. 6.40). Bleeding into the tubal lumen may produce a hematosalpinx (Fig. 6.41).

The placental tissue in tubal pregnancies is not different from that seen in the uterus, except for the expected high incidence of fetal vascular collapse (Fig. 6.42). Accordingly, while placental tissue usually is normal, it rarely may display those same diseases seen at any implantation site. Both hydatidiform moles and choriocarcinoma have occurred in the fallopian tube (Fig. 6.43). In addition, the normal trophoblastic functions that simulate neoplasia are routine (Fig. 6.44). While trophoblastic invasion of adjacent vessels is a physiologic function of implantation-site trophoblast, it may be more clinically important in ectopic gestations, as there is no surrounding myometrium to constrict the vessels when the implantation is disrupted (Fig. 6.45).

6.14

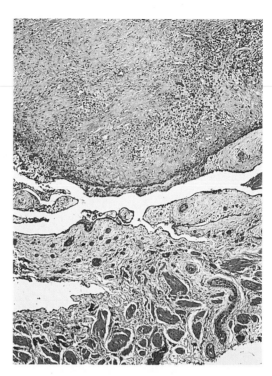

figure 6.36

This papillary frond (top) contains a focus of decidua that is being replaced by inflammation and fibrosis. Inflammation, fibrosis, and smooth-muscle-type cells (bottom) are present.

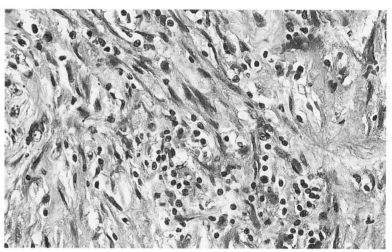

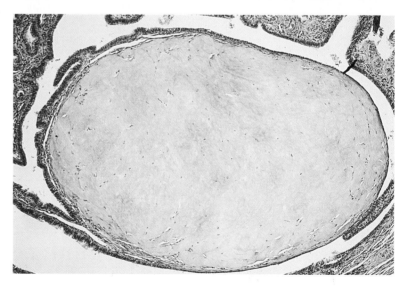

figure 6.37

This apparent tubal "myoma" is relatively acellular.

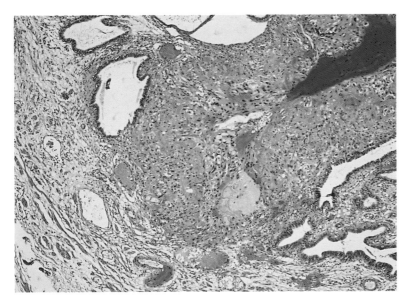

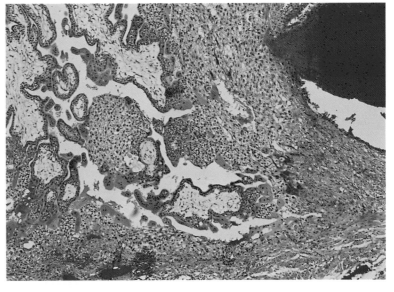

Trophoblast

Tubal wall

figure 6.38

A mass of trophoblast (left) has not only expanded the base of this papillary frond, but it also is extending into the tubal wall. The muscular component of the tubal wall (right) seen in the lower right portion of this photomicrograph is largely destroyed and perforated to the lower left.

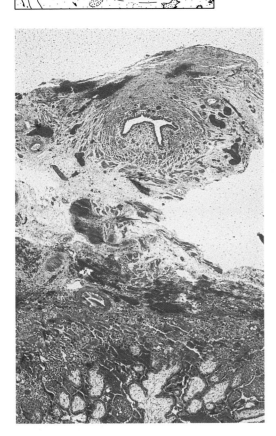

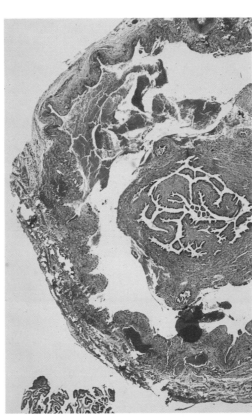

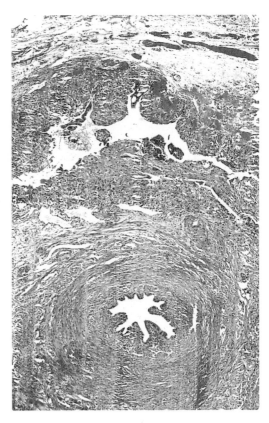

figure 6.39

Above lies a tubal lumen with investing tubal wall; below lies a well-advanced gestation (left). The tubal lumen and its wall are completely surrounded by a cleftlike space (center). At higher power, this cleftlike space is seen to have been produced by invading trophoblast (right).

fallopian tube

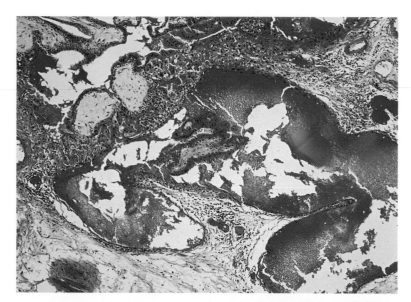

figure 6.40

To the lower right is a large blood-filled vascular channel that is filled to the upper left by multiple villi and their accompanying trophoblastic epithelium.

6.16

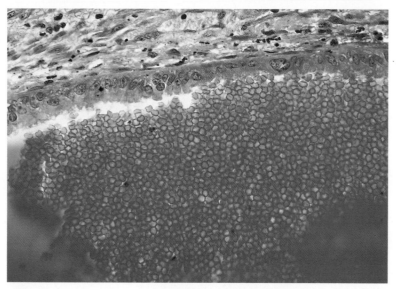

figure 6.41

The tubal lumen is filled with blood.

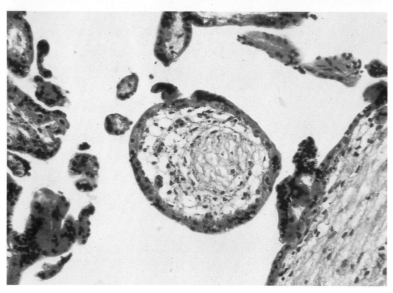

figure 6.42

Although the trophoblast is preserved, the stroma of this villus is fibrotic and lacks vascularity.

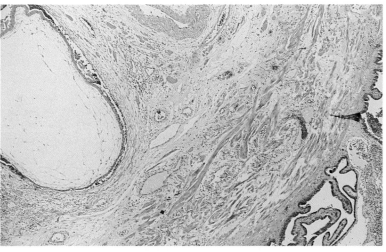

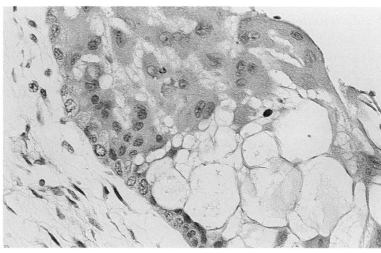

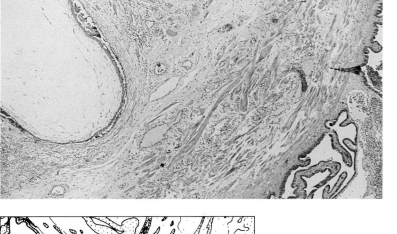

Wall of
fallopian tube

Hydropic villus

Lumen of
fallopian tube

figure 6.43

A hydropic villus with a central cistern (left) lies in a dilated vascular space in the wall of this fallopian tube. At higher power (right), abnormal trophoblastic proliferation is seen around the villus.

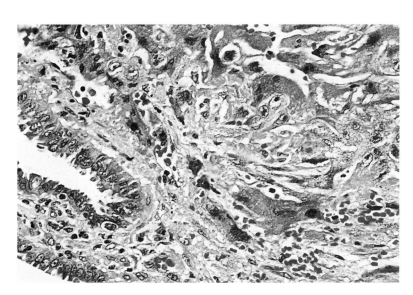

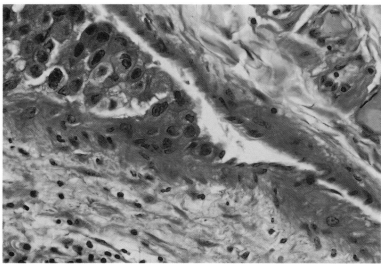

figure 6.44

Malignant trophoblast infiltrates the stroma of the lamina propria. Normal tubal epithelium lies to the left.

figure 6.45

Trophoblast invades the wall of this vessel and, in addition, tends to obstruct its lumen.

fallopian tube

In addition, the trophoblast may infiltrate the broad ligament, producing isolated mononuclear or multinuclear giant cells (Fig. 6.46). Occasionally, the formation of the cytotrophoblastic shell simulates neoplasia (Fig. 6.47).

In addition to the primary problem, the tube containing an ectopic gestation may also have transmural inflammation. When the inflammation is minimal, this consists of only perivascular infiltrates (Fig. 6.48). If rupture has occurred, then peritonitis will be present as well (Fig. 6.49). The pathology of tubal pregnancy includes (1) salpingitis isthmica nodosa, (2) chronic salpingitis, and (3) evidence of pre-existing surgical trauma. Each of these are thought to be factors that predispose to the development of tubal gestation.

Endometrial development is physiologic when ectopic implantation occurs, as long as the conceptus remains healthy, but the decidua is subject to poor development and early slough when the implantation dies and hormone levels fall. Therefore, both well-developed and abortive forms of decidualization, including the Arias-Stella phenomenon, are common (Fig. 6.50). Due to advances in imaging techniques, ectopic pregnancies are diagnosed with increasing accuracy (Fig. 6.51).

6.18

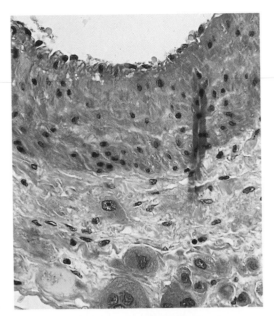

figure 6.46
Isolated trophoblastic giant cells occupy the soft tissue external to this arteriole, which itself is external to the tube.

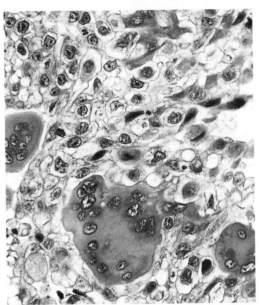

figure 6.47
Cytotrophoblast of the cytotrophoblastic shell is intermingled with trophoblastic giant cells. This is a physiologic structure.

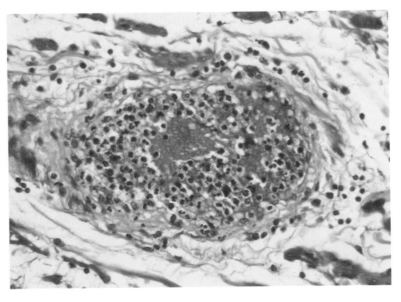

figure 6.48
Inflammatory cells are seen migrating through the vascular wall of this vessel in the soft tissue of the tube.

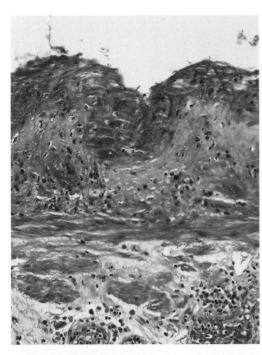

figure 6.49

The serosal surface seen in this photomicrograph has been denuded of epithelium, and expanded with edema fluid and an inflammatory infiltrate. This is typical of peritonitis.

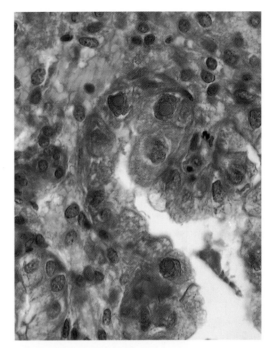

figure 6.50

Large, atypical nuclei with eosinophilic inclusions fill the enlarged secretory epithelial cells of this endometrial gland. This is a typical example of the Arias-Stella reaction.

6.19

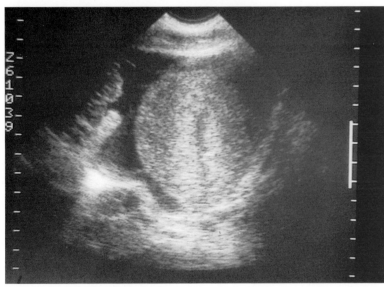

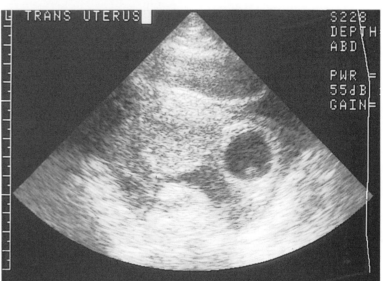

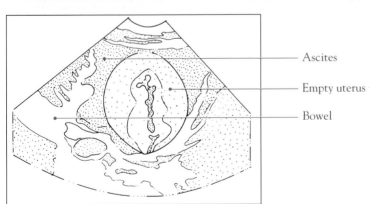

Ascites

Empty uterus

Bowel

Uterus

Gestational sac

Bowel

figure 6.51

Transverse transabdominal ultrasound image of the pelvis with a magnified view of the uterus (left) shows a small fluid collection within the uterine cavity surrounded by thickened endometrium. This is referred to as the decidual cast of an ectopic pregnancy. Transverse ultrasound view of the pelvis (right) shows a uterus that is displaced to the right of the midline. There is fluid in the cul-de-sac. A predominantly fluid filled mass is seen on the left representing the ectopic gestational sac. An embryonic pole is seen within the sac.

Infection

Classic pelvic inflammatory disease begins as an endosalpingitis that frequently becomes transmural (Fig. 6.52). The papillary fronds are swollen, edematous, and filled with acute and chronic inflammatory cells (Fig. 6.53); pus fills the lumen (Fig. 6.54). Initially, the transmural component consists of focal perivascular infiltrates, but eventually inflammation is present throughout the wall of the tube; with the development of peritonitis, the serosa of the broad ligament is inflamed as well (Fig. 6.55). Loss of surface epithelium from either the papillary fronds or the serosa may occur. As this acute phase is characterized by peritonitis and intraperitoneal pus, images of anatomic structures become more obscure (Fig. 6.56). Subsequently, the process localizes and becomes more discrete (Fig. 6.57), although intraperitoneal adhesions may result at any affected site (Fig. 6.58).

While in the acute phase, the tube is more likely to become obstructed at its ends and thus dilated in between. It fills first with pus, and later with clear fluid as the inflammation resolves (Fig. 6.59). Other changes that accompany resolution are infiltration of the fronds by "foam cells" (Fig. 6.60) and metaplastic repair of sloughed epithelium (Fig. 6.61). Subsequent healing may result in the formation of club-

6.20

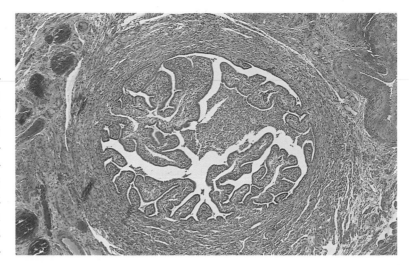

figure 6.52

Pus fills the lumen of this tube, and an inflammatory infiltrate fills and dilates the papillary fronds of the tube. The tubal wall and surrounding soft tissue are relatively spared.

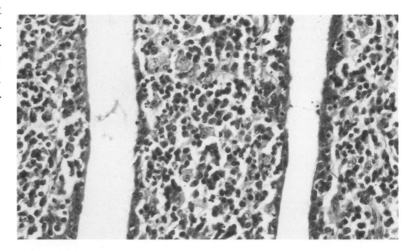

figure 6.53

The papillary fronds seen in this photomicrograph are dilated with edema fluid and filled with an inflammatory infiltrate. Varying degrees of epithelial loss are present.

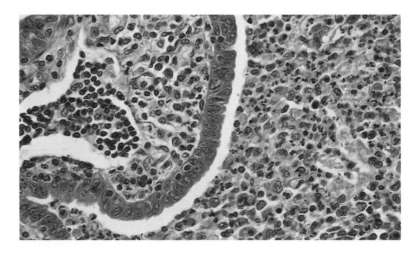

figure 6.54

A vessel within a papillary frond appears to be filled with inflammatory cells. Pus fills the lumen.

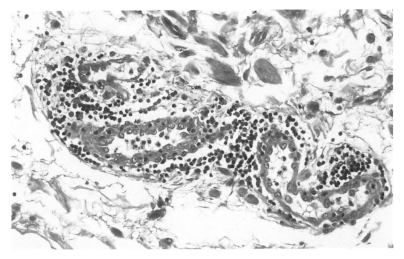

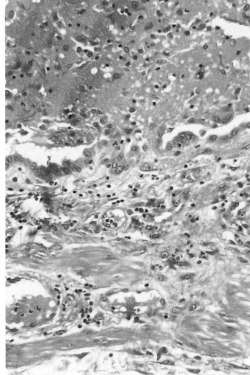

figure 6.55

A perivascular infiltrate (left) characterizes these vessels, which lie in edema-filled soft tissue. The tube (right) lies below. The epithelial surface of the serosa has been disrupted and is adherent to a mass of fibrin and inflammation. This will be an adhesion.

6.21

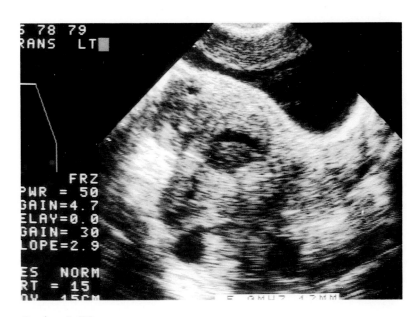

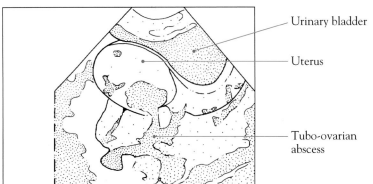

Urinary bladder

Uterus

Tubo-ovarian abscess

figure 6.56

Transverse transabdominal ultrasound view of the pelvis shows the uterus displaced anteriorly and to the right by a heterogeneous mass with mixed echogenicity. This represents a diffuse inflammatory process involving the adnexa and obliterating all the soft tissue planes of the pelvis.

fallopian tube

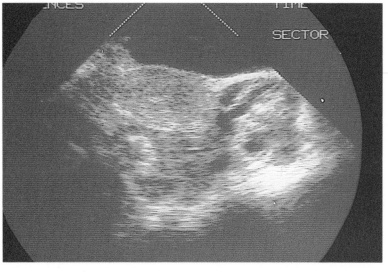

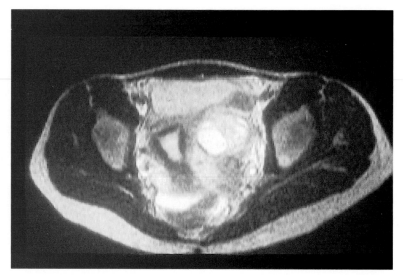

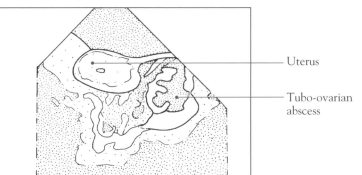

Uterus

Tubo-ovarian abscess

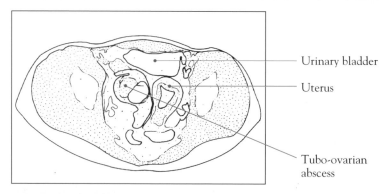

Urinary bladder

Uterus

Tubo-ovarian abscess

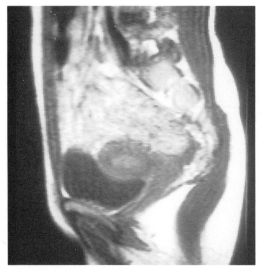

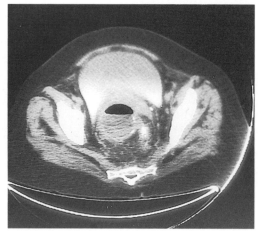

figure 6.57

Transverse transabdominal ultrasound view of the pelvis (top left) shows the uterus displaced to the right by a complex mass arising predominantly from the left adnexa. There are multiple internal septations and much debris within this mass which extends into the cul-de-sac. Axial T2-weighted MRI image of the pelvis (top right) shows the uterus displaced to the left of the midline by a right sided heterogeneous mass with mixed signal intensity. This represents a mixture of fluid and proteinaceous debris within an inflammatory mass. Saggittal T1-weighted MRI image of the pelvis (bottom left) shows the area posterior and superior to the urinary bladder filled by an ill-defined mass with high signal. This reflects the highly proteinaceous nature of the inflammatory debris. Axial CT view of the pelvis (bottom right) shows the urinary bladder filled with contrast. The uterus is displaced slightly to the left of midline by a fluid filled mass containing air within it. This represents an organized abscess, originating from the right adnexa, filling the cul-de-sac.

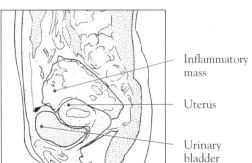

Inflammatory mass

Uterus

Urinary bladder

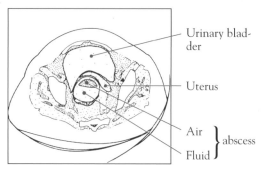

Urinary bladder

Uterus

Air } abscess
Fluid }

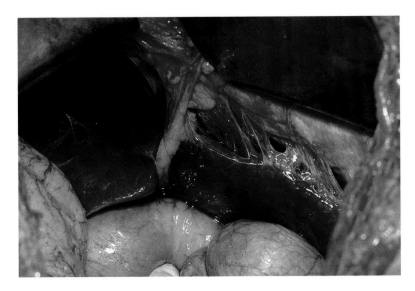

figure 6.58

These adhesions from the surface of the liver to the anterior abdominal wall characterize the Curtis-FitzHugh Syndrome, a manifestation of peritonitis secondary to pelvic inflammatory disease. (Courtesy of Dr. D. Bard).

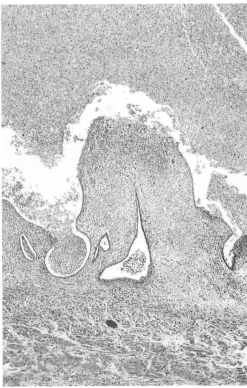

figure 6.59

Not only is this tubal lumen filled with pus, the papillary fronds are adherent, enlarged, and denuded of epithelium as a result of a destructive salpingitis.

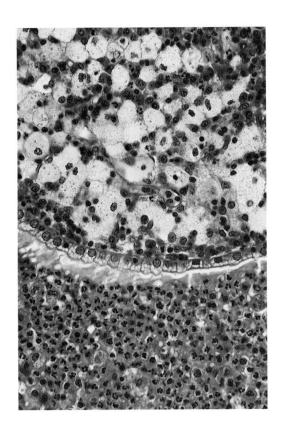

figure 6.60

Pus fills the lumen below. Foamy macrophages fill the stroma of the papillary frond above.

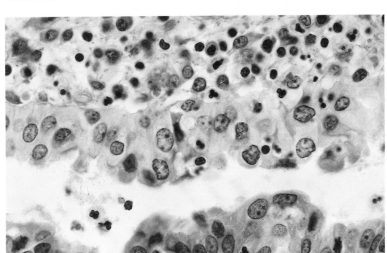

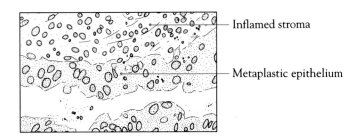

Inflamed stroma

Metaplastic epithelium

figure 6.61

Particularly above, this tubal epithelium is highly metaplastic and constitutes a repair process after loss of the original epithelium secondary to inflammation.

6.23

fallopian tube

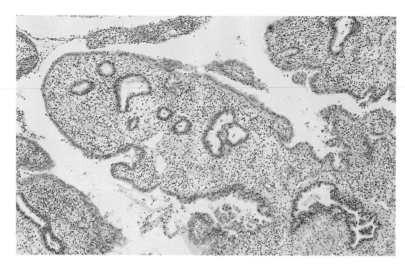

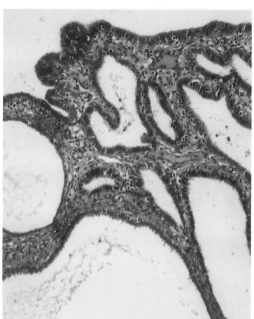

figure 6.62

This club-shaped structure is probably the result of the inflammation, dilatation, and adherence of two adjacent papillary fronds (left). In

this healing salpingitis (right), the papillary fronds to the left are clubbed. To the right they are adherent, producing an adenomatous pattern.

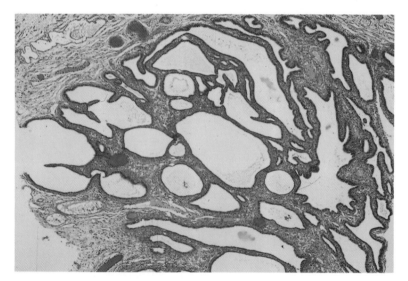

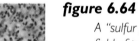

figure 6.63

The tubal lumen (left) has been converted into multiple dilated cystic spaces by the adherence of papillary fronds. A higher power view (right) shows multiple dilated and undilated spaces formed by adherent papillary fronds and lined by normal tubal epithelium.

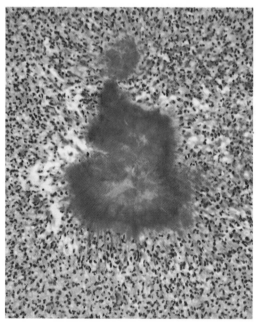

figure 6.64

A "sulfur granule," a huge colony of actinomyces, lies in the center of a field of pus. This unusual organism is associated with a pyosalpinx.

atlas of gynecologic pathology

shaped fronds or adherent ones (Fig. 6.62). If, secondary to sloughing of adjacent epithelial surfaces, papillary fronds adhere, and this is accompanied by persistent fluid in the tubal lumen and between the adherent fronds, then multiple cystic spaces will result in hydrosalpinx follicularis (Fig. 6.63).

IUD-related infections are more likely to consist of ovarian abscesses that secondarily involve the adjacent tube. Therefore, from the start, these infections are likely to look like transmural infections rather than like endosalpingitis. The tube will be severely involved where it is contiguous with the ovarian abscess, but it is almost totally uninvolved elsewhere, unless there is peritonitis. Of course, patients with IUDs also may experience routine pelvic inflammatory disease. Actinomyces is an unusual pathogen though it is found more frequently in IUD-associated pelvic infections (Fig. 6.64).

Granulomatous salpingitis may be secondary to a variety of entities, including foreign bodies, artificially introduced radiographic imaging substances, sarcoidosis, and tuberculosis (Fig. 6.65). The last is the most common.

Tubal tuberculosis usually is a part of systemic tuberculosis. The histology may be quite typical of tuberculosis, with dense chronic inflammation, caseation, and giant cells (Fig. 6.66); or, it may be adenomatous, with papillary frond adhesions having produced a complex pattern with glandlike spaces lined by tubal epithelium. The latter lacks atypicality, but the pattern may suggest neoplasia.

tubal epithelial abnormalities

HYPERPLASIA AND NEOPLASIA

In addition to the anomalous metaplasias referred to above, tubal epithelial abnormalities comprise a spectrum of hyperplasia and neoplasia. Highly associated with clinical circumstances that suggest estrogen stimulation (i.e., endometrial cancer), tubal epithelium may exhibit hyperplasia. In its simplest form, this consists only of piling up of the epithelium (Fig. 6.67). More dramatic examples possess intraepithelial glandlike spaces or epithelial papillae (Fig. 6.68). Nuclear atypicality and mitotic figures are rare, but occasionally may be observed. Although, classically, mitotic figures have been felt to suggest the presence of carcinoma in situ, such an entity is not well defined in the tube (Fig. 6.69).

The most common tubal tumor is the benign adenomatoid tumor. Usually detected incidentally at surgery, it is a firm white or yellowish nodule. Microscopically, it consists of cleftlike spaces lined by mesothelial or cuboidal epithelium, all embedded in a loose stromal reaction (Fig. 6.70). It requires no additional therapy.

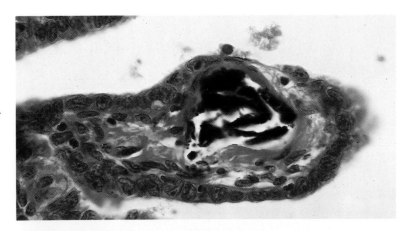

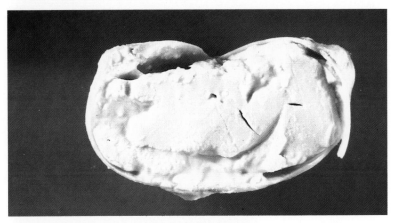

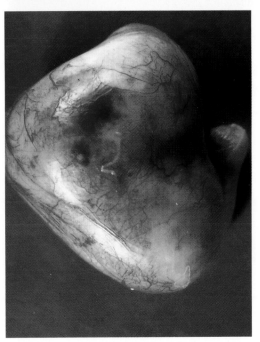

figure 6.65

An unidentified foreign body (top) has elicited local scarring and epithelial modification in this papillary frond. The caseous, or "cheesy," nature of the material in this tube (center) is strongly suggestive of tuberculosis. The dilated tube (bottom) seen in this photograph is consistent with almost any type of tubal infection or tumor.

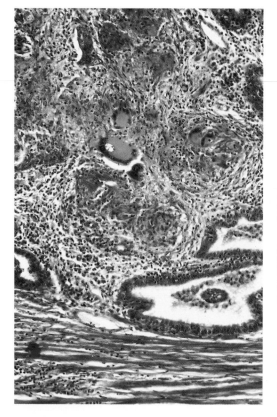

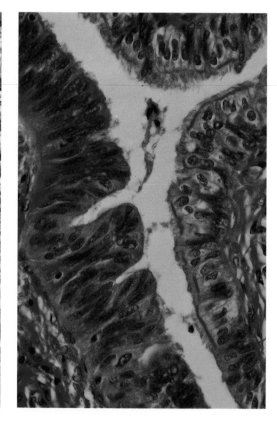

figure 6.66

Not only are typical tubercular granulomas present (left), but the papillary fronds are adherent and glandular spaces result. Typi-

cal Langhans' giant cells (right) are seen in a tubal stromal granuloma.

figure 6.67

Particularly to the left, this tubal epithelium is piled up and has some true papillae.

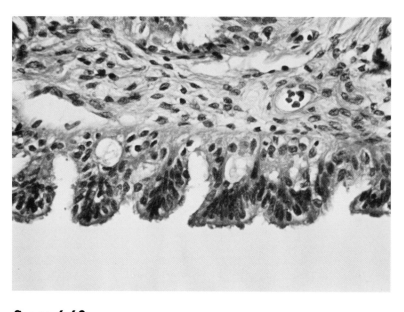

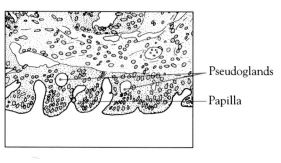

Pseudoglands

Papilla

figure 6.68

The papillary development of this epithelium is marked, producing a pseudoglandular pattern.

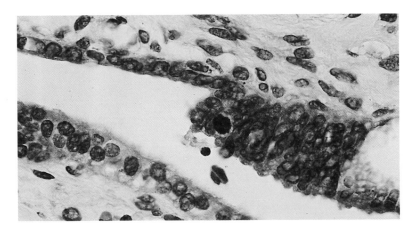
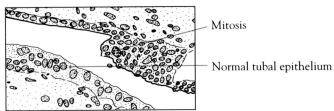

figure 6.69

Above, the epithelium is not only piled up, but there is a prominent mitotic figure within it. This suggests carcinoma in situ.

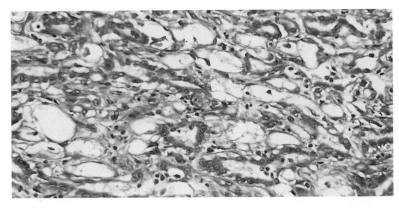

figure 6.70

This adenomatoid tumor (top) consists of multiple cleftlike spaces lined by flattened or cuboidal epithelium. Normal tubal epithelium (bottom) lies to the right. The tumor diffusely fills the stroma beneath this epithelium. Cuboidal and mesothelial epithelium lines the central cleft.

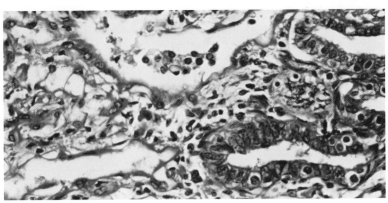

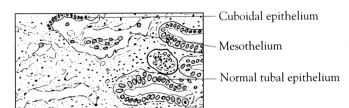

Primary tubal cancer is an unusual disease. The classic description of papillary, alveolar, and solid types reflects the fact that with increasing amounts of epithelial proliferation, the original papillary frond architecture is progressively wiped out (Fig. 6.71). Tubal cancer is, in fact, no different in cell type from epithelial neoplasms seen elsewhere in the upper genital canal, with papillary serous or endometrioid histologies predominating (Fig. 6.72). Primary tubal carcinoma tends to grow as an intraluminal mass for a prolonged period before invading the muscular wall of the tube, but it nearly always spreads into the upper abdomen long before such intramural invasion takes place (Fig. 6.73). It is treated like ovarian cancer.

The tubal epithelium also may participate in the general phenomenon when widespread intraabdominal papillary neoplasia is present (Fig. 6.74). This may consist of focal proliferation that represents little more than endometriosis, or it may consist of more aggressive clear-cut cancer. When the disease is sufficiently low grade to warrant the designation "borderline," tubal involvement does not suggest the need for adjuvant therapy.

As the stromal wall of the fallopian tube is developmentally identical to that of the rest of the genital canal, it produces neoplasms with similar histologies. Among these, the stromal sarcomas and mixed tumors probably are most frequent, although all of the mesenchymal lesions are extremely rare as primary tubal phenomena (Fig. 6.75). Like their counterparts elsewhere, these malignancies are highly aggressive and usually have spread extensively before a diagnosis is achieved.

Metastatic tumors

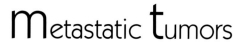

Metastatic tubal cancer usually is the result of spread from adjacent pelvic organs, but it may represent disease from more distant sites such as the stomach. In contrast to primary tubal cancer, it does not involve the lumen or the epithelium, but infiltrates the lymphatic and vascular channels of the lamina propria and tubal wall (Fig. 6.76). Even if the primary site is relatively local, this infiltrative pattern suggests a very poor prognosis.

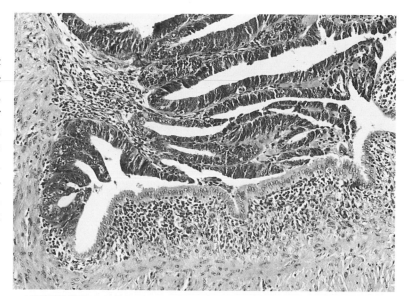

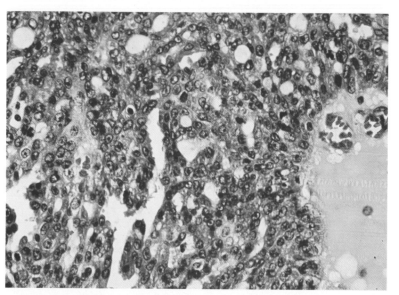

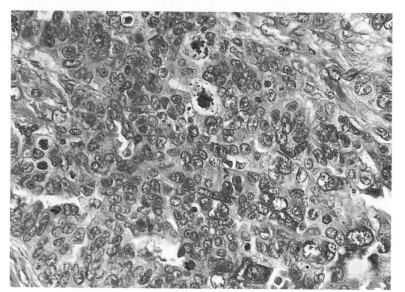

figure 6.71

Normal tubal epithelium (top) is seen below, but tubal carcinoma forms the papillary structures above. Papillary alveolar patterns (center) are formed by this relatively aggressive tubal cancer. A solid pattern (bottom) results from more aggressive cancer.

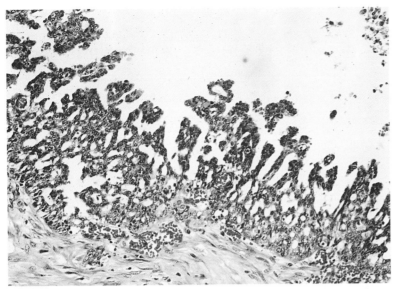

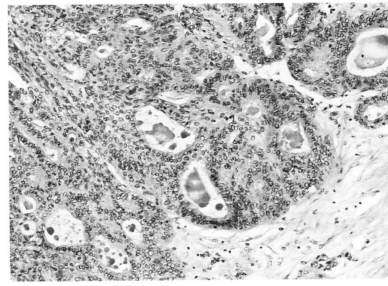

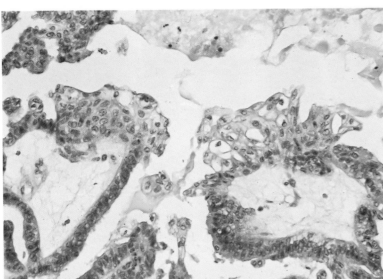

figure 6.72

This finely papillary tubal cancer (top left) is typical of high-grade papillary cancers of any genital site. This tubal adenocarcinoma (top right) could be located at any site from the endocervix to the peritoneal cavity. This papillary tubal cancer (bottom) has foci of squamous differentiation, associating it with adenosquamous lesions at all levels of the female genital canal.

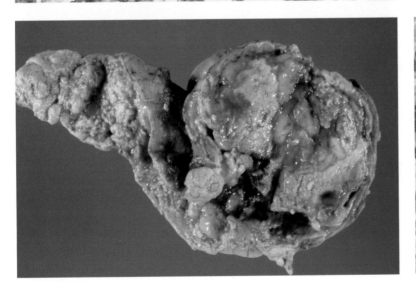

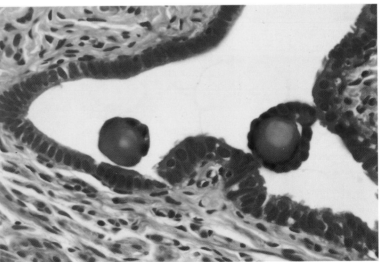

figure 6.73

Atypical tubal cancer has dilated and filled the tubal lumen without destroying the tubal wall.

figure 6.74

Tiny tubal papillae containing psammoma bodies are a part of the generalized process of papillary peritoneal proliferation that exists in this patient.

fallopian tube

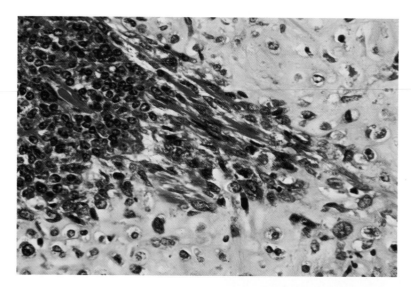

figure 6.75

Undifferentiated stromal sarcoma with a few rhabdomyoblasts merges with chondrosarcoma in this mixed mesodermal tumor of the tube.

6.30

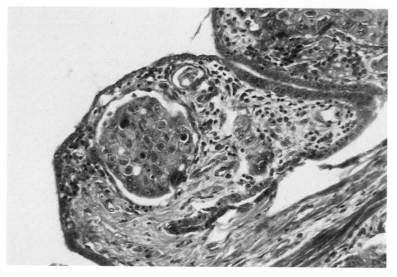

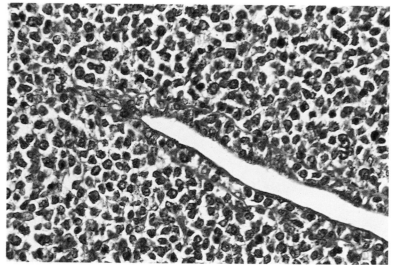

figure. 6.76

Metastatic adenocarcinoma (left) dilates the lymphatics within the papillary fronds of this fallopian tube. A malignant lymphoma (right) fills the

lamina propria of the papillary fronds of this tube. The epithelium is intact, although it is significantly distorted by the underlying tumor.

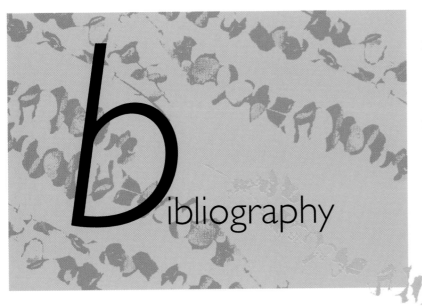

b ibliography

Budowick M, Johnson TRB Jr.,
Genadry R, et al: The
histopathology of the
developing tubal ectopic
pregnancy. *Fertil Steril* 34:169,
1980.

Novak E, Everett HS: Cyclical and
other variations in the tubal
epithelium. *Am J Obstet
Gynecol* 16:499, 1928.

Novak E, Woodruff JD: *Novak's
Gynecologic and Obstetric,*
8th ed. Philadelphia,
WB Saunders, 1979.

O'Rahilly R: The embryology and
anatomy of the uterus. In
Norris HJ, Hertig AT (eds.):
The Uterus. Baltimore,
Williams & Wilkins, 1973.

Pauerstein CJ: *The Fallopian Tube:
A Reappraisal.* Philadelphia,
Lea & Febiger, 1974.

Pauerstein CJ, Croxatto HB, Eddy
CA, et al: Anatomy and
pathology of tubal pregnancy. *Obstet Gynecol* 67:301,
1986.

Rock JA, Parmley TH, King TM,
et al: Endometriosis and the
development of tuboperi-
tonei fistula after tubal ligation. *Fertil Steril* 35:16, 1981.

Sampson JA: Post-salpingectomy
endometriosis (endosalpin-
giosis). *Am J Obstet Gynecol*
20:443, 1930.

Seibel MM: Infection and infertility. In DeCherney AH (ed.):
Reproductive Failure. New
York, Churchill Livingstone,
1986.

Siegler AM: *The Fallopian Tube.* Mt.
Kisco, NY, Futura Publishing
Co., 1986.

Stern J, Buscema J, Parmley TH,
et al: Atypical epithelial proliferations in the fallopian
tube. *Am J Obstet Gynecol*
140:309, 1981.

Sweet RL: Etiology, diagnosis, and
management of acute and
chronic pelvic inflammatory
disease. In Osofsky HL (ed.):
*Advances in Clinical Obstetrics
and Gynecology,* vol 2.
Baltimore, Williams &
Wilkins, 1984.

Thrasher TV, Richart RM: Ultra-
structure of the Arias-Stella
reaction. *Am J Obstet Gynecol*
112:113, 1972.

Ovary

development

Development of the ovary begins during the fourth, fifth, and sixth weeks of embryonic life, when the germ cells migrate into the medial wall of the urogenital ridge. In response, the coelomic epithelium begins to proliferate, contributing to the development of both the ovarian hilum and the ovarian cortex (Figs. 7.1 and 7.2). If aberrant germ cells migrate to other subcoelomic epithelial sites, anomalous gonads may form at these sites (Fig. 7.3). If no germ cells migrate into the primordial gonadal area, or if they migrate into it then subsequently die, lesser degrees of gonadal development will take place, giving rise to ovarian streaks. These consist of a small but variable amount of gonadal stroma immediately beneath the coelomic epithelium. Interstitial- or hilus-type cells are prominent in the medullary area of streaks, suggesting that they are stimulated by gonadotropins (Fig. 7.4).

When development is normal, the invading germ cells induce an early component of the surface epithelial proliferation that produces rudimentary tubules analogous to, but not as discretely organized as, the sex cords of the testis. In the ovary, these rudimentary structures never develop fully but instead become the rete ovarii, tubules lined by flattened or cuboidal cells. Occasionally, rete tubules of coelomic epithelial origin are associated with mesonephric tubule remnants, which are distinguishable by their well-developed investment of supporting stroma (Fig. 7.5). Separately, or in association with these tubular structures, nerve target-organ cells analogous to the interstitial cells of the testis, termed the hilus cells in the ovary, may be seen (Fig. 7.6). They are insignificant throughout most of the reproductive life of the human female, but may exhibit hyperplasia in postmenopausal women and rarely may be the site of tumor formation. In hyperplasia, the interstitial cells may

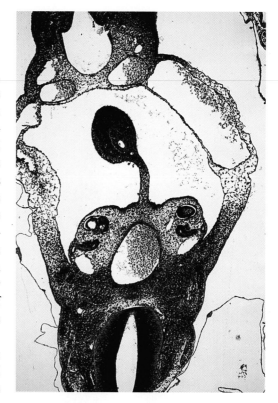

figure 7.1

The neural tube lies below. The hind gut is suspended by its mesentery in the middle of the coelomic cavity. Between it and the neural tube lies the dorsal aorta, between the two urogenital ridges containing mesonephric glomeruli and the wolffian duct. On the medial surface of the urogenital ridge, the surface epithelium is thickening at the site of the future gonad.

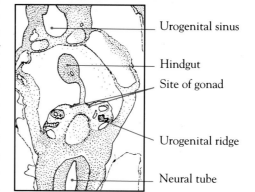

- Urogenital sinus
- Hindgut
- Site of gonad
- Urogenital ridge
- Neural tube

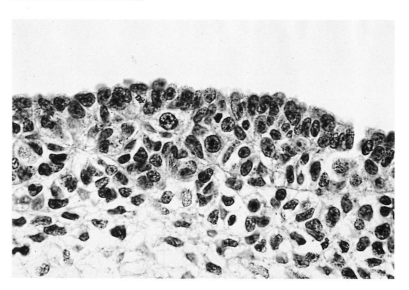

figure 7.2

Large germ cells have entered the epithelial compartment. Both epithelium and stroma are proliferating.

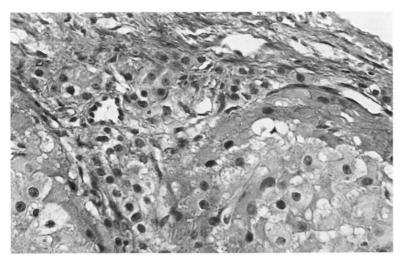

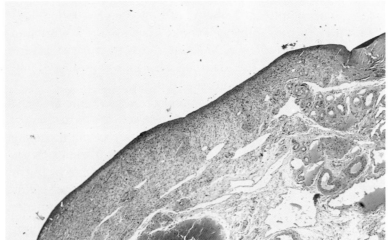

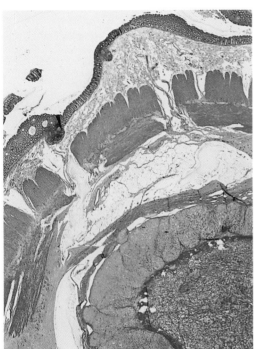

figure 7.3

In the middle, a triangular-shaped collection of luteinized theca interna cells separates two larger collections of granulosa (top). At lower power, both collections are seen to lie in the mesentery of the small bowel (bottom).

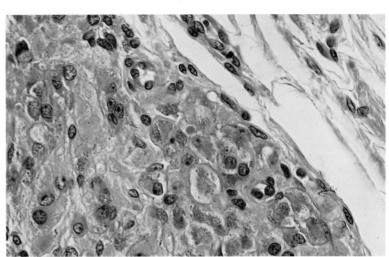

figure 7.4

In this cross section of an ovarian streak (top), ridgelike elevation of the coelomic epithelium is secondary to the thin collection of gonadal stroma beneath it. In this streak (bottom), a nodule of hilus cells lies immediately beneath the gonadal stroma.

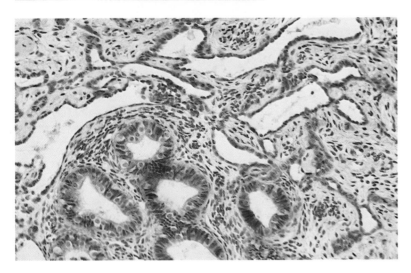

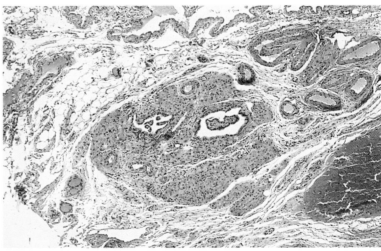

figure 7.5

Rete tubules of coelomic epithelial origin lie above, while tubules more consistent with a mesonephric origin lie below.

figure 7.6

Photomicrograph of rete tubules embedded in a nest of hilus cells.

7.3

ovary

contain significant amounts of brown pigment (Fig. 7.7). Although pure hilus cell tumors are usually a postmenopausal occurrence, in adolescent girls the hilar structures occasionally give rise to arrhenoblastomas consisting of both tubular-type elements and interstitial cells.

Subsequent proliferation of the coelomic epithelial cells and the invading germ cells results in the formation of a thick cortical layer on the medial surface of the urogenital ridge (Fig. 7.8). Beginning in the second trimester, the medullary mesenchyme of the urogenital ridge begins to penetrate this cellular mass, dividing it into nests of epithelial and germ cells (Fig. 7.9). This process proceeds from the medulla to the surface of the ridge (Fig. 7.10). Interstitial-type cells are prominent in this mesenchyme in the second trimester but disappear by term (Fig. 7.11). As the nests of epithelial and germ cells successively divide, primordial follicles are formed. This occurs first in the medulla and later near the surface of the gonad (Fig. 7.12). Primordial follicles consist of a single germ cell completely surrounded by a single layer of epithelial cells. Occasionally, two germ cells are contained within the same follicle.

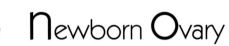

7.4 Newborn Ovary

By birth, the development of primordial follicles is almost but not quite completed, so that some undivided nests of epithelial and germ cells are still immediately beneath the surface epithelium. In the medullary portion, almost all of the germ cells are in the form of primordial follicles (Fig. 7.13). The high levels of maternal hormone circulating in the newborn may cause significant development of some follicles, resulting in follicular cysts and, rarely, histologic evidence suggesting ovulation. Some of these cysts may produce

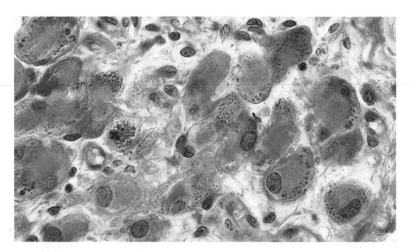

figure 7.7
These enlarged hilus cells are in a focus of hilus cell hyperplasia in a postmenopausal ovary. Note the prominent brown granules in the cytoplasm of some cells.

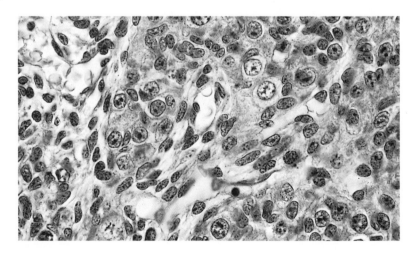

figure 7.8
The medial surface of this urogenital ridge is now a thickened mass suspended from the bulk of the ridge by a mesovarium.

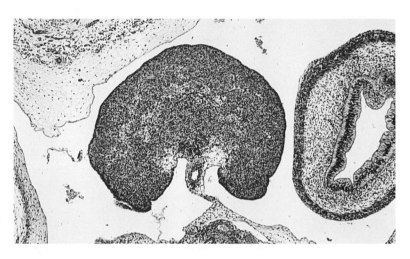

figure 7.9
Near the gonadal medulla, the lighter-colored mesenchyme is penetrating the mass of germ cells and epithelial cells and dividing them into smaller groups.

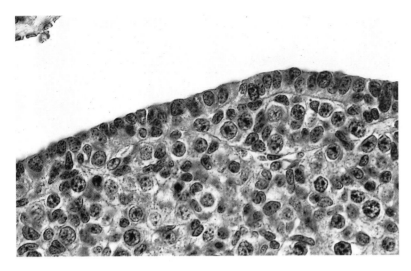

figure 7.10

At the periphery of the gonad in this photomicrograph, the mixture of germ cells and epithelial cells is as yet undivided.

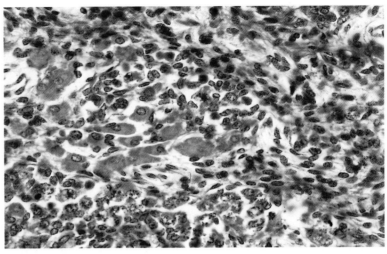

figure 7.11

Large, eosinophilic, interstitial-type cells are seen in the mesenchyme of this developing gonad.

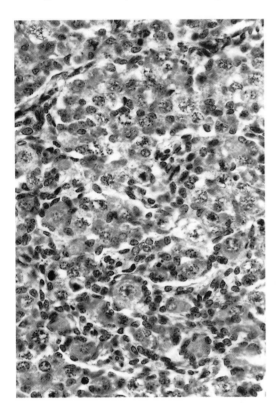

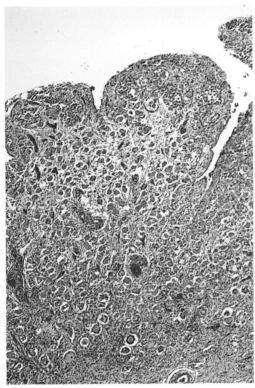

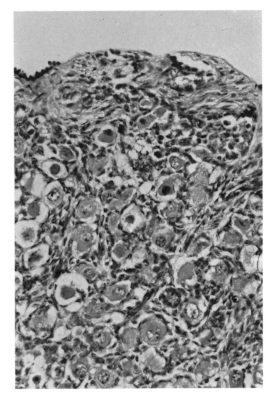

figure 7.12

In the top half of this photomicrograph, nearer the cortex of the developing ovary, the germ cells and epithelial cells are mixed in an amorphous mass. In the bottom half of the picture, nearer the medulla, a few large germ cells are specifically invested by a layer of epithelial cells. These are the first primordial follicles.

figure 7.13

In this newborn ovary (left), a gradual progression can be seen from the surface at the top to the medulla below. Nests of cells are present above, while single primordial follicles are seen in the medulla. In this higher power view (right), superficial nests of mixed epithelial and germ cells lie near the surface, but, below, the germ cells are being individually sequestered.

ovary

clinically important symptoms such as pain, bleeding, or large masses (Fig. 7.14). Most are operated upon, but usually they will regress as maternal hormone levels decline.

Normal functional histology

Between birth and maturity, the primary change is one of follicular atresia so that the adult gonad consists of a surface epithelium (the mesothelial peritoneal epithelium) and an underlying stroma (the theca) derived from the mesenchyme of the urogenital ridge (Fig. 7.15). The theca is usually bilayered in appearance, with a more fibrous superficial layer overlying a more cellular ovarian stromal layer. Multiple primordial follicles are embedded in this ovarian stroma, or theca; in the hilum of the ovary are found the rete ovarii and hilus cells (Fig. 7.16).

OLLICULAR DEVELOPMENT

Only with puberty does regular follicular development begin, although, occasionally, follicular cysts develop in prepubertal ovaries as a result of sporadic follicular development. The primordial follicles possess only a single layer of flattened pregranulosa cells investing the oocyte, but when the oocyte begins to secrete a glycoprotein coat—the zona pellucida—the surrounding cell layer becomes multicelled and is known as the granulosa (Fig. 7.17). When a large enough mass of granulosa cells has developed, a fluid-filled space—the antrum—develops eccentrically in the granulosa, displacing the oocyte to a position on one side of the follicle. At the site of the oocyte, the intrafollicular layer of granulosa is piled up to form a local collection, the cumulus oophorus; the zona pellucida is prominent at this time (Fig. 7.18).

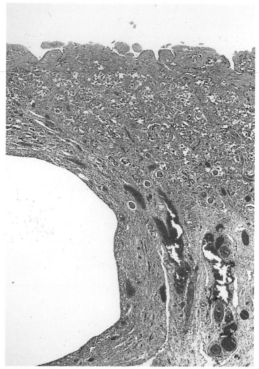
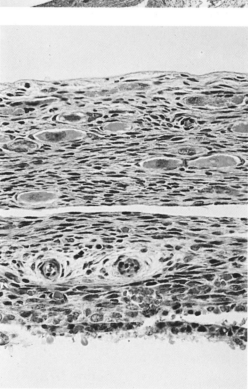
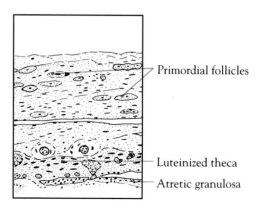

figure 7.14

Photomicrograph of a neonatal ovary with a prominent follicle in the medullary portion of the cortex (top). This section of a large cyst in a newborn ovary (bottom) reveals primordial follicles near its surface and an atretic granulosa layer below. Just above the atretic granulosa is luteinized theca interna. (Courtesy of Dr. Grover Hutchins.)

— Primordial follicles

— Luteinized theca
— Atretic granulosa

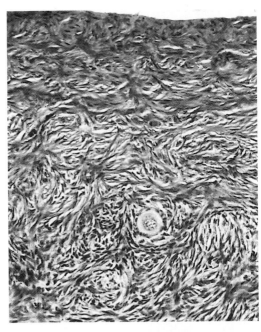

figure 7.15

The more fibrous component of the stroma lies above and the typically ovarian stroma lies below. A primordial follicle occupies its customary position near, but below, the junction of the two.

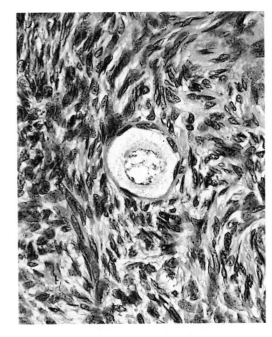

figure 7.16

A single oocyte is surrounded by flattened pre-granulosa cells. This is a typical primordial follicle.

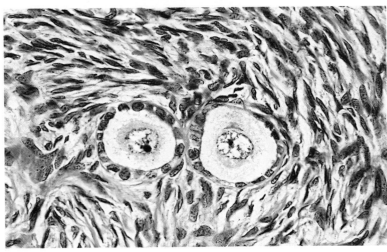

figure 7.17

Both oocytes (left) are surrounded by cuboidal cells that are more numerous than the pregranulosa cells seen in Figure 7.16. The one on the left is further along in the process than the one on the right. A fully

developed granulosa layer (right) is present in this oocyte, which has a definable zona pellucida.

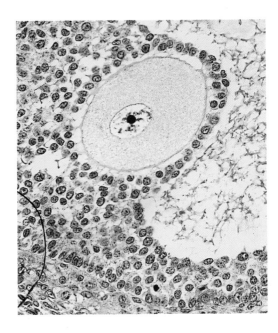

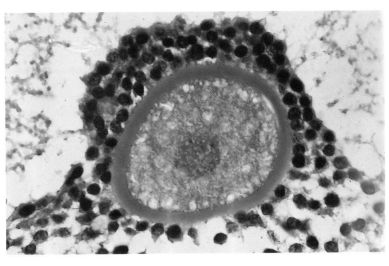

figure 7.18

This large oocyte (left) is contained within a piled-up mass of granulosa, the cumulus oophorus, on one side of the antral space that has developed within the follicle. This cumulus (right) is not well preserved, but the zona pellucida is dramatic.

ovary

The granulosa cell layer, as well as the theca interna, contains mitoses (Fig. 7.19). The granulosa is an epithelium that lacks vasculature, but it does contain small fluid collections around which the granulosa cells orient themselves, producing a so-called *Call-Exner* body (Fig. 7.20). The theca around the follicle becomes organized into a layer of thecal cells, which immediately surrounds the follicle and the more distant thecae cells. The cells in the layer closest to the follicle, the theca interna, become epithelial in character and develop a significant amount of steroid-hormone-producing cytoplasm (see Figs. 7.19 and 7.20). This process is called luteinization, because the cells look yellow grossly (Fig. 7.21). The cells of the more peripheral theca, the theca externa, are histologically unchanged. With each cycle, many follicles progress to this antrum stage of development and contribute to hormone production. Only one undergoes ovulation; the rest undergo atresia. This process is well illustrated by endovaginal ultrasound (Fig. 7.22).

OVULATION

Ovulation consists of the rupture of the selected follicle and the extrusion of the cumulus oophorus containing the oocyte. Immediately after ovulation, the ovulatory follicle collapses. This produces the picture of a collapsed cyst lined by a thick layer of granulosa, more or less opposed to a similar layer of granulosa from the opposite wall of the cyst. However, the follicle soon reseals, redistends, and again becomes cystic. The granulosa layer is redundant and arranged in a scalloped manner. The cells of the granulosa layer become luteinized even more dramatically than those of the theca

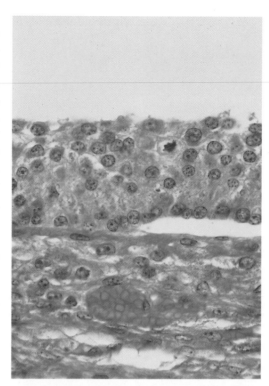

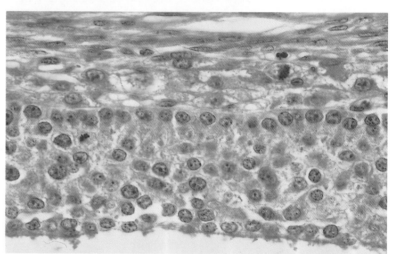

figure 7.19

The granulosa layer (top) is slightly separated from the theca interna below, which contains a capillary at the level that separates the theca interna from the theca externa. A mitosis is present in the granulosa. The theca externa (bottom) above merges into theca interna, which contains a mitotic figure. The granulosa is below.

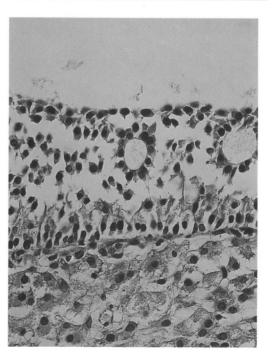

figure 7.20

Two Call-Exner bodies are sharply outlined by a rosette-like arrangement of granulosa cells. The theca interna lies below.

7.8

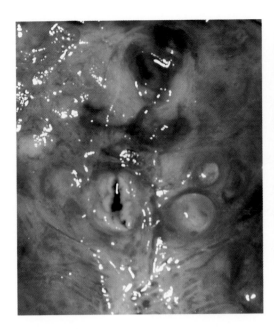

figure 7.21

The grossly yellow appearance of these ovarian follicles is consistent with dramatic luteinization.

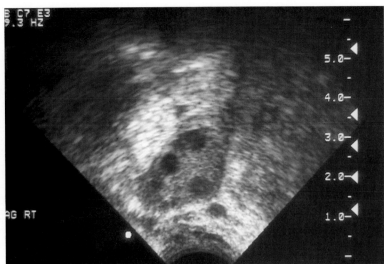

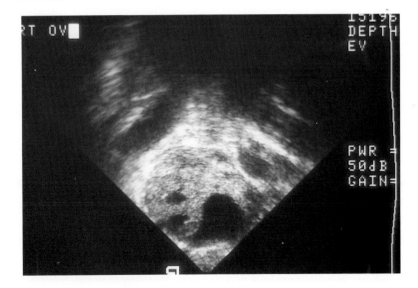

Bowel gas

Follicles

Ovary

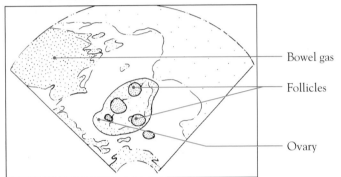

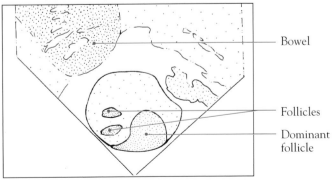

Bowel

Follicles

Dominant follicle

figure 7.22

Sagittal endovaginal ultrasound view of the right ovary (top) shows multiple hypoechoic follicles in the periphery of the ovary. The uterus is not included due to the limited field of view of the endovaginal study. Coronal endovaginal ultrasound view of the right ovary (bottom) shows multiple small follicles within the ovary. A larger cyst, representing the dominant follicle, is seen at the periphery.

7.9

externa (Fig. 7.23). However, this latter layer further differentiates. At this stage, the follicle is referred to as the corpus luteum because of its grossly yellow color (see Fig. 7.21).

As mentioned above, the granulosa cell layer, an epithelium, is not vascularized routinely, but after the 16th or 17th day of a normal cycle, the luteinized granulosa cell layer is invaded by capillary blood vessels from the adjacent theca. During the 17th cycle day, these capillaries reach the antral space and hemorrhage freely into the lumen of the corpus luteum (Fig. 7.24). This free hemorrhage may on occasion be uncontrolled and may produce a clinically important rupture of the corpus luteum. However, under normal circumstances, the hemorrhage is limited, and fibroblastic invasion of the antral space begins immediately. When implantation occurs, the central coagulum in this antral space is normally organized by cycle day 21. (Fig. 7.25). Ultrasonically, the complex wall of the corpus luteum may be apparent (Fig. 7.26).

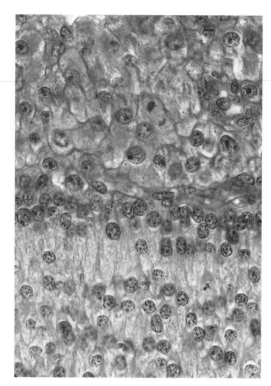

figure 7.23
The granulosa cells below are becoming dramatically luteinized in comparison to the small, pre-ovulatory granulosa cells. A mitotic figure is present in the theca interna above.

7.10

Theca

Granulosa

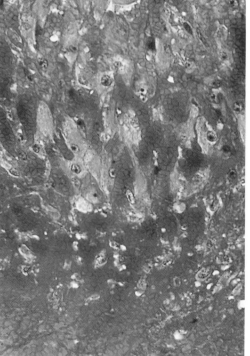

figure 7.24
Capillaries penetrate the granulosa layer above and freely hemorrhage into the antral space below.

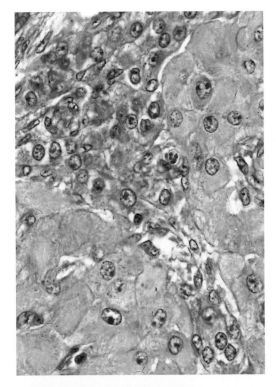
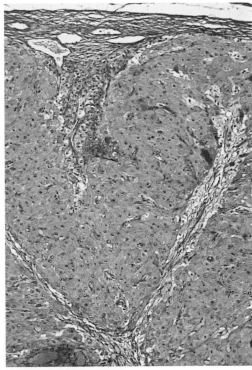

figure 7.25

To the left and right (left) are masses of luteinized granulosa cells separated by less dramatically luteinized theca interna cells. This is a mature corpus luteum. This lower power view of the corpus luteum (right) seen in the previous view illustrates the scalloped appearance of the granulosa cell layer. In addition, fibroblastic proliferation has organized the central space around which the scalloped granulosa cell layer is arranged.

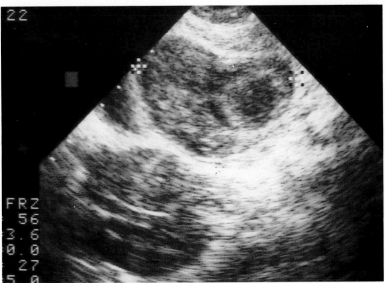

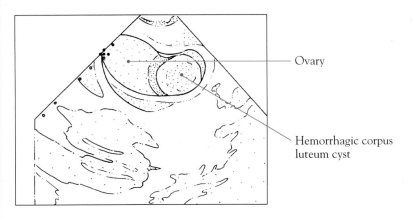

Ovary

Hemorrhagic corpus luteum cyst

figure 7.26

Transverse transabdominal ultrasound exhibits the complex multilayered wall of a corpus luteum cyst by illustrating its alternating hypoechoic and hyperechoic circles.

ovary

PREGNANCY

If implantation does in fact take place, additional luteinization of the corpus luteum in response to placental hormones is the result, and both the theca lutein and the granulosa lutein cells become large polygonal cells that produce progesterone throughout the course of pregnancy. This process is sufficiently dramatic that the corpus luteum of pregnancy is usually recognizable histologically (Fig. 7.27).

In the ovary during pregnancy, anovulatory follicles also demonstrate theca luteinization (Fig. 7.28). Occasionally, this is so exaggerated that one or both ovaries swell with multiple theca lutein cysts. This is particularly likely to occur if exogenous gonadotropins have been used to induce ovulation, resulting in multiple ovulations and a multiple pregnancy. Clinical recognition of this phenomenon has been greatly facilitated by the advent of imaging techniques that do not employ x-rays (Fig. 7.29).

Beyond the luteinization that takes place in the perifollicular theca, isolated stromal cells may luteinize in pregnancy (Fig. 7.30). If this is diffuse and massive or focal, but extensive enough to constitute a tumor, it may be responsible for testosterone production and is termed a *luteoma* (Fig. 7.31).

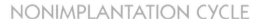

NONIMPLANTATION CYCLE

In the absence of implantation, the corpus luteum degenerates over time. Beginning as soon as day 21, intracellular vacuoles begin to accumulate in the granulosa cells. This results in so-called *mulberry cell* formation (Fig. 7.32), which is a prelude to cell death. The granulosa and theca lutein layer shrink (Fig. 7.33). Frequently, they are replaced by lipid and then are hyalinized (Fig. 7.34). Hemosiderin, the residue of the follicular hemorrhage, may persist. As the hyalinized corpus luteum or corpus albicans maintains its scalloped appearance, the scar of an old corpus luteum is recognizable (Fig. 7.35). These scars may persist for many months but eventually are reabsorbed. Rarely, as the corpus luteum is organized, the central coagulum liquefies rather than organizes, and a true corpus luteum cyst is formed (Fig. 7.36). This structure may persist as a corpus albicans cyst and may

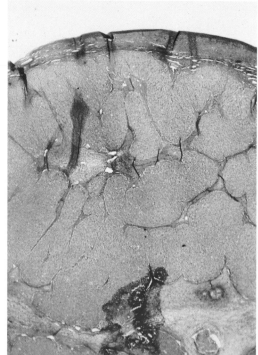

figure 7.27

This huge corpus luteum almost entirely fills one pole of the ovary. In this case, it was associated with a first-trimester pregnancy.

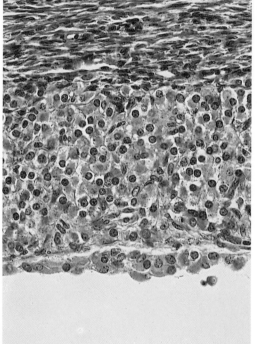

figure 7.28

It can be seen by the fragmentary, degenerating granulosa cell layer below that this follicle is atretic, but the theca interna is nevertheless well luteinized.

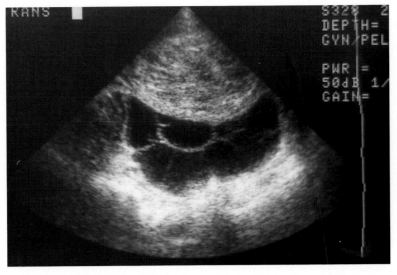

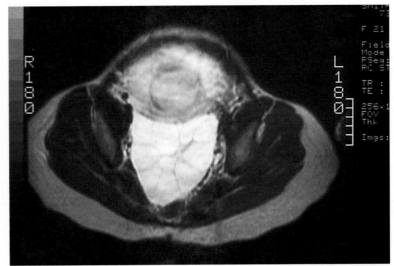

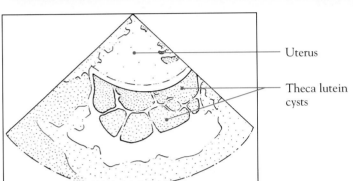

Uterus

Theca lutein cysts

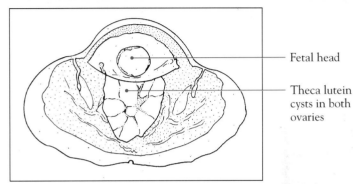

Fetal head

Theca lutein cysts in both ovaries

figure 7.29

Axial transverse ultrasound image of the pelvis (top left) presents the uterus anteriorly as an ovoid structure. The cul-de-sac is filled by a multiseptated mass representing large theca lutein cysts in both ovaries. Axial T-2 MRI weighted image of the pelvis (top right) shows a gravid uterus in cross section with the fetal head filling the uterine cavity. A septated mass fills the cul-de-sac representing theca lutein cysts in both ovaries. The fluid content of the cysts gives rise to their high signal intensity. Sagittal T-2 weighted MR image of the pelvis (bottom) shows the gravid uterus filling the anterior abdo-men and pelvis. The ovaries, filled with large theca lutein cysts, are crowded into the cul-de-sac.

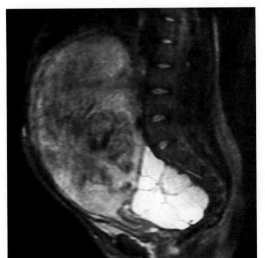

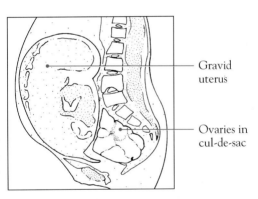

Gravid uterus

Ovaries in cul-de-sac

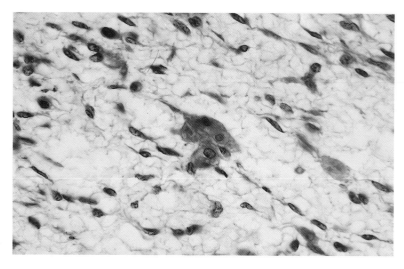

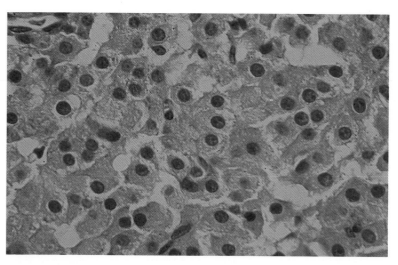

figure 7.30

Isolated stromal cells demonstrate luteinization in this ovary associated with pregnancy.

figure 7.31

A luteoma in the ovary of this pregnant woman was a solid tumor producing testosterone, and was composed of luteinized stromal cells.

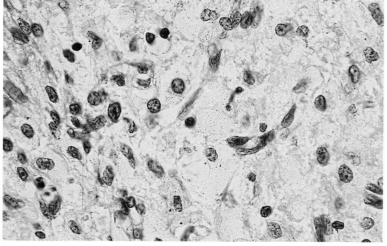

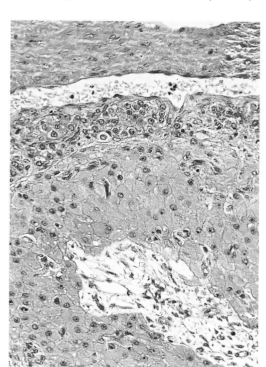

figure 7.33

Both the theca interna layer and the granulosa cell layer are less prominent than the corresponding tissue seen in the early corpus luteum (see Fig. 7.25). The central space is well organized.

figure 7.32

Large, "foamy" cells in the granulosa layer represent cells becoming vacuolated prior to degeneration.

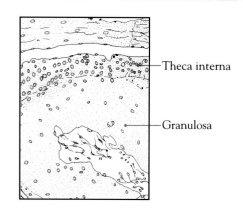

Theca interna

Granulosa

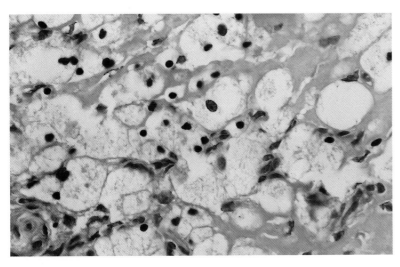

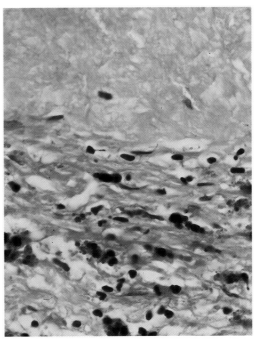

figure 7.34

Lipid (left) has replaced the granulosa cell layer in this photomicrograph. A well-developed hyaline scar (right) above has replaced the granulosa cell layer. Hemosiderin is present in the central space below.

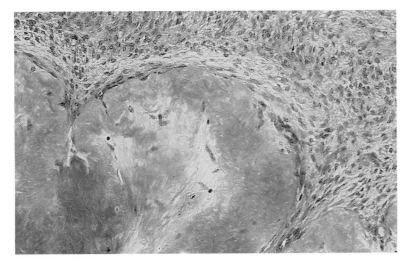

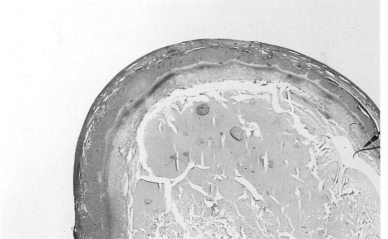

figure 7.35

This corpus albicans possesses a well-preserved scalloped appearance, which illustrates its origin.

figure 7.36

This corpus luteum (top) is not scalloped and has no central organization. Instead, a fluid-filled space results in the formation of a true cyst lined by luteinized granulosa. At higher power (bottom), the cyst wall seen in the previous view illustrates the granulosa cell layer, lacking the normal scalloped configuration associated with follicular collapse.

ovary

be present in the ovary for prolonged periods of time (Fig. 7.37). Even more rarely, an old corpus albicans will demonstrate focal calcification (Fig. 7.38).

The follicles not selected for ovulation regress rapidly if any cycle does not result in conception. Moreover, the granulosa disintegrates (Fig. 7.39). A hyaline scar develops that is smaller and less convoluted than the same structure associated with the corpus luteum (Fig. 7.40). It is reabsorbed over weeks to months and usually disappears completely.

If ovulation does not occur for any reason including oral contraceptives, Stein-Leventhal disease, or chronic ill health, ovarian morphology displays some combination of the following features: the ovarian cortex appears thickened and contains variable numbers of follicles in different stages of maturation or atresia (Fig. 7.41); evidence of ovulation is rare. Many of the follicles are characterized by prominent luteinization of the theca interna, and there may or may not be significant luteinization of other stromal cells (Fig. 7.42). Alternately, the ovary may contain large amounts of theca with prominent individual cell luteinization and few poorly developed follicles, an event that is commonly termed *hyperthecosis*. Rarely, functional ovarian tumors appear to develop

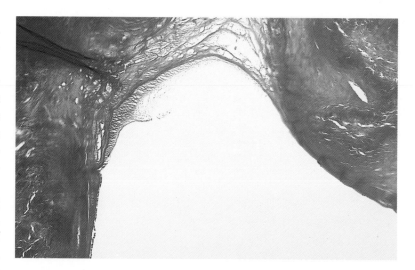

figure 7.37
A cystic space, rather than an organized scar, occupies the center of this corpus albicans.

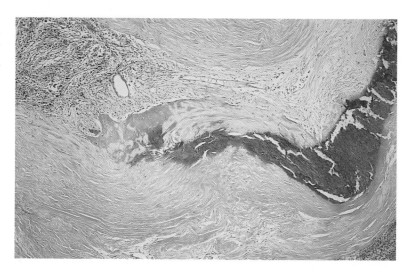

figure 7.38
Focal calcification is occurring in this old corpus albicans.

atlas of gynecologic pathology

in such a background. In the condition known as the edematous ovary syndrome, stromal cell luteinization also may be prominent (Fig. 7.43). This condition, which is of unknown etiology, consists of an enlarged swollen ovary with prominent edema.

POSTMENOPAUSAL OVARIES

After the menopause, ovaries are, by definition, devoid of follicles; however, it is well to remember that occasional ovulation occurs in ostensibly postmenopausal women (Fig. 7.44). In the absence of follicles, the ovary can no longer feed upon the pituitary and hypothalamus. Therefore, the gonado-tropin level rises, stimulating the postmenopausal ovary. This manifests routinely in the thickening of the theca, sometimes resulting in a picture that is not different from the hyperthecosis described above. Isolated cells or nests of stromal cells may be luteinized (Fig. 7.45).

In addition, the hilus cells appear to respond to the gonadotropins, and significant hilus cell hyperplasia may develop with prominent Reinke crystalloids (Fig. 7.46). Most hilus cell tumors are postmenopausal developments.

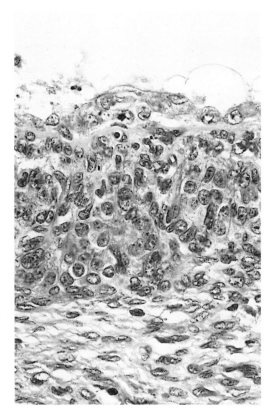

figure 7.39

Fragmentation and loss of the granulosa above illustrate atresia in this follicle. The cells of the theca interna also are shrinking.

7.17

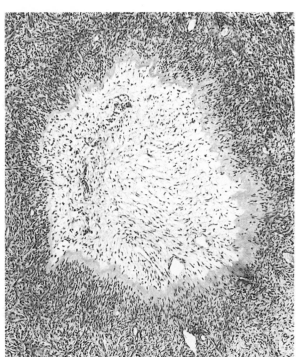

figure 7.40

This hyaline scar, much less dramatic than that of a corpus albicans, lines an atretic follicle.

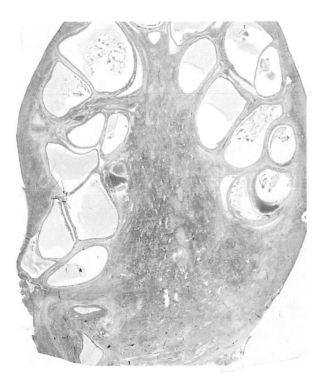

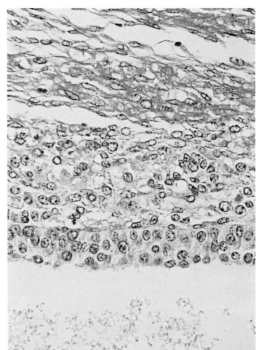

figure 7.42

The granulosa (top) is not well developed in this follicle in an anovulatory ovary, but the theca interna is well luteinized. This ovary (bottom) contains isolated nests of luteinized stromal cells unassociated with follicles. Follicular development is not prominent elsewhere in this ovary.

figure 7.41

Multiple follicles fill the cortex of this ovary associated with the polycystic ovary syndrome.

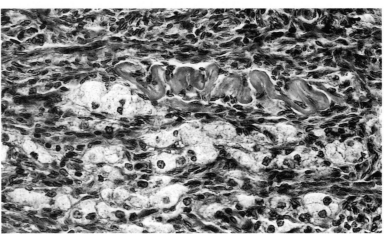

figure 7.43

In an enlarged edematous ovary, stromal cells scattered throughout the gonad, without follicular association, are nevertheless luteinized.

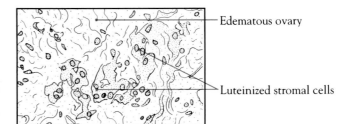

Edematous ovary

Luteinized stromal cells

atlas of gynecologic pathology

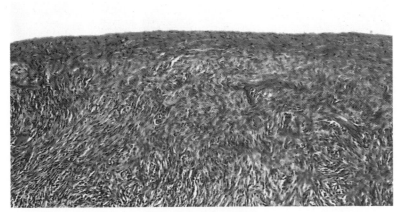

figure 7.44

This postmenopausal ovary has a thickened cortex, but no primordial follicles.

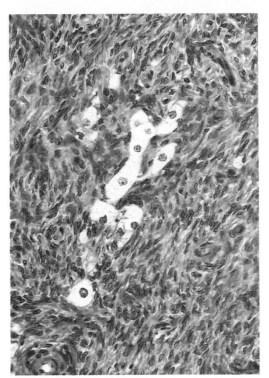

figure 7.45

Isolated stromal cells are luteinized in this postmenopausal ovary, presumably in response to elevated gonadotropins.

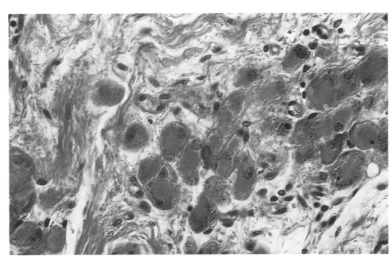

7.19

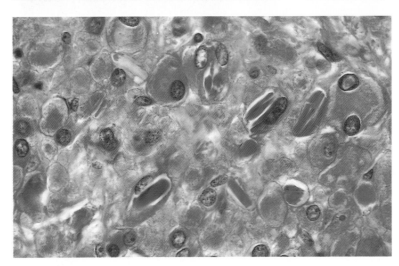

figure 7.46

Hilus cells (top) are dramatically enlarged in the hilum of this postmenopausal ovary. Prominent Reinke crystalloids (bottom) are present in this focus of hilar cell hyperplasia.

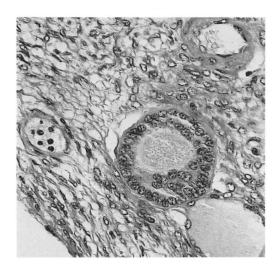

figure 7.47

Photomicrograph of a developing follicle amid edematous, inflamed ovarian stroma. The disruption of this tissue is such that its nature is no longer clear-cut.

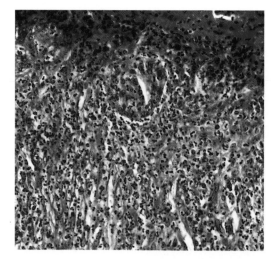

figure 7.48

Peritonitis on this ovary's surface is associated with such dramatic cortex inflammation that almost no ovarian structure is recognizable. At the top center is a focus of epithelium that is being destroyed.

7.20

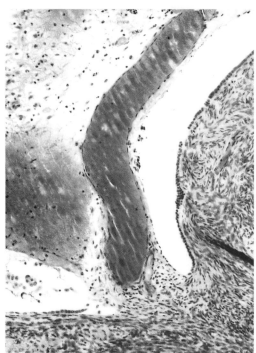

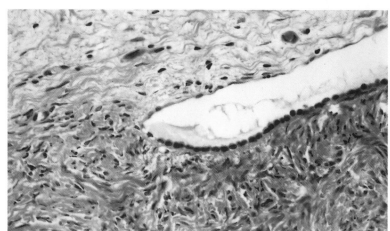

figure 7.49

A postinflammatory (left) adhesion arises from the ovarian surface in this photomicrograph. It contains an infiltrate and prominent capillaries. Where this adhesion (right) has resulted in covering of the surface epithelium, that epithelium is proliferating and becoming cuboidal.

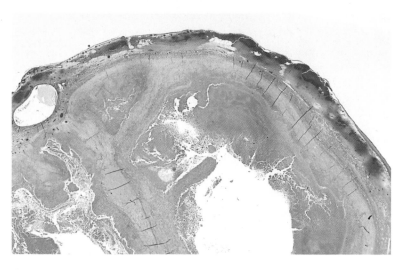

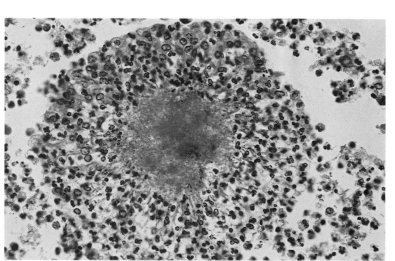

figure 7.50

A pus-filled abscess cavity occupies the medullary area of this ovary, with a dilated, expanded ovarian cortex around it (left). A typical sulfur granule, with an inflammatory infiltrate organized radially around it, occupies the center of this ovarian abscess (right).

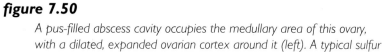

Infection

Infection in the ovary is uncommon. Except in extreme cases the structure is resistant to the effects of tubo-ovarian abscesses related to pelvic inflammatory disease. When, in such extreme cases, the ovarian stroma is edematous and filled with infiltrate, an identifiable ovary may not be present. Only an isolated germ cell reveals that the ovary is being viewed (Fig. 7.47). This process is more obscuring than destructive, however. Although some cases appear to be associated with ovarian destruction, pelvic inflammatory disease almost never results in castration (Fig. 7.48). Subsequently, peritoneal adhesions are common; when these adhesions cover the ovarian surface, the result is proliferation and metaplasia of the ovarian surface epithelium (Fig. 7.49). True intraovarian abscesses are rare. They have been described in association with IUDs and in circumstances where the ovaries are infected post-hysterectomy. In both cases, it has been postulated that bacteria are deposited into the ovary when its surface is broken by the process of ovulation, and thus the abscess is within the corpus luteum. This conjecture is based on the absence of a corpus luteum in such ovaries. In any case, edematous, distorted ovarian tissue in such cases surrounds a typical abscess cavity. If the abscess is associated with an IUD, then actinomyces may be present (Fig. 7.50).

Ovarian Pregnancy

Ovarian implantation is a rare event that also has been ascribed to intrafollicular fertilization (Fig. 7.51). However, because the invading trophoblast destroys the actual site of implantation, this is usually very difficult to document, and others have suggested that ectopic ovarian implantations probably occur in decidual foci on the ovarian surface. It is desirable to distinguish invasive gestational trophoblastic disease in the ovary from choriocarcinoma resulting from germ cell neoplasia, as treatment and prognosis may differ.

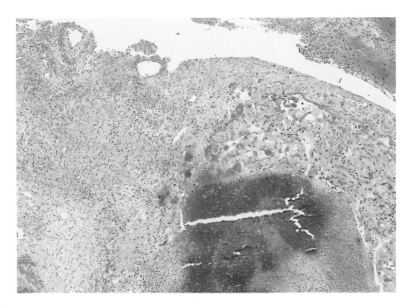

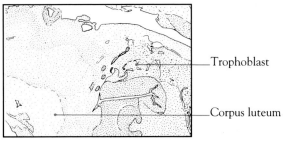

figure 7.51

Immature trophoblast associated with a large focus of hemorrhage occupies one pole of this ovary. A degenerating corpus luteum lies to the left, in this example of an ovarian implantation.

7.21

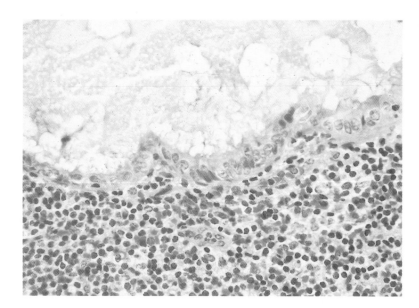

figure 7.52

Mucinous epithelium lines the inclusion cyst in this pelvic lymph node.

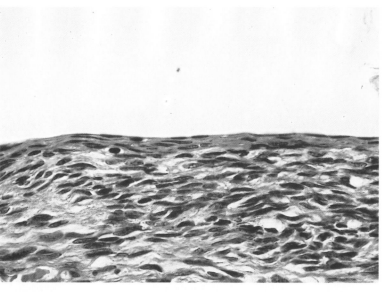

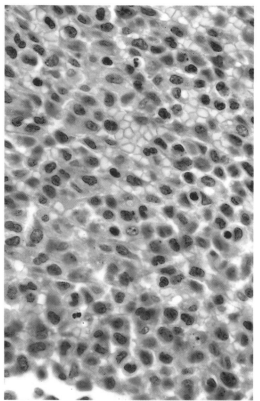

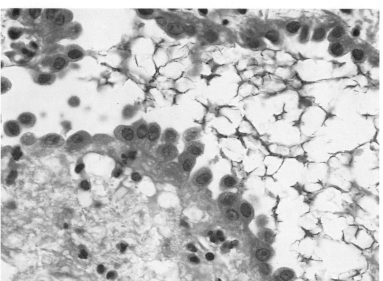

figure 7.53

A few flattened mesothelial cells (top left) are barely apparent on the surface of this normal ovary. This ovarian surface (bottom left) is proliferating in response to peritoneal blood from a ruptured ectopic pregnancy. The mesothelial cells are cuboidal or round, with prominent eosinophilic cytoplasm. This sheet of reactive mesothelial cells (right) illustrates what reactive mesothelium looks like when tangentially sectioned.

atlas of gynecologic pathology

Surface Epithelial Variation

The ovarian surface is a portion of the broader peritoneal surface. It is modified by the subepithelial stroma, but generally it is most accurately viewed as part of a field that includes the rest of the pelvic and abdominal peritoneum, and less commonly the pleura. Epithelial inclusions in pelvic and abdominal lymph nodes are more remote extensions of the same field (Fig. 7.52). When this epithelial surface is resting, its cells are mesothelial, but when it is proliferating, the cells become cuboidal, with a moderate amount of eosinophilic cytoplasm (Fig. 7.53). Many stimuli serve as irritants, and thus produce such proliferations.

In the premenopausal ovary, ovulation is a regular source of disruption of the surface (Fig. 7.54). When healing occurs, surface epithelium may be included into the cortex, resulting in cortical inclusion cysts. Inflammatory processes may produce similar inclusions on other peritoneal surfaces. Epithelial inclusions regularly occur in the pelvic and para-aortic lymph nodes, for unknown reasons.

In addition to proliferating, peritoneal inclusions characteristically undergo metaplasia, thus resulting in a variety of cell types in inclusions (Figs. 7.55 to 7.57). Prominent among these are ciliated, serous, mucinous, and squamous cell types; all of these epithelia occur in more distant peritoneal inclusions (Fig. 7.58; see Fig. 7.52). Mixtures including the native mesothelial cell types are common. Particularly within the ovary, but elsewhere as well, it is common for proliferating epithelium to be associated with stromal proliferation or metaplasia (Fig. 7.59). Recent insights suggest that the stromal response may in fact be primary.

ENDOMETRIAL-LIKE REACTIONS

Regurgitant menstruation is common in cycling women; in industrialized societies, there also is a certain degree of exposure to foreign bodies that reach the peritoneal cavity from the lower genital canal. Talc crystals are common contaminants of the pelvis in North America. When these or other irritants reach the ovarian surface, they elicit a local inflammatory reaction that may contain foreign body giant cells engulfing the crystalline foreign particles (Fig. 7.60). In an estrogenic environment, the stromal reaction to any irrita-

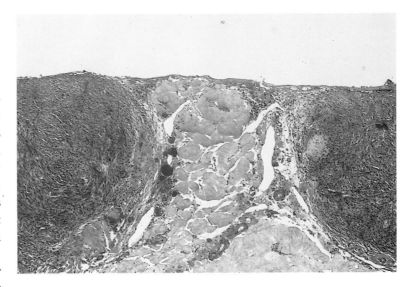

figure 7.54

The ovarian cortex is interrupted by the scar of an old corpus luteum that penetrates to the surface at this former ovulation site.

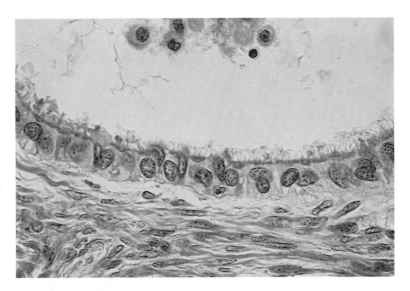

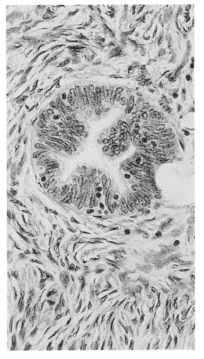

figure 7.55

Well-developed ciliated epithelium lines this cortical inclusion cyst (top). Serous epithelium typical of the tube lines this cortical inclusion cyst (bottom).

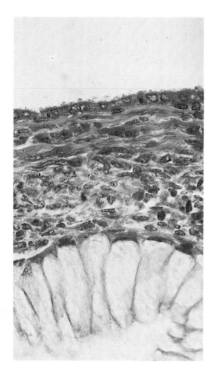
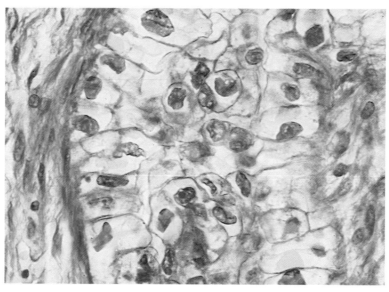

figure 7.56

In this epithelial inclusion in the ovarian cortex (left), prominent mucinous epithelium is seen. Well-developed squamous epithelium (right), fills this inclusion cyst in the ovarian cortex.

7.24

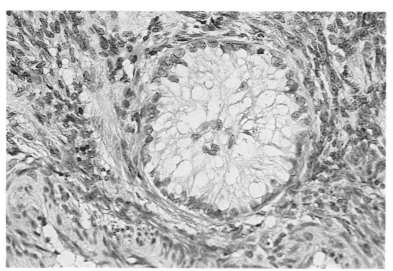
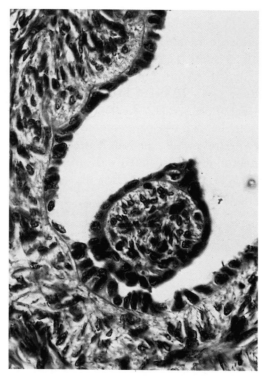

figure 7.57

In this very unusual cortical inclusion cyst (left), the epithelia appear to be reproducing Sertoli cell types. In this epithelial inclusion in the ovarian cortex (right), a small papilla is lined with both mesothelial- and tubal-type cells, as is the rest of the inclusion.

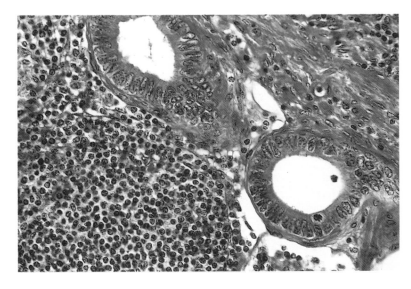 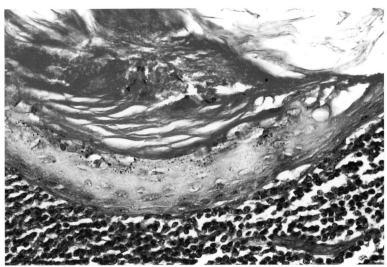

figure 7.58

Tubal-type epithelium lines the inclusion cyst in this pelvic lymph node (left). Fully mature squamous epithelium (right) is present in this epithelial inclusion cyst in a pelvic lymph node.

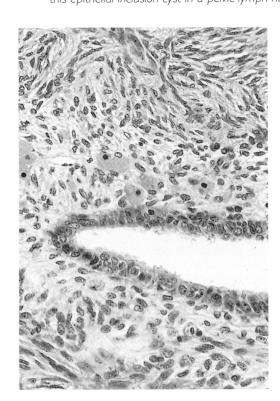

figure 7.59

This epithelial inclusion cyst in the ovarian cortex is associated with a prominent stromal reaction that may be endometrial in nature. Macrophages are prominent.

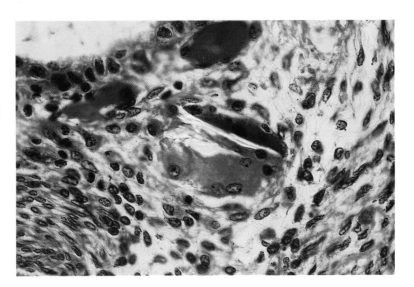

figure 7.60

Giant cells containing apparent crystalline structures are present in this focus of stromal reaction around an epithelial inclusion.

ovary

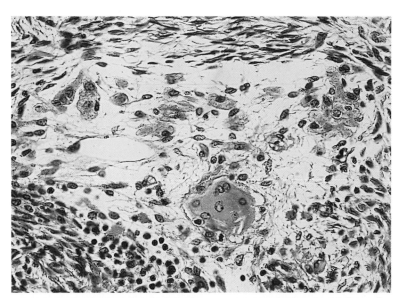

figure 7.61

The stromal reaction around this giant cell is more clear-cut. Its resemblance to endometrial stroma is apparent, as are the macrophages.

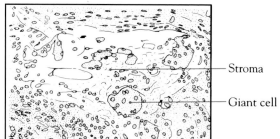

Stroma

Giant cell

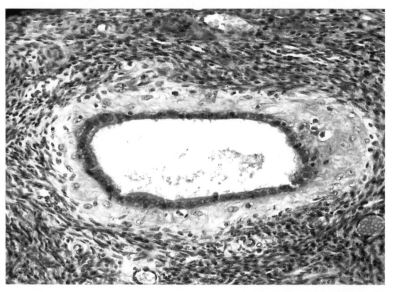

7.26

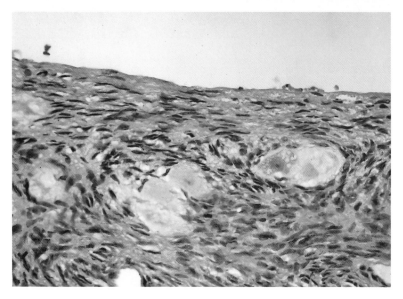

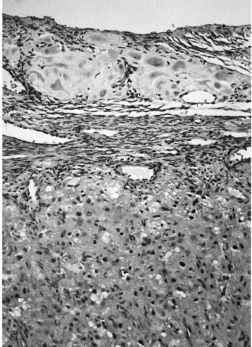

figure 7.62

Decidualization (top left) has occurred in the stroma around this epithelial inclusion in an ovary associated with pregnancy. Isolated stromal cells in this ovarian cortex (bottom left) display decidualization. A corpus luteum of pregnancy (right) lies below in this photomicrograph. Immediately beneath the ovarian surface, small nodules of decidua have formed.

tion may be endometrial in nature (Fig. 7.61). For this reason or others, microscopic foci of endometrial-type tissue are ubiquitous within the field described above, including the pelvic lymph nodes. In the presence of progestational influences such as pregnancy, these foci become decidualized and present as microscopic subepithelial nodules of decidua (Fig. 7.62). If muscle metaplasia occurs in these nodules, they may produce local deposits of smooth muscle (Fig. 7.63); when these are generalized, leiomyomatosis peritonealis disseminata may result (Fig. 7.64).

Conversely, when normal cycles are occurring, endometrial tissue in these foci tends to function and to produce hemorrhage, necrosis, and an inflammatory reaction (Fig. 7.65). The result is local inflammation, scarring with hemosiderin residues, and the loss of tissue surfaces. Adhesions may occur (Fig. 7.66). Histologically, endometriosis goes through a regular progression that may be identified in the ovarian cortex or elsewhere in the pelvis or abdominal cavity. First the stroma is scarred and obliterated, leaving only epithelial inclusions (Fig. 7.67). When the epithelial inclusions are lost, only scars containing multiple capillaries persist (Fig. 7.68). When necrosis is massive, lipid residues

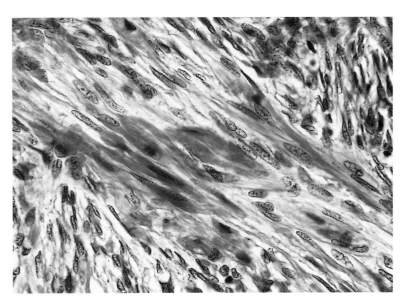

figure 7.63

A small collection of smooth muscle cells occupies this site beneath the epithelium in the ovarian cortex.

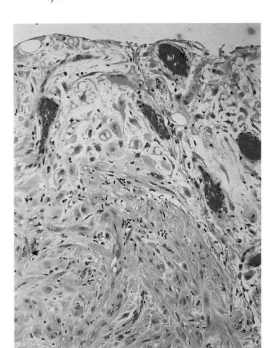

figure 7.64

In this example of leiomyomatosis peritonealis disseminata, the stroma contains decidual cells immediately beneath the surface epithelium. Below is a well-developed nodule of smooth muscle.

7.27

ovary

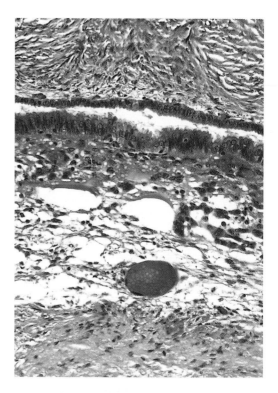

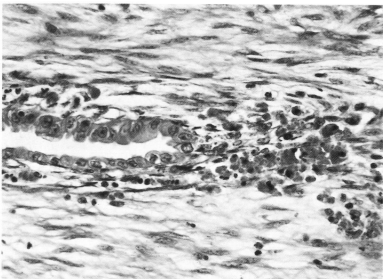

figure 7.65

In this example of endometriosis in the ovarian cortex (left), breakdown and hemorrhage are occurring in response to normal cyclic function. In this focus of endometriosis (right), the stroma contains an inflammatory reaction and hemosiderin-laden macrophages because of prior "menstruation." Scarring is taking place both above and below.

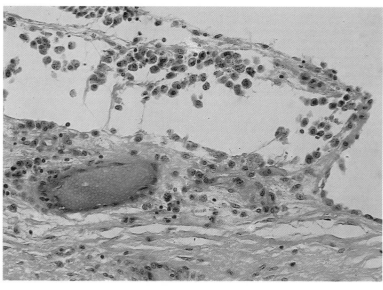

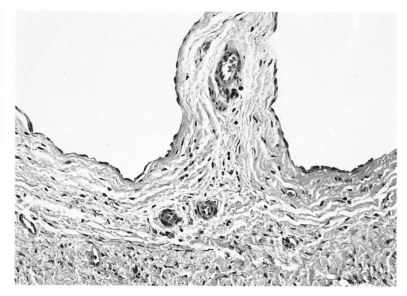

figure 7.66

The ovarian adhesion in this case of endometriosis (left) consists only of scar with hemosiderin-laden macrophages and prominent capillaries.

In this much older and better organized adhesion (right), no evidence of the prior inflammatory process is present.

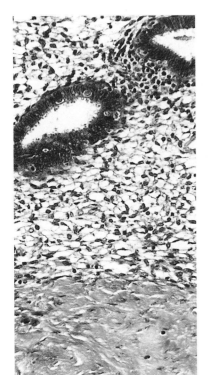
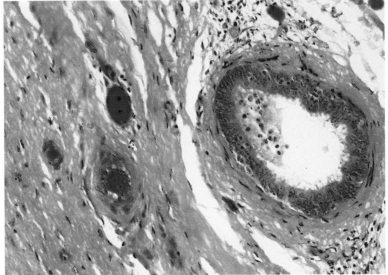

figure 7.67

Photomicrograph showing endometriosis above is partially replaced below by prominent scar (left). At another site (right), all of the stroma has been scarred and only an epithelial inclusion and capillaries remain.

figure 7.68

Prominent deposits of hemosiderin and massive capillaries (left) fill this adhesion associated with endometriosis. This scar in the ovarian cortex (right) is associated with endometriosis elsewhere.

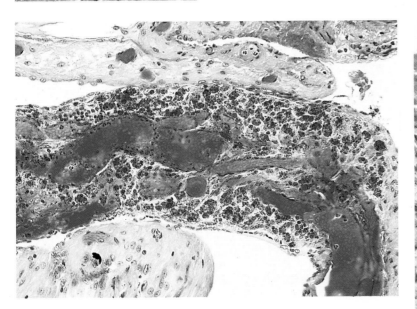
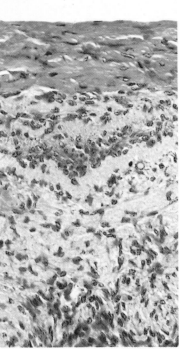

may result in cholesterol clefts; focal calcification is common in these tissues (Fig. 7.69).

Endometriosis within the ovary, more so than at other sites, tends to form functioning cysts. (Fig. 7.70). These may result in large collections of blood within the ovarian tissue. The cysts go through the progression described above for endometriosis in general, and some epithelial cysts in ovaries are remnants of endometriosis (Fig. 7.71). The magnetic resonance signals from endometrioma are heterogeneous (Fig. 7.72).

7.30

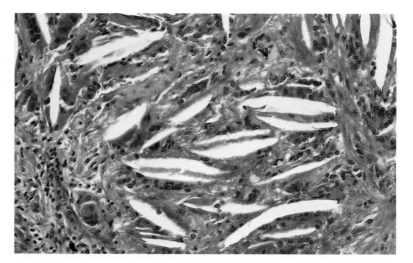

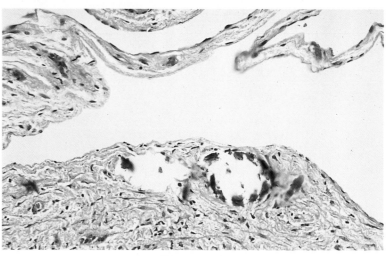

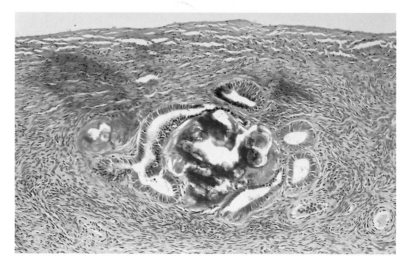

figure 7.69

Multiple cholesterol clefts (top) are surrounded by giant cells, where the necrosis produced by endometriosis is being organized. The focus of calcification in this scar (center) is typical of what is seen in old endometriosis. In this nest of cortical inclusions (bottom) a scarred stroma contains calcification. This may or may not represent a tiny focus of old endometriosis.

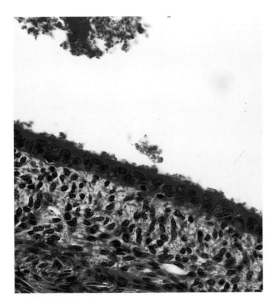

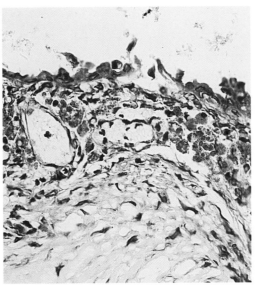

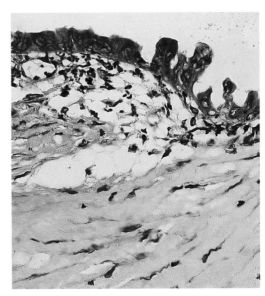

figure 7.70

Both epithelium and stroma line this ovarian cyst.

figure 7.71

In this ovarian cyst (left), function has occurred and hemosiderin-laden macrophages fill the stroma beneath the epithelium. Scar lies below. In this endometrioma (right), all of the stroma to the right has been scarred, but to the left a small portion of stroma persists.

— Stroma

— Scar

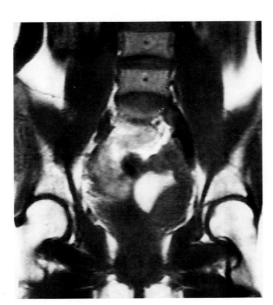

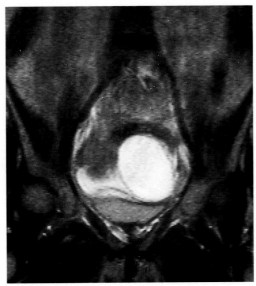

figure 7.72

Coronal T-1 weighted MR image of the pelvis (left) shows a mass in the posterior pelvis with a bright signal along its medical aspect and a medium intensity signal laterally. The bright signal is attributed to recent areas of hemorrhage within the mass. Coronal T-2 weighted MR image of the pelvis (right) shows diffuse increase in the signal intensity of the left adnexal mass, which on this imaging sequence indicates the fluid nature of the mass.

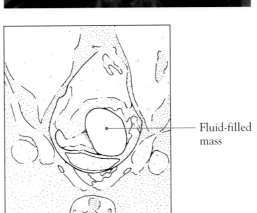

— Recent hemorrhage

— Fluid-filled mass

ovary

SURFACE REACTIONS

Most of the reactions described so far tend to occur within the ovarian cortex, but other types of reactions seem to be surface phenomena (Fig. 7.73). Usually papillary, they are characterized by mesothelial and serous cell types and may produce complex surface patterns. The difference between these and the other types of response described above is unexplained. When menopause occurs, if estrogen deficiency is the result, epithelial and stromal reactions in all the pelvic tissues tend to become quiescent. Foreign bodies may continue to elicit inflammatory reactions, however, and, if endogenous or exogenous estrogen is present, the reactions described above continue to occur unmodified by progesterone unless it is supplied exogenously. Because estrogen and irritation both produce proliferations and metaplasias in the field in which pelvic neoplasias arise, they may be viewed as providing the background for, but not necessarily the etiology of, that neoplasia.

epithelial tumors

Conveniently, neoplasms arising on the ovarian and other peritoneal surfaces are described in standard formats, in terms of cell type. However, such descriptions invariably are misleading, because in reality neoplasms usually have a mixture of cell types. They often have a pattern, such as papillary, that is associated with a cell type, such as mucinous, that is classically associated with another pattern, such as cystic. In addition, the amount and nature of the associated stroma may be anomalous. The result is a bewildering array of histologies. Therefore, the following convenient description is only a crude guide.

SEROUS TUMORS

The term *serous* has been used to describe ovarian or peritoneal tumors with flattened mesothelial cell types, ciliated tubal cell types, or secretory tubal cell types (Fig. 7.74). Tumors composed of flattened mesothelial cells, termed adenomatoid tumors, occur in the ovary and elsewhere in the genital canal (Fig. 7.75). The fact that the tumor cell type is morphologically identical to the normal peritoneal cell indicates its benignity. Uncommonly, one sees ovarian or pelvic neoplasms that resemble proliferative peritoneal reactions but lack cytologic atypicality and mitoses (Fig. 7.76). The malignant potential of these lesions is uncertain. When mesothelial cell tumors are characterized by obvious atypicality, they are highly malignant, usually involving all the intraabdominal surfaces and the omentum massively (Fig. 7.77).

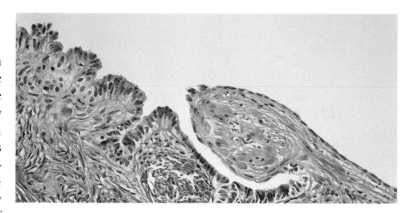
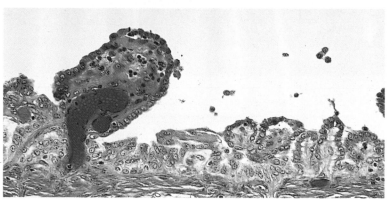

figure 7.73

The ovarian surface (top) is papillary, and the papillae are lined by an epithelium that is tubal in appearance in contrast to the flattened mesothelial epithelium to the right. Multiple micropapillary projections from the ovarian surface (bottom) are covered by a proliferating epithelium.

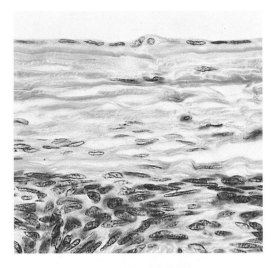

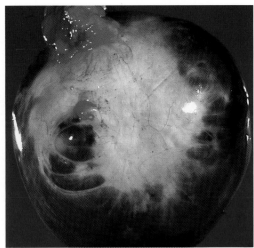

figure 7.74

This ovarian cyst (left) is lined by a flattened mesothelial epithelium except in the very center, where a single ciliated cell is seen. The rest of the cyst wall is scarred. This (right) is the typical gross appearance of benign cystic lesions in the ovary.

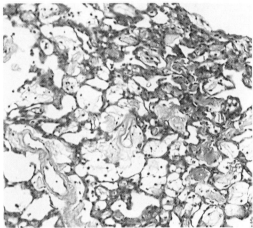

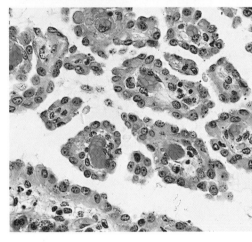

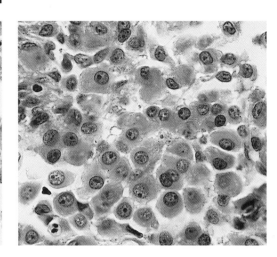

7.33

figure 7.75

This ovarian tumor is composed of flattened mesothelial-type cells forming clefts and spaces.

figure 7.76

This papillary ovarian tumor (left) contains an epithelium that consists of cells reminiscent of the proliferating mesothelium seen

in Fig. 7.53. A higher power view of the cells in this tumor (right) reveals little atypicality and no mitoses.

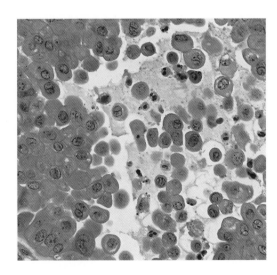

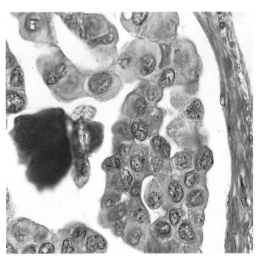

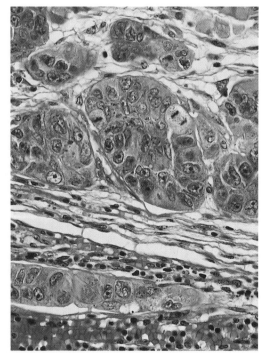

figure 7.77

The proliferating mesothelial-type cells in this tumor are grossly atypical, with multiple mitoses present (left). In this mesothelial cell tumor (center), there is much nuclear atypicality but one small focal calcification.

The tumor is in a lymphatic channel. In this example (right), multiple mitoses are present, together with nuclear atypicality. The tumor is present in a pelvic lymph node.

Tumors composed of tubal-type cells, ciliated or secretory, are usually cystic in the benign form. Many so-called serous cystadenomas are possibly only inclusions resulting from inflammation or endometriosis. But some are sufficiently papillary and are sufficiently associated with a stromal reaction to suggest neoplasia (Fig. 7.78). When the stromal reaction is the major component of the tumor, these tumors are termed *cystadenofibromas* or *fibroadenomas* (Fig. 7.79). Papillary serous proliferations, which lack individual cell atypicality or mitoses but nevertheless are widespread in the pelvis or abdominal cavity, are termed borderline when they are piled up with micropapillae and appear destructive, if not invasive, of local tissues (Fig. 7.80). Focal calcifications—so-called psammoma bodies—are common in the papillary tumors. These lesions are characterized by a prolonged, but in many cases persistent, course and only rarely are lethal. More aggressive serous lesions are common (Fig. 7.81). These possess a papillary, cystic or solid structure, and are characterized by highly atypical cells that are only remotely tubal or any

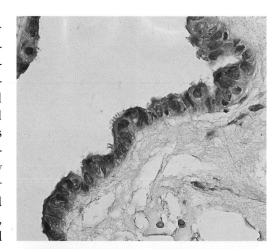

figure 7.78

This papillary cystic lesion in the ovary is lined by tubal-type epithelium with some flattened mesothelial component. The cells are well differentiated and recognizable, and there are no mitoses.

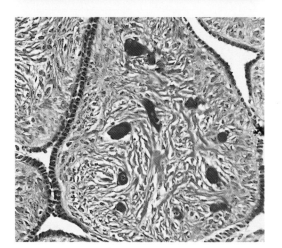

figure 7.79

In this cystic ovarian tumor (top), the papillae are sufficiently large as to be apparent on gross examination. This microscopic view (bottom) illustrates that the tumor is composed primarily of stroma, with a normal tubal-type epithelial lining.

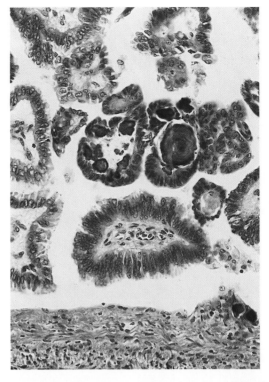

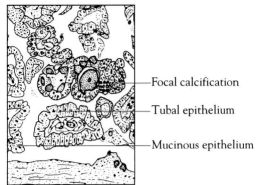

Focal calcification

Tubal epithelium

Mucinous epithelium

figure 7.80

This papillary ovarian tumor is lined by an epithelium that is recognizably tubal, but it is very proliferate with many focal calcifications. There are only very rare mitotic figures. Notice the focus of mucinous epithelium on the papillae to the lower left.

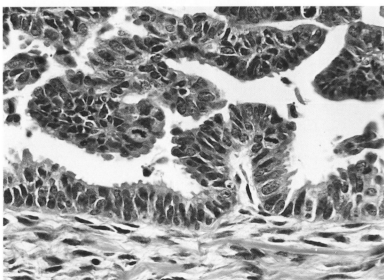

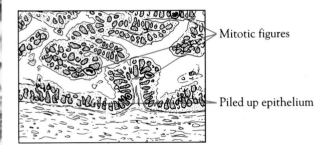

Mitotic figures

Piled up epithelium

figure 7.81

This papillary ovarian tumor is covered with an epithelium that is piled up and multilayered, and contains multiple mitotic figures. It is only dimly reminiscent of the tube.

ovary

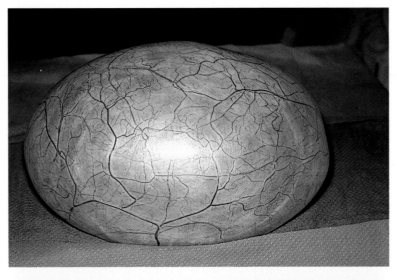

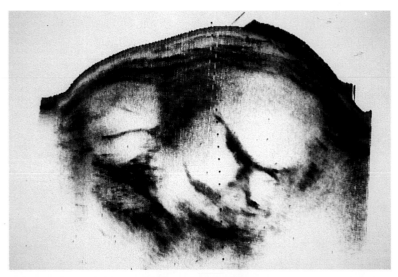

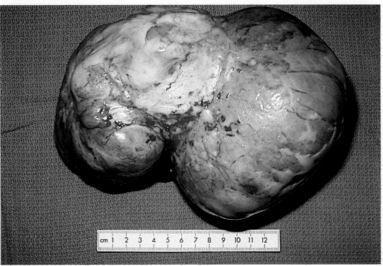

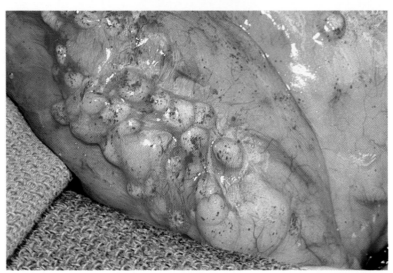

figure 7.82

This large smooth cystic mass from a paraovarian site (top left) is typical of benign serous cysts. (Courtesy of Dr. D. Bard.) Sagittal transabdominal ultrasound (top right) reveals the multiple cysts of an ovarian tumor produced by a neoplasm that is more likely to be malignant than the one seen at top left. The lobulated external appearance of

this mass (bottom left) reveals a more complex architecture consisting of both cystic and solid areas suggesting malignancy. (Courtesy of Dr. D. Bard.) The solid white masses forming in this mesentery (bottom right) are indicative of high grade malignancy. (Courtesy of Dr. D. Bard.)

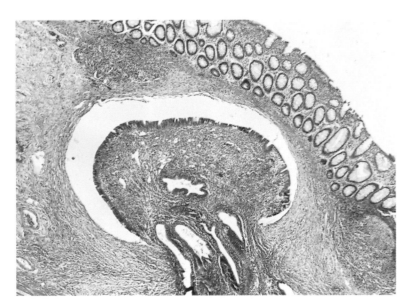

figure 7.83

This focus of endometriosis appears to be invading a lymphatic channel in the submucosa of the bowel. Notice that the pattern is mildly hyperplastic.

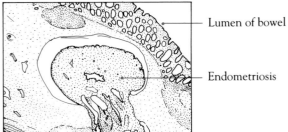

— Lumen of bowel

— Endometriosis

atlas of gynecologic pathology

other type. Gross and radiologic examination may allow one to speculate where in this spectrum a tumor lies (Fig. 7.82). Speculation must always be confirmed by histology.

Both mesothelial- and tubal-type cell neoplasms tend to be extraovarian and involve other peritoneal surfaces early on. This is in contrast to endometrioid, clear cell, mucinous, and Brenner tumors, which tend to develop initially as intraovarian lesions. Although this is subject to many exceptions, the most interesting one is that it may be more accurate if stated in reverse. That is, tumors arising in intraovarian locations may tend to be endometrial, clear cell, mucinous, or squamous.

ENDOMETRIOID, CLEAR CELL TUMORS

Endometriosis, with its tendency to form intraovarian cysts, has been described above. Some examples of endometriosis, however, are highly aggressive and invade adjacent tissues extensively, producing significant local damage. They may invade the wall of the bowel or grow on the right leaf of the diaphragm, penetrate to the chest, and involve the pleura; histologically, these cases often have a pattern that is at least mildly hyperplastic (Figs. 7.83 and 7.84). If endometriosis were being described today, such cases might well be called borderline malignant. Historically, endometrioid carcinomas were those documented to arise in endometriosis (Fig. 7.85). Currently, the term is used for adenocarcinomas consistent with those observed more routinely in the endometrial cavity. All the variations seen at that site also may be observed in the ovary (Fig. 7.86). The typical endometrial tumor is multilobulated and initially intraovarian (Fig. 7.87).

Clear cell tumors are not known to occur in low-grade forms, but their frequent association with endometriosis has suggested an origin from this type of tissue. Consisting of sheets of clear cells or glandular or papillary patterns, they are not different from similar lesions in the endometrium or vagina (Fig. 7.88). So-called *hobnail* cells in the papillary or glandular portion are prominent nuclei lacking an investing cytoplasm (Fig. 7.89).

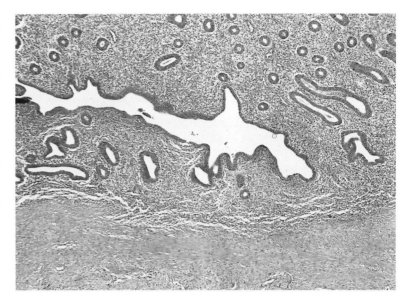

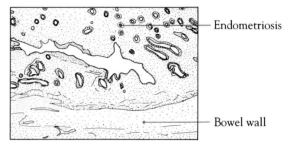

Endometriosis

Bowel wall

figure 7.84

More normal proliferative-type endometrium is present to the upper right, but in the lower left this endometriosis in the bowel wall is hyperplastic.

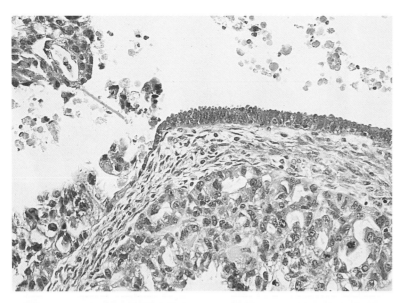

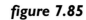

figure 7.85

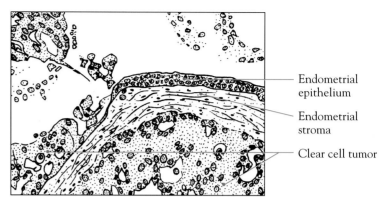

This clear cell carcinoma is arising in a preexisting endometrial cyst. Such evidence of direct origin in endometriosis has been required for the designation of endometrioid carcinoma in the past.

Endometrial epithelium

Endometrial stroma

Clear cell tumor

figure 7.86

This well-differentiated endometrial carcinoma (top left) consists of endometrial-type glands that are closely packed. This highly malignant solid (top right) tumor was a more typical endometriod adenocarcinoma in other fields. Both the glandular epithelium and the stroma in this tumor (bottom left) appear endometrial in nature, but the glands are not well formed in all areas and are losing their differentiation. This ovarian tumor (bottom right) contains well-differentiated squamous and glandular elements, typical of similar lesions in the endometrium.

7.38

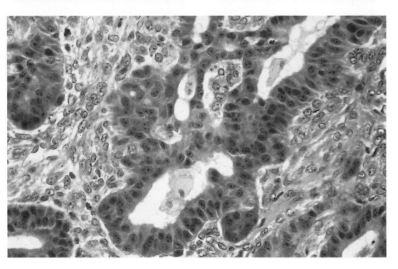

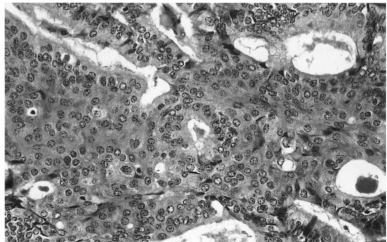

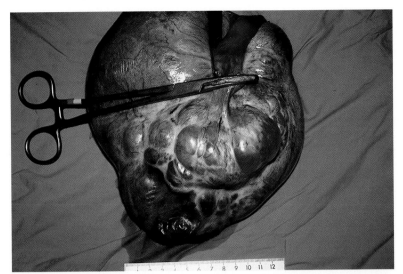

figure 7.87

Though the tumor is large and multilobulated, its surface is intact, which is consistent with an intraovarian origin for this adenocarcinoma. (Courtesy of Dr. D. Bard.)

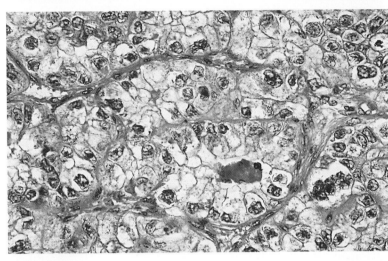

figure 7.88

This clear cell carcinoma of the ovary is typical of that seen in the endometrial cavity or elsewhere in the genital canal. The pattern here is glandular.

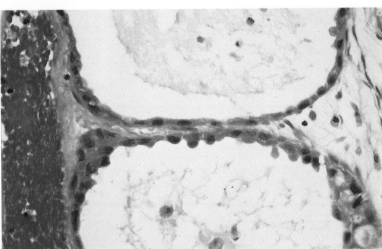

figure 7.89

In the cyst above, prominent nuclei project from the epithelium, producing a so-called hobnail appearance.

MUCINOUS TUMORS

Mucinous tumors tend to be intraovarian, and to consist of multilocular cysts. Cystadenomas are lined by epithelium that is entirely consistent with that in the endocervical canal (Fig. 7.90). Such a comforting sign of good behavior has to be confirmed in multiple sections, however, as mucinous tumors characteristically possess focal areas of dedifferentiation in otherwise benign or low-grade neoplasms. Mucinous tumors of low-grade potential take two forms. The intraovarian cystic ones usually are cured by simple surgery. They possess a piled-up, micropapillary, or tufted epithelium that lacks mitoses (Fig. 7.91). Goblet-type cells may be prominent. In the other form, pseudomyxoma peritonei, the course is usually long, but likely to be eventually fatal, as free movement in the peritoneal cavity is gradually obliterated. These lesions possess an epithelium that lacks the individual cell atypicality or the mitoses that characterize more aggressive malignancy, but neither is it entirely consistent with endocervical epithelium (Fig. 7.92). In the most common variation, the nucleus is enlarged and elevated in the cell rather than in its more normal basal position. The clinical picture of pseudomyxoma peritonei is also produced by low-grade mucinous tumors of the appendix (Fig. 7.93). These tumors have a similar histology.

Less well differentiated mucinous lesions tend to be composed of cells with larger, darker nuclei and more basophilic cytoplasm (Fig. 7.94). Mitotic figures are present. Occasionally, primary ovarian mucinous tumors will infiltrate the ovarian stroma as individual cells result in a pattern resembling Krukenberg's tumor. In such a case, areas of myxomatous stroma are mingled with denser stromal foci containing nests of mucinous cells. Individual mucinous cells

7.40

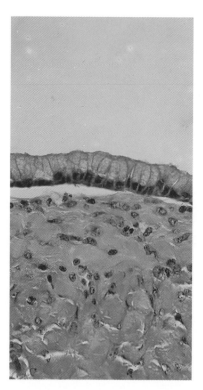

figure 7.90

Normal-appearing mucinous epithelium lines the wall of this mucinous cystadenoma.

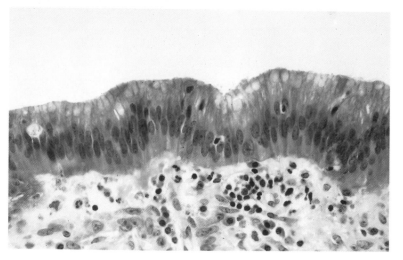

figure 7.91

In this borderline tumor, the mucinous epithelium has lost a significant portion of its differentiation, only partially resembling normal mucinous epithelium. Mitoses are not present, but the epithelium is piled up and papillary in some sites.

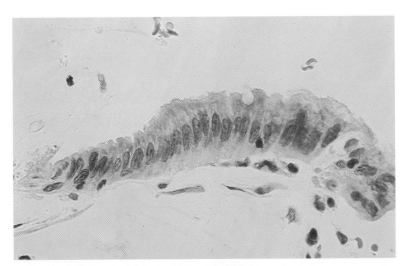

figure 7.92

The epithelium in this example of pseudomyxoma peritonei is clearly mucinous, but it is not perfectly differentiated. The nuclei are enlarged and elevated in the cell.

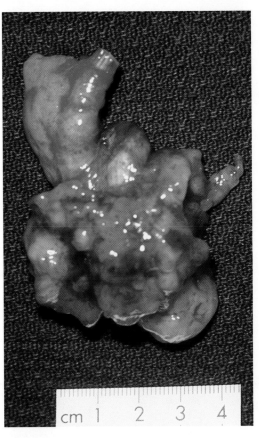

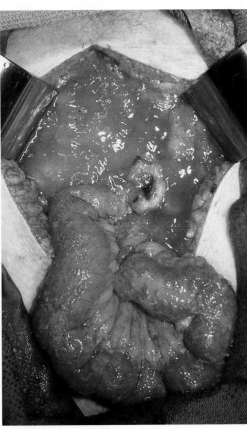

figure 7.93

The tip of the appendix (left) is occupied by a mucin producing tumor. This is the characteristic location. The peritoneal cavity (right) is filled with mucin and all surfaces are involved. (Courtesy of Dr. D. Bard.)

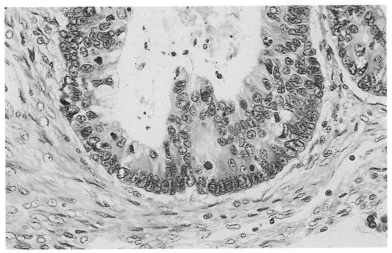

figure 7.94

This epithelium is barely recognizable as mucinous. It is papillary, piled up, and contains both nuclear atypicality and multiple mitotic figures.

ovary

may assume a signet-ring appearance (Fig. 7.95). Despite the capacity of primary mucinous tumors to produce this picture, a more distant primary tumor must always be ruled out.

Any epithelial ovarian tumor may be associated with an important stromal component, but mucinous ones are most likely to possess a hormone-producing stromal component. In serous tumors the stroma, if prominent, is likely to be fibrotic, giving rise to fibroadenomas; but in mucinous lesions the stroma is more often thecal in appearance, or even luteinized (Fig. 7.96). This can occur in low- or high-grade examples and is quite common in primary or metastatic tumors of the Krukenberg type. In contrast, CA-125 production is characteristically associated with serous tumors but occasionally occurs in mucinous ones (Fig. 7.97).

BRENNER TUMORS

Mucinous tumors frequently contain foci of squamous metaplasia, which has led to the view that Brenner tumors arise in this way. This undoubtedly occurs in some cases but not necessarily in all. Brenner tumors, however, like mucinous lesions, tend to result in hormone-producing stromal reactions. They consist of nests of squamous cells, embedded in ovarian stroma (Fig. 7.98). In some cases, the epithelial nests are cystic and a layer of mucinous epithelium lines the cystic lumen, further contributing to the view that these lesions are mucinous in origin (Fig. 7.99). On other occasions, the epithelium lining Brenner tumors is transitional in appearance (Fig. 7.100). If the epithelium appears proliferative but

7.42

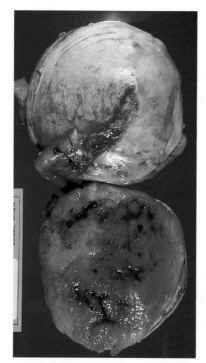
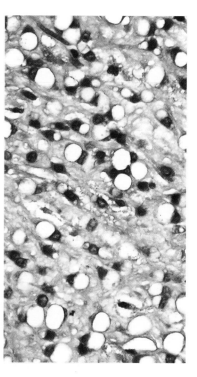

figure 7.95

This solid ovarian tumor (left) appeared confined to the gonad. The tumor (right) is made of benign mucinous cells infiltrating the stroma, producing a signet-ring appearance. (Courtesy of Dr. Ibrahim Ramsey.)

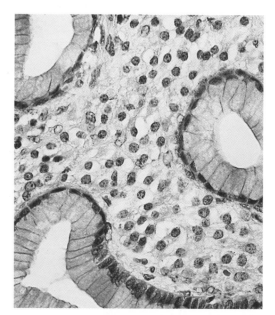

figure 7.96

This mucinous cystadenoma (top) is associated with a prominent stromal reaction consisting of luteinized cells. This photomicrograph (bottom) demonstrates one of the many exceptions to the rule in ovarian tumors, as a prominent luteinized stromal reaction is associated with a serous rather than a mucinous epithelium.

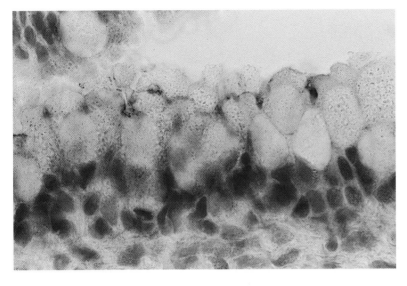

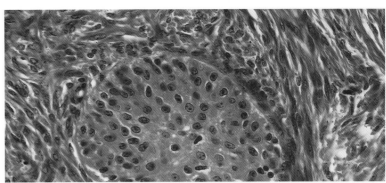

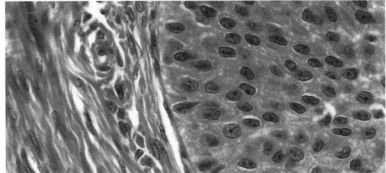

figure 7.97

This immunoperoxidase stain for CA-125 demonstrates the antigen in a characteristic site on the surface of the epithelium. (Courtesy of Dr. H. Hardadottir and T. O'Brien.)

figure 7.98

A nest of benign squamous epithelium is embedded in ovarian theca (top). A higher power view (bottom) illustrates the benign nature of the squamous epithelial nest.

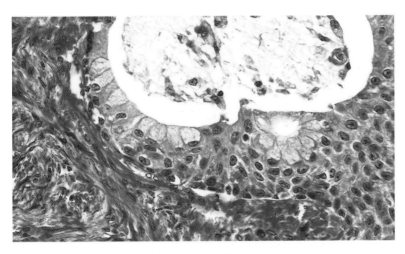

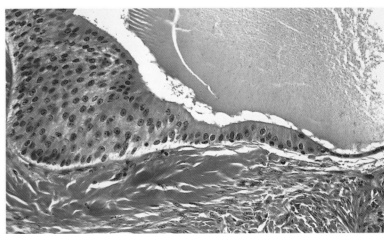

figure 7.99

This cystic epithelial nest in a Brenner tumor is lined by mucinous-type epithelium supported by squamous metaplasia.

figure 7.100

Transitional-appearing epithelium lines this cystic space in a Brenner tumor.

invasion is not occurring, then a proliferative Brenner tumor exists and these lesions may have some potential for malignancy (Fig. 7.101). True malignant Brenner tumors are rare. They are composed of clear-cut malignant squamous epithelium that looks like epidermoid carcinoma of the cervix (Fig. 7.102).

GONADAL EPITHELIAL TUMORS

Consistent with the origin of gonadal epithelium from the coelomic epithelium, epithelial tumors of gonadal epithelial type also occur in the ovary. These tumors specifically look like epithelial tumors with an incidental stromal component, and merge with a group of stromal tumors (to be described below) that look primarily stromal, with an epithelial component.

Granulosa cell tumors occur in microfollicular and macrofollicular forms (Fig. 7.103) as well as in the form of cords of granulosa-type cells (Fig. 7.104). As long as the individual cells are well differentiated, all of these patterns are associated with a benign course and with the production of hormones in the surrounding stroma. Occasionally, they are luteinized and produce progesterone (Fig. 7.105). To the

7.44

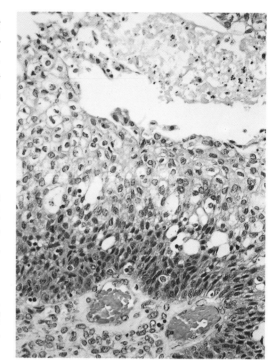

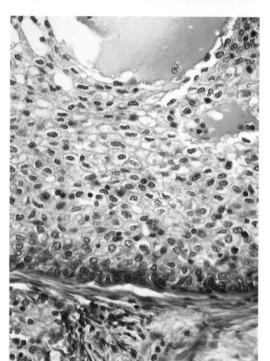

figure 7.101

The epithelium in this Brenner tumor is proliferate and papillary, but no invasion appears to be taking place (top). A higher power view (bottom) reveals relatively normal maturation in this squamous epithelium.

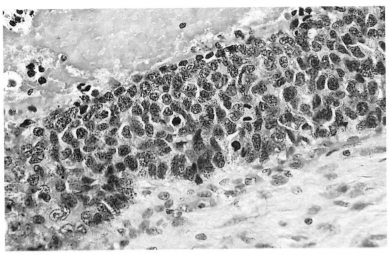

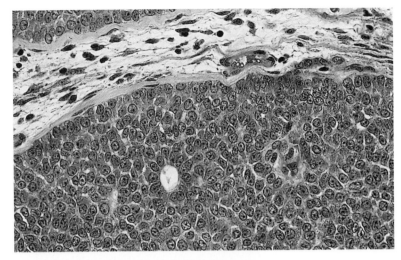

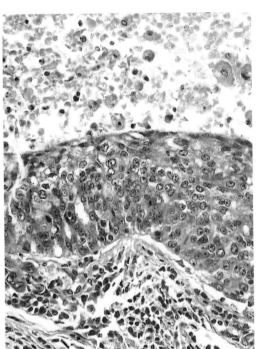

figure 7.102

The epithelium lining the cystic spaces in this ovarian tumor is consistent with carcinoma in situ of the cervix (top). More clear-cut squamous differentiation is apparent in this example (bottom).

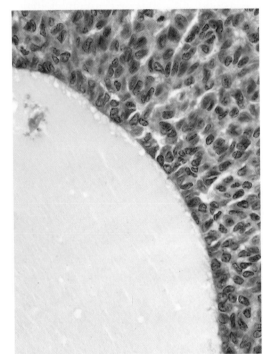

figure 7.103

Small granulosa-like epithelial cells (top) are arranged in nests containing small follicular spaces typical of the microfollicular pattern. In this case (bottom), the same cells are lining a large macrofollicular space.

7.45

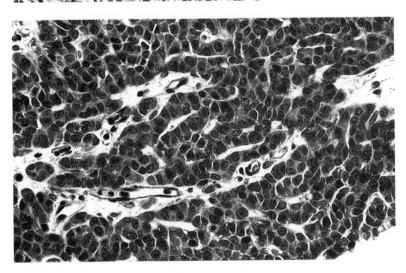

figure 7.104

Similar cells are producing solid cords in this granulosa cell tumor.

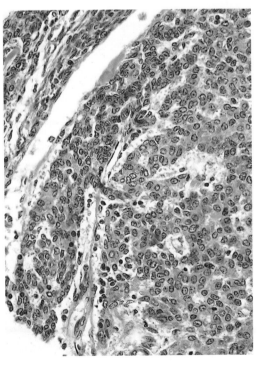

figure 7.105

To the left and above in this photomicro-graph, the granulosa cells are small and dark. To the right and below, they are larger and contain more eosinophilic cytoplasm, indicating luteinization.

ovary

extent that the cells are not well differentiated, a more malignant course may occur (Fig. 7.106). If an undifferentiated small-cell tumor with a follicular pattern is termed a *granulosa cell tumor,* the lesion will behave poorly.

When the epithelial cells resemble closely Sertoli's cells of the testicular tubule, the stromal reaction is likely to consist of Leydig-type cells, and a Sertoli-Leydig cell tumor exists (Fig. 7.107). These neoplasms are benign, but are associated in some cases with malignant colonic polyps in the Peutz-Jeghers syndrome (Fig. 7.108). Less well differentiated tubular tumors may also possess interstitial-type cells, and these lesions have some malignant potential (Fig. 7.109). True arrhenoblastomas consisting of tubules and associated interstitial cells sometimes arise in the ovarian hilum from the rete structures in young girls; these are usually benign.

7.46

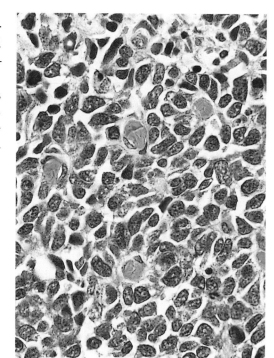

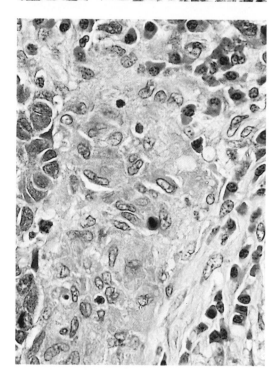

figure 7.106

An apparent follicular pattern (top) is produced by the arrangement of these tumor cells around capillaries, but the cells are grossly atypical, only superficially resembling the granulosa. At another site (bottom), this highly malignant, infiltrative tumor is associated with a dramatic stromal granulomatous reaction.

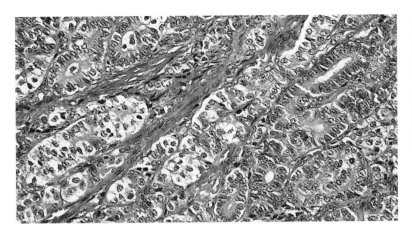

figure 7.107

Tubules containing well-developed Sertoli-type cells (left) lie to the lower left, while to the right the epithelium is less well differentiated. Tubules lined by Sertoli-type cells in this tumor (right) are also associated with a stroma containing interstitial or Leydig-type cells.

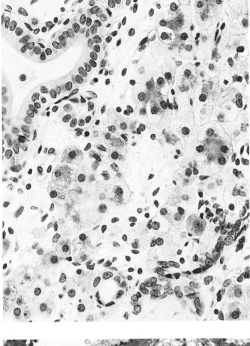

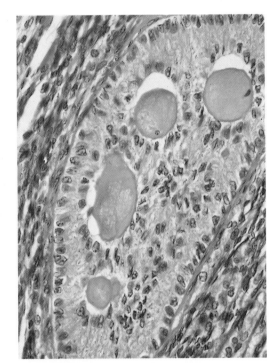

figure 7.108

This tumor with annular tubules is the type often associated with Peutz-Jeghers syndrome.

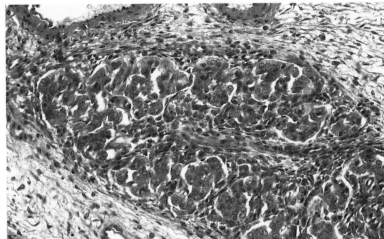

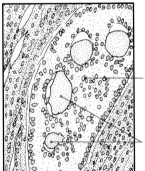

Sertoli-type epithelium

Lumina of tubules

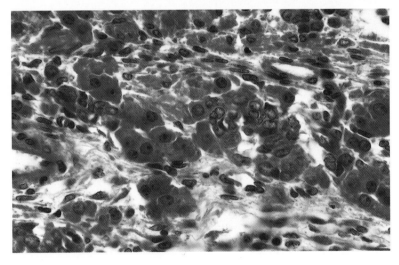

figure 7.109

Nests of epithelial cells form only rudimentary tubules in a stroma that contains interstitial or Leydig-type cells (top). A higher power view reveals the Leydig's cells (bottom).

ovary

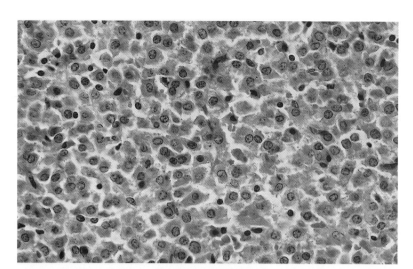

figure 7.110

Sheets of hilus-type cells are the only feature of this tumor.

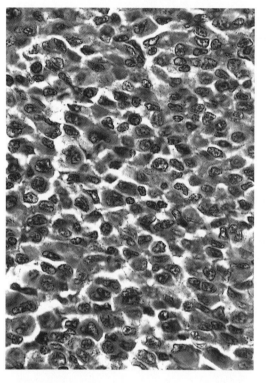

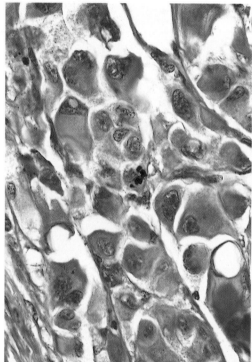

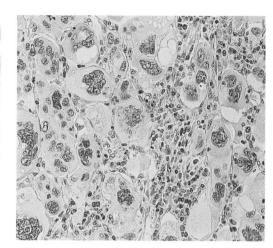

figure 7.111

This ovarian tumor (left) consists largely of small cells lacking any specific differentiation. In the same undifferentiated ovarian tumor in another field (center), the cells are quite large. In this undifferentiated ovarian tumor (right), the cells are super large, with huge collections of multiple nuclei.

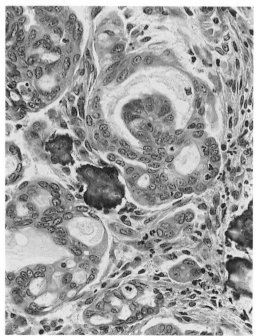

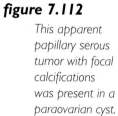

figure 7.112

This apparent papillary serous tumor with focal calcifications was present in a paraovarian cyst.

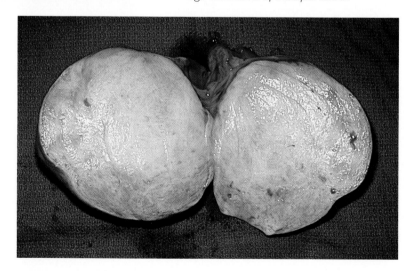

figure 7.113

The glistening white surfaces of this cut fibroma are typical. The yellowish areas suggest histologic variation. (Courtesy of Dr. D. Bard.)

atlas of gynecologic pathology

Hilus cell tumors, in which no epithelial elements are present but only sheets of hilus cells, occur largely in older women (Fig. 7.110).

A general theme in all of the above descriptions is that when the cell type accurately recapitulates a cell type in the normal genital canal, the tumor is benign. When the cells differ from this normal parent cell type, then at least some malignant potential exists. It further follows that highly malignant dedifferentiated tumors of all epithelial cell types tend to resemble each other and that the most undifferentiated cases are indistinguishable. Roughly, dedifferentiated tumors in the genital canal can be divided into types composed of small cells and types composed of huge, highly anaplastic cells that produce a variety of bizarre patterns (Fig. 7.111).

It is worth reiterating that, because the coelomic epithelium is identical to the surface epithelium of the ovary and only differs quantitatively from it, all the epithelial metaplasias and neoplasias described as ovarian may arise at other peritoneal or mesothelial sites. The most prominent example of this is endometriosis, but other examples cumulatively are not rare. An interesting example is the so-called paraovarian cyst. Although usually benign, these structures may give rise to malignant tumors typical of the ovary (Fig. 7.112).

Stromal tumors

Stromal tumors of the ovary reproduce all of the stromal tissues and patterns seen elsewhere in the genital canal. As in the case of the epithelial tumors described above, the following description is standardized and, thus, oversimplified. Fibrothecomas—stromal tumors that resemble ovarian stroma—are, grossly, firm, white to yellow masses (Fig. 7.113) that may be bilateral and inordinately large (Fig. 7.114). His-

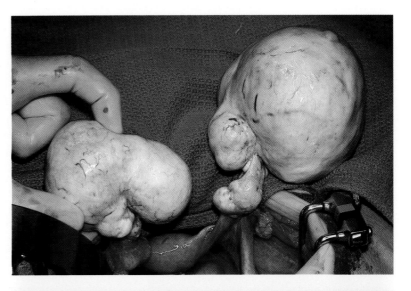

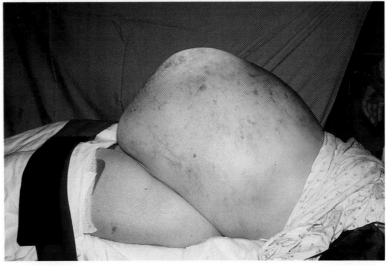

figure 7.114

These bilateral white masses (top) present the typical gross appearance of fibromas. This large abdominal mass (bottom) originally interpreted as a cystic lesion turned out to be a fibroma.

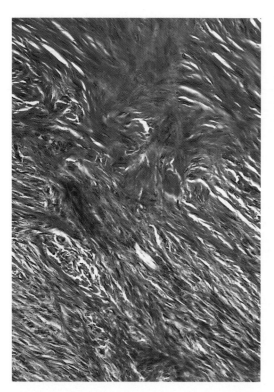

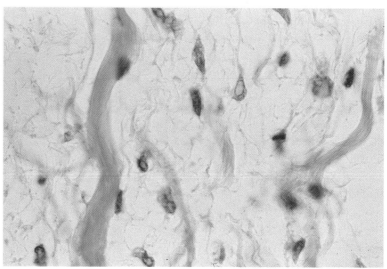

figure 7.115

In this fibrotheco-ma (left), the thecal tissue lies below and the fibrous portion lies above. This relatively acellular fibrothecoma (right) was characterized by large strips of extracellular matrix which give the neoplasm its most dramatic histologic features.

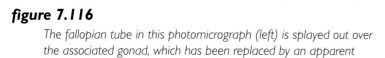

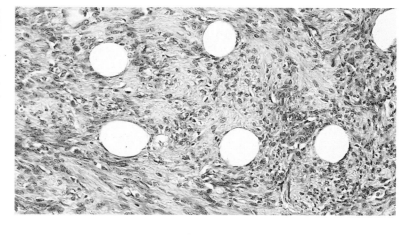

figure 7.116

The fallopian tube in this photomicrograph (left) is splayed out over the associated gonad, which has been replaced by an apparent myoma. In this apparent ovarian myoma (right), there are foci of degeneration and lipid-containing cells.

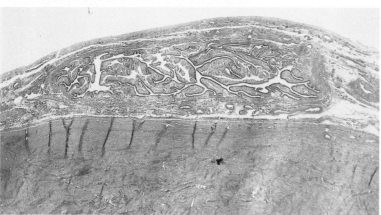

figure 7.117

This ovarian thecoma contains foci of luteinized thecal cells.

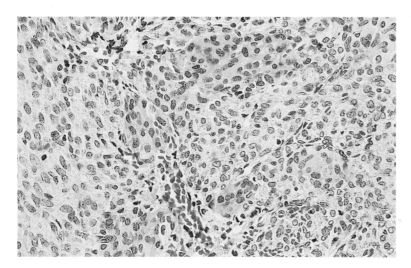

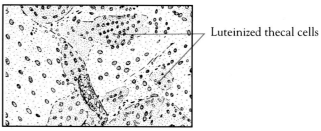

Luteinized thecal cells

tologically, they present a spectrum of fibrous or ovarian stromal-like appearance (Fig. 7.115). Less often the organization and cell type are suggestive of myoma (Fig. 7.116). Fibrothecomas tend to be estrogen producers. They may be luteinized in whole or in part (Fig. 7.117). Tumors that appear predominantly stromal may show focal epithelial differentiation that results in cords resembling granulosa or tubules resembling Sertoli epithelium (Fig. 7.118). Depending on the specific pattern and cell type, this will result in a neoplasm that looks like a granulosa theca cell tumor or a stromal tumor with tes-

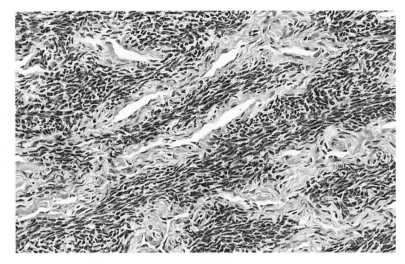

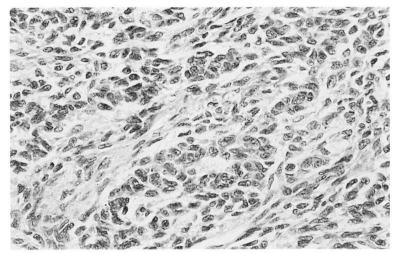

7.51

figure 7.118

The theca in this fibrothecoma (top) is arranged in cords reminiscent of granulosa cell tumors, although these cells are still obviously stromal. In this case (bottom), the cords of stromal cells are achieving some epithelial differentiation.

ticular tubules (Fig. 7.119). In addition, stromal tumors that possess foci of testicular-type tubular differentiation frequently will possess interstitial cells; these lesions are androgen producers. Thus, granulosa theca cell tumors or Sertoli-Leydig cell tumors may arise as stromal lesions as well as epithelial ones.

The ovarian stroma may give rise to the so-called *lipoid cell tumor,* which possesses cells resembling those of the adrenal cortex (Fig. 7.120). These have been called adrenal rest tumors, although true adrenal rest tumors probably do not occur in the ovary and are vanishingly rare in the retroperitoneal space. Adrenal rests do occur in the mesosalpinx and occasionally are multiple in the retroperitoneal space (Fig. 7.121).

More malignant ovarian stromal tumors, including all varieties of stromal sarcomas and mixed mesodermal tumors, are shown in Figure 7.122. Mitosis is a critical feature

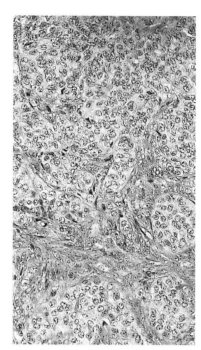
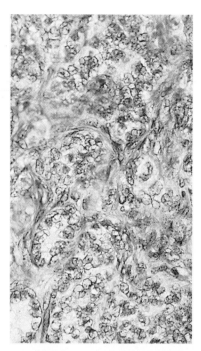
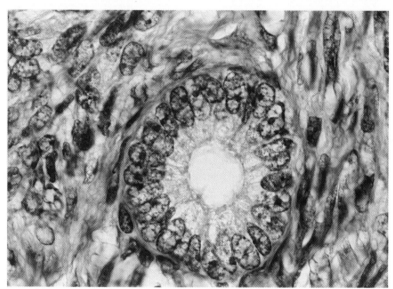

figure 7.119

In this photomicrograph (top left), stromal-type tissue appears above, but below it is differentiating into rudimentary tubules. A single well differentiated tubule (bottom) is seen in a tumor that is also composed of stroma and poorly differentiated tubules. The stromal nature of the main portion of this tumor (top right) is suggested at the lower right. At the bottom, particularly on the left, the tumor cells are differentiating into Sertoli-like tubules.

7.52

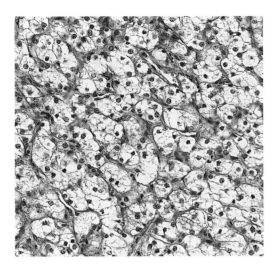

figure 7.120

This tumor consists of cells that resemble those in the adrenal cortex.

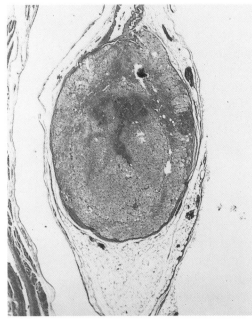

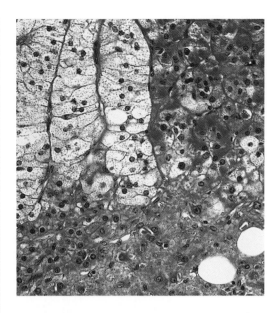

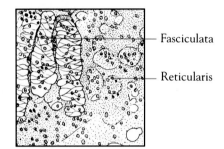

Fasciculata

Reticularis

figure 7.121

This adrenal rest (left) lies in the mesos-alpinx, external to the ovary. A higher power view (right) shows cells consistent with those of the zonae reticularis and fasciculata of the adrenal cortex.

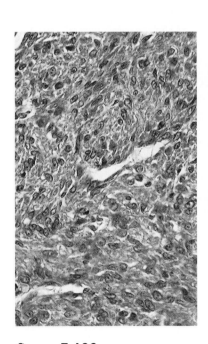

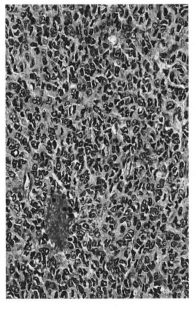

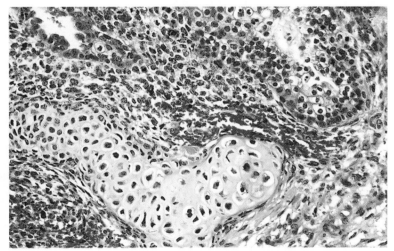

figure 7.122

This theca-like ovarian tumor (left) was associated with significant atypicality and numerous mitoses. A tumor (center) containing tissues similar to those seen in low-grade endometrial stromal lesions or stromatosis replaced this ovary. Poorly developed cartilage below (right) is associated with malignant epithelium above in this malignant mixed tumor.

(Fig. 7.123) in these tumors which have a bleak prognoses and are usually detected late. Like germ cell tumors, they may develop explosively and present as an acute abdomen. Lymphomas are usually secondary in the ovary, but primary lesions are seen (Fig. 7.124). Rarely, malignant stromal tumors arise from other peritoneal surfaces as well (Fig. 7.125).

ascites

Significantly large ovarian tumors may be associated with ascites. Benign tumors become ascitic by producing more fluid flow into the peritoneal cavity than can be immediately removed by the outflow lymphatics in the right leaf of the diaphragm. Malignant tumors become ascitic not only by producing excessive fluid flow into the peritoneal cavity but also by obstructing the outflow lymphatics in the right leaf of the diaphragm (Fig. 7.126). This type of widespread ovarian disease may also be responsible for a Sister Mary Joseph's nodule (Fig. 127).

7.54

germ Cell tumors

Germ cell pathology in its broadest sense probably covers much reproductive pathology, but in the ovary there is a less extensive spectrum, the most important components of which are the germ cell tumors. The encapsulation of more than one germ cell in a single follicle has been alluded to. Dysgenetic gonads, or foci in gonads, which consist of large nests of granulosa cells and intermixed germ cells, have been termed *gonadoblastomas* (Fig. 7.128). In many cases, these probably represent only anomalies, but in some cases they are large and almost certainly are neoplastic. The granulosa cells and germ cells are mixed in a variety of patterns, some of which contain structures resembling Call-Exner bodies. Degeneration and focal calcification are prominent features.

If gonadoblastomas are not true tumors, they are nevertheless gonads in which germ cell tumors are likely to develop. The germ cell tumors are conveniently divided into dysgerminomas, extraembryonal teratomas, and embryonal teratomas. However, all of these may occur in mixtures.

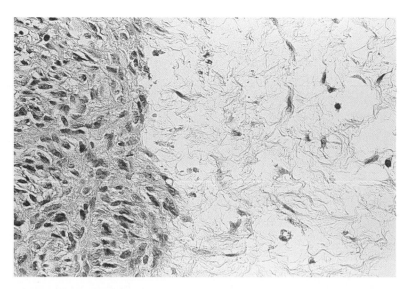

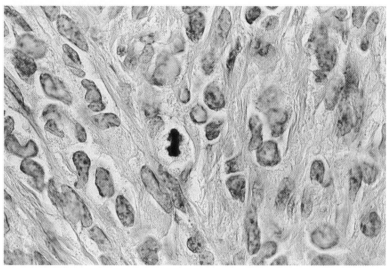

figure 7.123

Both thecal type tissue, on the left, and fibrous type tissue, on the right, are represented in this tumor (top) and both possess cells with enlarged atypical mitotic figures. The concerns aroused by cellular atypia (bottom) are confirmed by numerous, enlarged atypical mitotic figures.

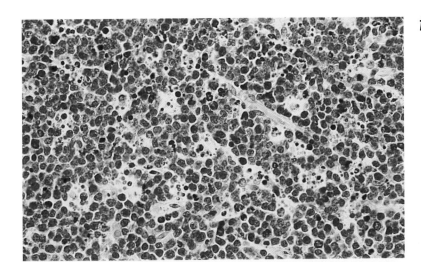

figure 7.124

Burkitt's lymphoma was apparently primary in this ovary.

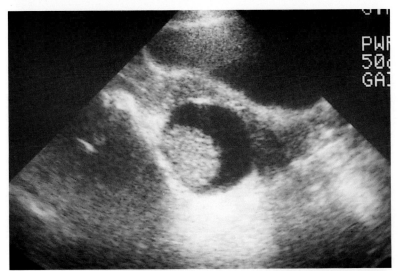

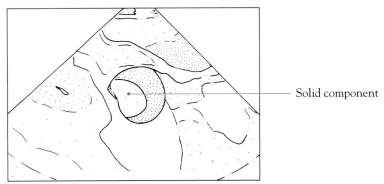

Solid component

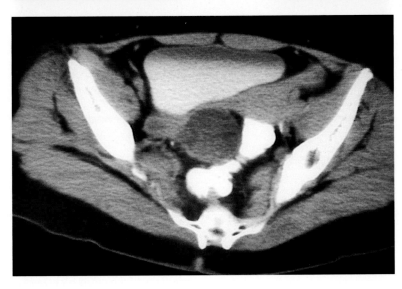

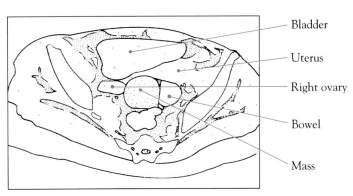

Bladder

Uterus

Right ovary

Bowel

Mass

figure 7.125

Sagittal transabdominal ultrasound of the pelvis taken to the right of the midline (top) shows the pelvic mass with a thick anterior border and a solid component arising from the posterior wall. Artifacts from bowel gas are seen posterior to this mass. Axial CT view of the pelvis

(bottom) shows the urinary bladder opacified by intravenous contrast. The uterus is displaced to the left of the urinary bladder by a mass separating the uterus from the right ovary. Due to its density, it is doubtful that the mass is completely cystic.

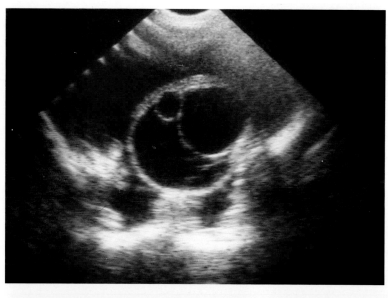

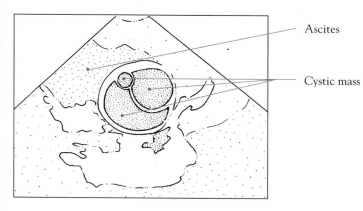

Ascites

Cystic mass

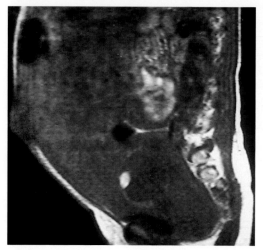

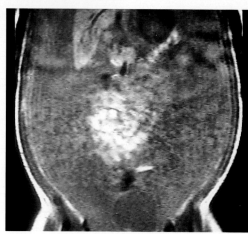

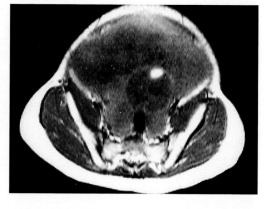

figure 7.126

Transverse transabdominal ultrasound view of the pelvis (top) shows a septated cystic mass within the pelvis surrounded by ascites. Sagittal T-1 weighted MR image of the abdomen and pelvis (bottom left) shows severe ascites cause protrusion of the abdomen. The borders of the fluid filled pelvic mass are barely delineated by its capsule. A focus of bright signal is seen along the anterior aspect representing a focus of hemorrhage. Axial T-1 MRI image of the pelvis (bottom right). The cystic pelvic mass is surrounded by ascites, making it difficult to outline. The bright focus of hemorrhage demarcates the anterior border of the mass. Coronal T-1 weighted MR image of the abdomen (bottom center) demonstrates the extent of the of the ascites. The liver and loops of small bowel are displaced medially by the fluid which appears to fill the whole abdomen and pelvis.

Bowel

Ascites

Fluid

Hemorrhage
} Mass

Liver

Ascites

Bowel

Mass

atlas of gynecologic pathology

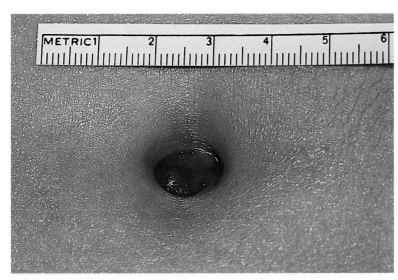

figure 7.127

Widespread intraperitoneal ovarian cancer produced this discolored umbilicus. A Sister Mary Joseph's nodule may result from any type of peritoneal carcinomatosis. (Courtesy of Dr. D. Bard.)

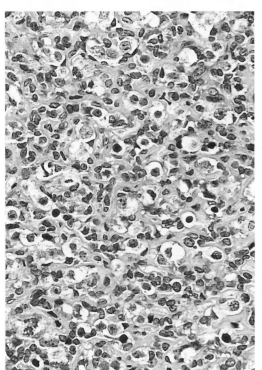

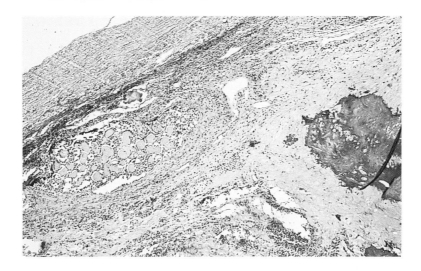

Epithelial cell

Call-Exner body

Germ cell

figure 7.128

Germ cells and epithelial cells (left) are mixed in an amorphous mass reminiscent of the embryonic ovary in this example of gonadoblastoma. In this nest (right), the epithelial cells are forming Call-Exner bodies. Necrosis and calcification (bottom) replace a portion of this gonadoblastoma.

DYSGERMINOMAS

Grossly, dysgerminomas tend to be white or yellow masses with a characteristic multilobulated form (Fig. 7.129). Microscopically, they consist of cords and nests of large germ cells, separated by a supporting stroma (Fig. 7.130). Characteristically, the stroma between the germ cell nest is infiltrated with round cells that resemble lymphocytes or plasma cells. When dysgerminomas consist of thin strands of germ cells infiltrating inflamed necrotic stroma, they can be difficult to distinguish from lymphomas or undifferentiated carcinomas (Fig. 7.131). Giant cells may be seen; occasionally, these are clearly trophoblast, which is important since choriocarcinoma in a germ cell tumor is a considerably greater therapeutic challenge than uncomplicated dysgerminoma (Fig. 7.132). Dysgerminomas are highly sensitive to cytotoxic therapies; therefore, even if they have extended, the prognosis may be good. If the presence of trophoblast is proven with positive HCG titers, complex chemotherapy is required.

EXTRAEMBRYONAL TERATOMAS

Among the extraembryonal teratomas are choriocarcinomas and the various forms of yolk sac tumor. Histologically, choriocarcinoma of germ cell origin is not different than choriocarcinoma of gestational origin, but it is less responsive to single-agent chemotherapy (Fig. 7.133). Historically, these lesions have had a terrible prognosis, but currently they are responding to multiagent chemotherapy. Because of this clinical difference, it is useful to distinguish gestational choriocarcinoma from that of a germ cell tumor by identifying other forms of teratoma, if possible.

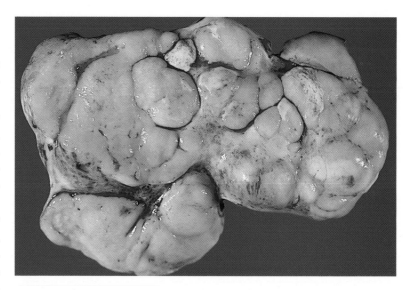

figure 7.129

This multilobulated ovarian tumor has the characteristic form and yellowish color of dysgerminoma. (Courtesy of Dr. D. Bard.)

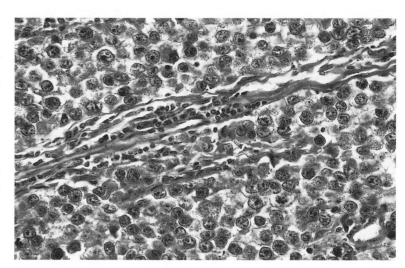

figure 7.130

Above and below lie nests of large germ cells, separated by a strand of stroma across the middle. Lymphocytes and plasma cells infiltrate this stroma.

7.58

atlas of gynecologic pathology

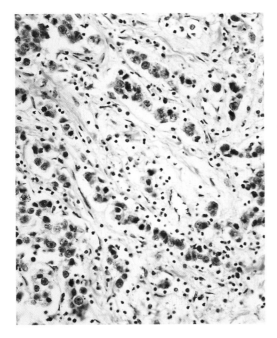

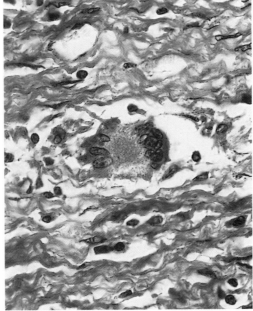

figure 7.132

Giant cells are seen in this dysgerminoma (top). One can speculate that this represents syncytiotrophoblast. The trophoblastic nature of this giant cell in a dysgerminoma (bottom) is more clear-cut.

figure 7.131

Isolated strands of germ cells infiltrate the lymphocyte-filled stroma in this tumor.

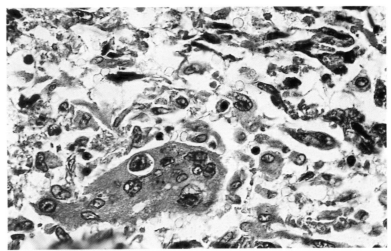

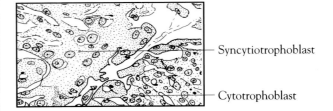

figure 7.133

Both cytotrophoblastic and syncytiotrophoblastic cell populations characterize this ovarian choriocarcinoma.

— Syncytiotrophoblast

— Cytotrophoblast

ovary

Among the yolk sac tumors, the rarest form is the polyvesicular vitelline tumor (Fig. 7.134). Large and small cysts lined by endodermal epithelium are embedded in the undifferentiated mesenchyme. Often the cyst appears to be at least partially divided into two chambers, one lined by cuboidal endodermal-type epithelium and the other by mesothelial-type epithelium. This is consistent with the development of the early yolk sac, in which the secondary yolk sac is segregated from the primary one. In the investing mesenchyme are small epithelial buds, which develop into the larger vesicles that give the tumor its name (Fig. 7.135).

The most common picture produced by the yolk sac tumors is that of the endodermal sinus tumor proliferating endodermal epithelium lines, cleftlike spaces, and sinuses (Fig. 7.136). Bright, eosinophilic globules termed *teratoid bodies* contain γ-fetoprotein. Characteristically, one side of the cystic sinus is indented by a capillary containing stromal projection, so that an apparent glomerulus is formed. This is the Schiller-Duval body (Fig. 7.137).

When the yolk sac tumor has a particularly prominent epithelial component and the lesion is therefore dramatically cellular, it is termed an embryonal carcinoma (Fig. 7.138). When, very rarely, blastocystic-type structures are found, the tumor may be termed a polyembryoma.

All of these patterns are routinely mixed in most extraembryonal teratomas, and the specific designations are more convenient than accurate (Fig. 7.139). All of the yolk sac tumors are highly malignant. They grow explosively and frequently present as acute abdominal emergencies. Complex chemotherapy has been successful in some cases.

7.60

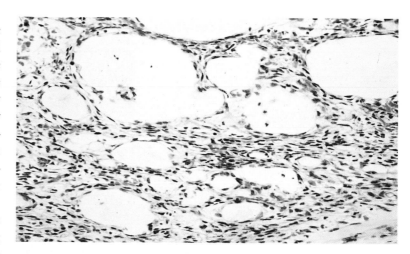

figure 7.134

Multiple cystic spaces characterize this polyvesicular vitelline tumor. Epithelial buds in the surrounding mesenchyme are only dark spots at this power.

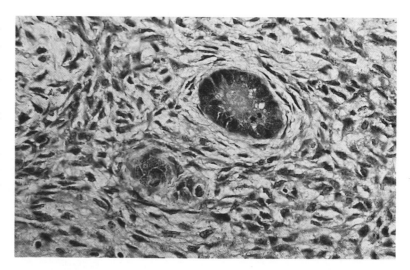

figure 7.135

At higher power, these epithelial buds are composed of embryonic epithelium that will result in ever-enlarging cysts in the mesenchyme.

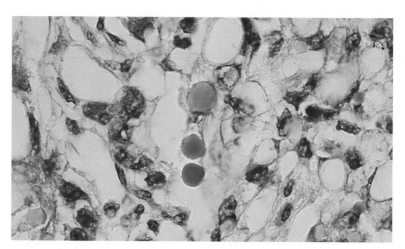

figure 7.136

Cleftlike spaces characterize this endodermal sinus tumor. Three prominent teratoid bodies are seen in the center.

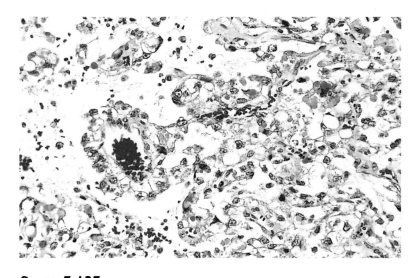

figure 7.137

A Schiller-Duval body lies just to the left of center in this extraembryonal teratoma.

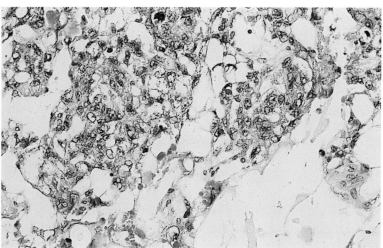

figure 7.138

Considerably more cellularity characterizes this extraembryonic teratoma, which has more epithelium and less mesenchyme than the tumor seen in Figure 7.136.

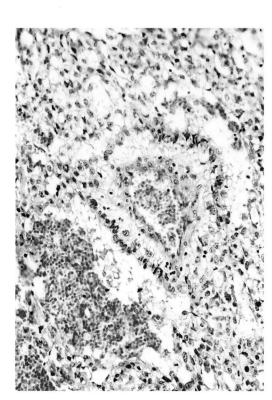

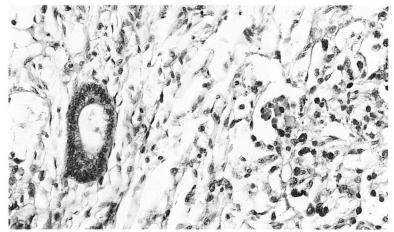

figure 7.139

This Schiller-Duval body (left) was seen in a highly cellular tumor, more reminiscent of embryonal carcinoma than the classic endodermal sinus pattern. To the right (right), the pattern is that of endodermal sinus; however, to the left, an endodermal tube of the type characterizing the polyvesicular vitelline pattern is seen.

EMBRYONAL TERATOMAS

Among the embryonal teratomas, certainly the most common is the benign cystic teratoma, or dermoid cyst. Early on, these contain cystic spaces lined by embryonic ectoderm supported by mesoderm. The ectoderm differentiates into both the mature type of epidermis and supporting epidermal appendages, as well as nervous tissue, including brain and sometimes retina (Fig. 7.140). When choroid plexus is present, the cyst within benign cystic teratomas may contain spinal fluid, but most often these spaces are lined by epidermis and its appendages so that the cyst contains hair, desquamated keratin, and sebaceous gland secretion (Fig. 7.141). When this material erodes the stratified squamous epithelium of a portion of the cyst, it elicits a dramatic giant cell reaction in the underlying mesoderm (Fig. 7.142). Cholesterol clefts can occur. Dissection of adjacent soft tissue by the oily material may result, with rupture of the cyst into the peritoneal cavity.

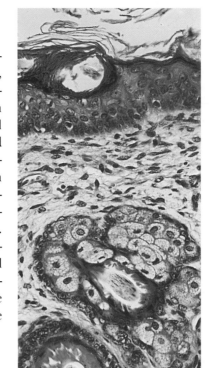

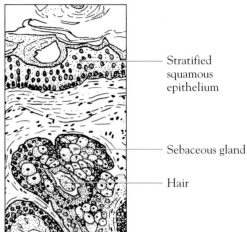

Stratified squamous epithelium

Sebaceous gland

Hair

7.62

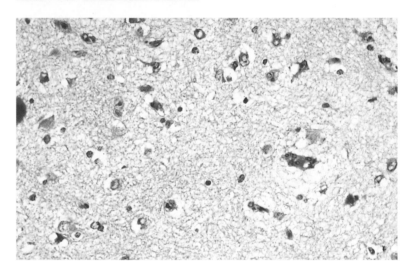

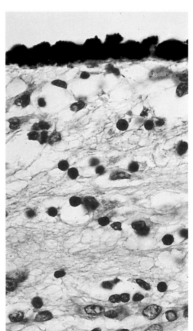

figure 7.140

A mature, stratified squamous epithelium (top), possessing a stratum corneum and hair follicles with sebaceous glands, is present. The mature neural tissue (center) seen in this photomicrograph is compatible with brain. This pigmented neuroepithelium (bottom) is typical of the developing retina.

atlas of gynecologic pathology

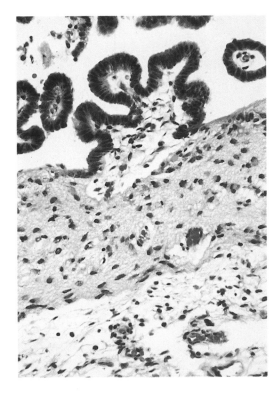

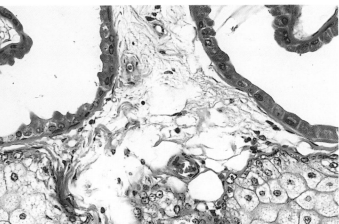

figure 7.141

A small focus of mature choroid plexus (left) lies above the equally mature-appearing brain tissue in this photomicrograph. Normal sebaceous glands (right) below are adjacent to well-developed apocrine sweat glands above.

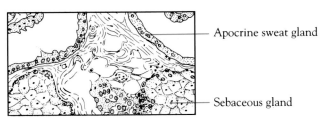

Apocrine sweat gland

Sebaceous gland

figure 7.142

The wall of this dermoid cyst (left) is being dissected by sebum and hair that have broken through the stratified squamous epithelium lining most of the cyst. An identical reaction (right) is occurring in response to the inclusion of two hairs in an abdominal skin scar.

7.63

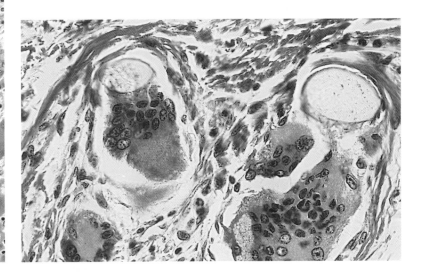

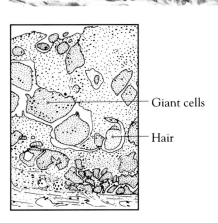

Giant cells

Hair

ovary

The mesoderm in the wall of the tumor usually differentiates into fat, connective tissue, and muscle (Fig. 7.143). With time, it becomes scarred and collagenous in appearance. Mesoderm also may produce cartilage, bone, and teeth (Fig. 7.144). Endoderm in dermoid cysts usually produces respiratory epithelium (Fig. 7.145). Both thyroid tissue and carcinoids may result, and both types of tissue may be responsible for clinical symptoms (Fig. 7.146). In the majority of cases, most of the body tissue in a dermoid cyst is concentrated into a grossly visible nodule known as Rokitansky's protuberance (Fig. 7.147).

Although rare, secondary malignancy may occur in dermoid cysts, usually after menopause. The most common type is squamous cell cancer arising in the stratified squamous epithelium.

Radiologic imaging of benign cystic teratomas produces characteristic pictures. X-Rays frequently show calcification or well formed teeth (Fig. 7.148), whereas ultrasound's characteristic bright echoes may obscure the limits of the mass (Fig. 7.149). Magnetic resonance imaging enhances the lipid in the cyst and shows it as bright signals on T-1 weighted images (Fig. 7.150).

7.64

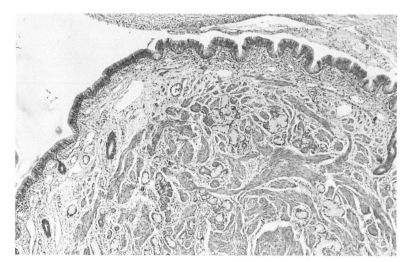

figure 7.143

Mature muscle and connective tissue lie below respiratory epithelium in the wall of this benign cystic teratoma.

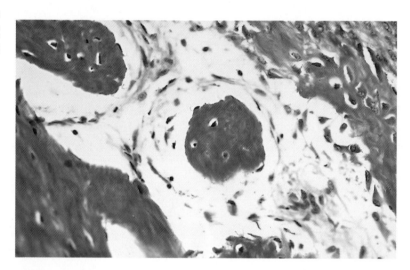

figure 7.144

Bone is developing in this teratoma, but it is not yet calcified.

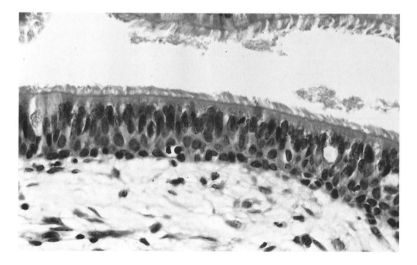

figure 7.145

This respiratory epithelium has well-developed cilia on its surface.

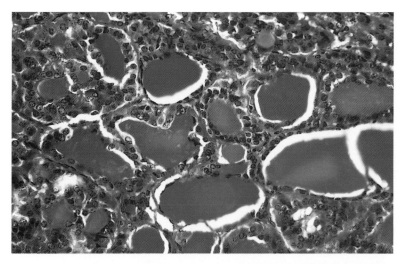

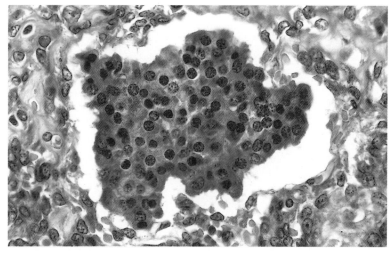

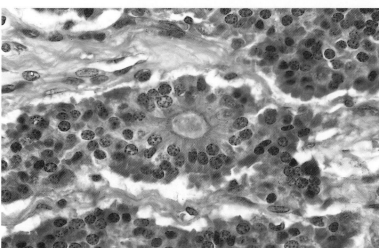

figure 7.146

Thyroid tissue made up the majority of this ovarian teratoma (top left). This carcinoid in a benign cystic teratoma (top right) is characterized by nests and cords of typical cells. Retraction from the surrounding stroma is common. In this case (bottom), the cord contains an acinar structure formed by radially arranged epithelial cells.

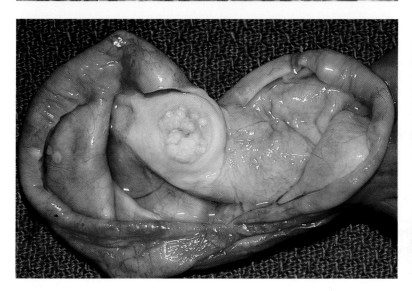

figure 7.147

This classic example of Rokitansky's protuberance is the site of tooth formation.

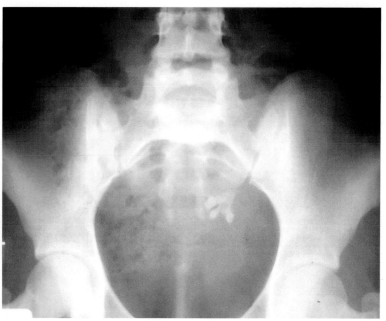

figure 7.148

X-Ray film of the pelvis shows there is a soft tissue mass in the left pelvis with borders that are difficult to delineate on the film. However, the presence of teeth within the mass suggests a benign cystic teratoma.

ovary

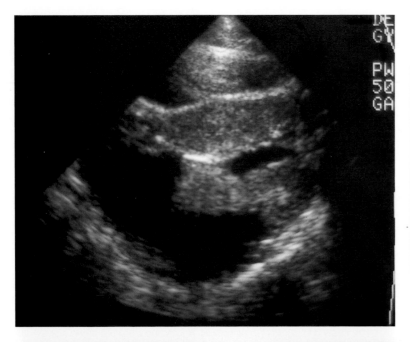
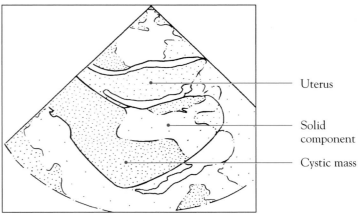

Uterus

Solid
component

Cystic mass

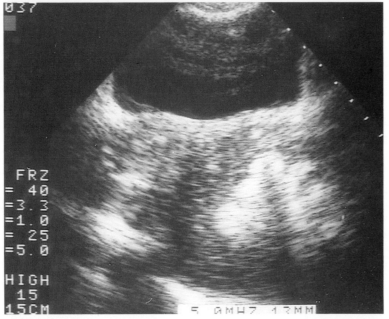
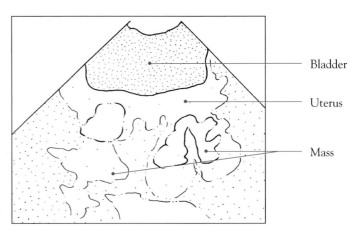

Bladder

Uterus

Mass

figure 7.149

Transverse transabdominal ultrasound view of the pelvis (top) shows the uterus displaced anteriorly by a predominantly cystic mass representing a benign cystic teratoma. The cluster of echoes on the left side of the mass indicates the location of its solid component. The uterine fundus (bottom) is displaced to the right by a very dense cluster of

echoes representing the surface of the mass. The remainder of the mass and its borders are difficult to delineate because of shadowing from the dense contents of the mass. This is referred to as the "tip of the iceberg" sign.

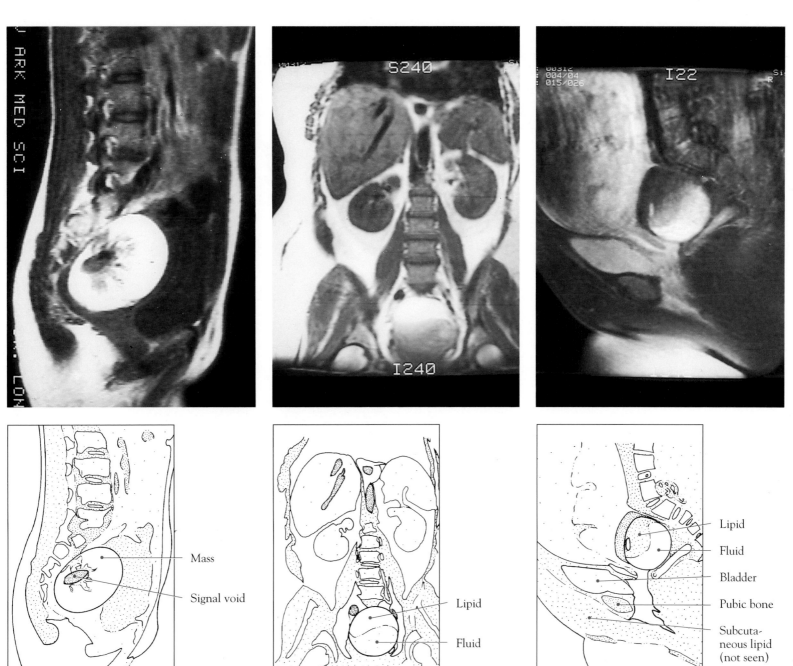

figure 7.150

Sagittal T-1 weighted MRI image of the pelvis (left) shows the center of the pelvic mass. The signal void within the mass corresponds to cartilage, bone, or teeth which are present. The intense signal produced by the lipid component of the mass is characteristic on MRI. Coronal T-1 weighted MRI image of the abdomen and pelvis (center) shows a pelvic mass through the posterior pelvis. The bright lipid signal is obvious along the superior half of the mass. The inferior half is occupied by a lower signal corresponding to the more fluid component of the mass. Sagittal T-2 weighted MRI image of the pelvis with fat suppression (right) shows the pelvic mass with its lipid component suppressed by the choice of imaging sequence. Note similar suppression of the subcutaneous tissues. The fluid component of the mass is now enhanced, similar to the urine within the urinary bladder.

Immature embryonal teratomas consist of embryonic-type tissues, as in benign cystic teratomas, but the tissues are not fully differentiated. The most common components of immature teratomas are mesenchymal connective tissues, ectodermal skin, and nervous tissue (Figs. 7.151 and 7.152). Endodermal respiratory-type epithelium is seen less often. Nervous tissue is ubiquitous and is particularly useful in grading. Abortive neural tubes consisting of neural ectoderm merge with large sheets of partially differentiated neural tissue (Fig. 7.153). The larger the percentage of undifferentiated neural tissue in an immature teratoma, the higher the grade. Metastatic deposits of this neural ectoderm throughout the peritoneal cavity are known as gliosis (Fig. 7.154). This alarming picture is not always lethal, as some teratomas

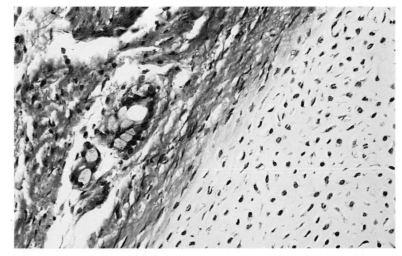

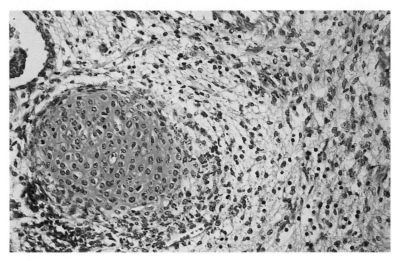

figure 7.151

In this immature teratoma (top), the cartilage is not well organized but looks close to mature. In this somewhat more immature example (bottom), an attempt is being made to form cartilage.

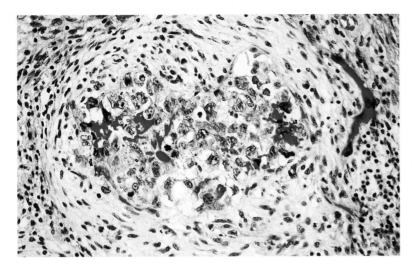

7.69

figure 7.152

In this highly immature teratoma (left) chondrosarcoma
is suggested. The skin and
appendages (right) are characteristic of embryonic skin
just acquiring hair follicles.

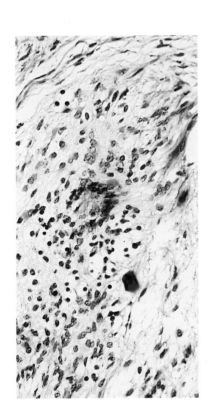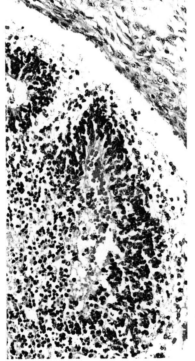

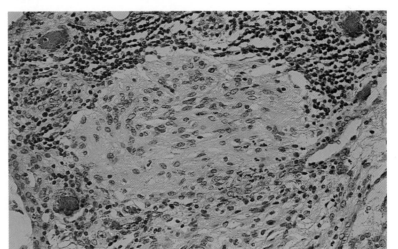

figure 7.154

An omental nodule of immature neural tissue is associated with an
intense inflammatory reaction in this example of gliomatosis.

figure 7.153

Small collections of neural ectodermal cells (left) are arranged in a
tubular configuration and embedded in more fully developed neural
tissue, which is nevertheless immature. Neuroectoderm (right) is producing poorly formed neural tubes in this case, which shows no signs
of maturing.

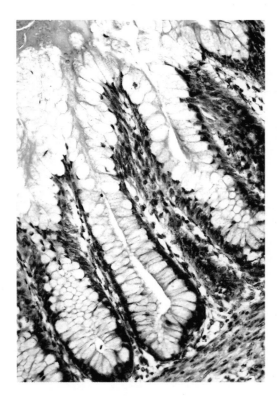

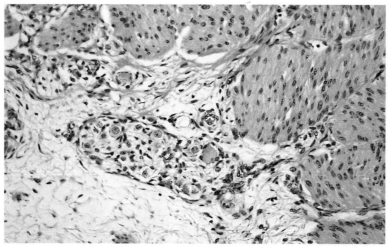

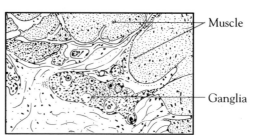

Muscle

Ganglia

figure 7.155

This example of apparently mature gastrointestinal epithelium (left) lines a segment of seemingly normal bowel in this otherwise immature teratoma. Normal muscle (right) and associated peripheral autonomic ganglion cells are seen here. Normal ganglion cells (bottom) are seen here in the same case.

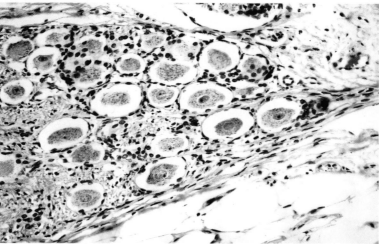

figure 7.156

Both the bilaterality and the multilobulated appearances of this metastatic breast cancer are typical. The bilaterality is of course due to the systemic nature of metastatic disease. The multilobulated but intact surface is due to multiple foci of intraovarian disease. (Courtesy of Dr. D. Bard.)

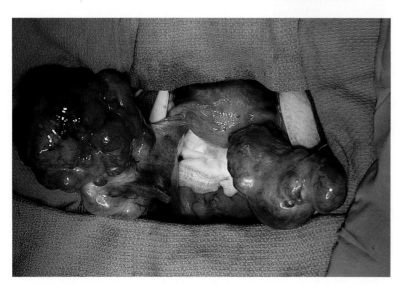

atlas of gynecologic pathology

eventually differentiate fully and then behave in a benign manner. Remarkably mature components are sometimes seen in immature teratomas, suggesting this capacity for spontaneous maturation (Fig. 7.155).

Metastatic Cancer

Metastatic cancer to the ovary is often bilateral (Fig. 7.156). The histology is variable, but two patterns are classic. Metastatic breast disease may be very subtle and consist of single-cell or "Indian file" cords of tumor cells, radially arranged in the ovarian cortex (Fig. 7.157). This pattern is believed to result from the obstruction of the arcade of lymphatics in the cortex. Gastrointestinal tumors are the other large group of tumors that metastasize to the ovary. They present in the medulla or subcortically, unlike primary ovarian cancer (Fig. 7.158). They also can produce the second classic pattern of metastatic cancer to the ovary, that of Krukenberg. When metastatic but mucin-producing tumors infiltrate the ovarian stroma as single cells, they create a mass with alternating patches of dense cellularity and loose myxomatous ovarian stroma (Fig. 7.159). The latter are portions of stroma infiltrated by more mucin than tumor cells. The former are collections of stroma and tumor cells, which may be the site of significant hormone production. If the mucin in the tumor cells pushes the nucleus to one side, a so-called signet-ring appearance results (Fig. 7.160).

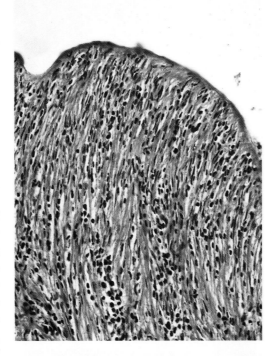

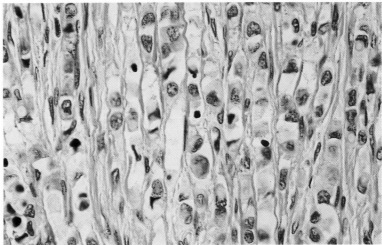

7.71

figure 7.157

Metastatic lymphoma is producing an "Indian file" infiltrative pattern in this photomicrograph of the ovarian cortex (top). Metastatic breast cancer cells (bottom) are arranged in long lines perpendicular to the surface of the ovarian cortex.

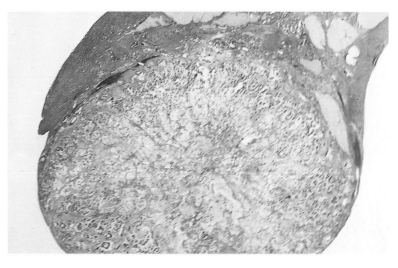

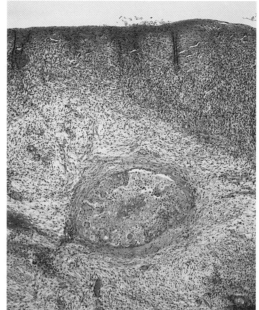

figure 7.158

This nodule of metastatic cancer (left) occupies the medulla of the ovary. The cortex extends above, out of the field of view. Photomicrograph (right) of metastatic cancer in the ovarian medulla, beneath the cortex.

7.72

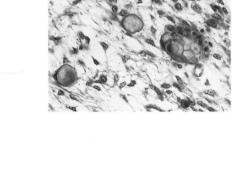

figure 7.159

A mixture of tumor cells and thecal cells lies above a relatively acellular myxomatous stroma.

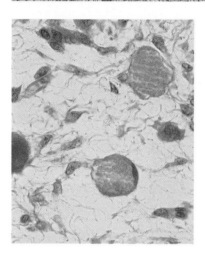

figure 7.160

A well-developed signet-ring cell is one of several tumor cells in this field.

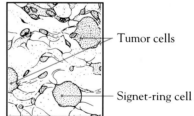

Tumor cells

Signet-ring cell

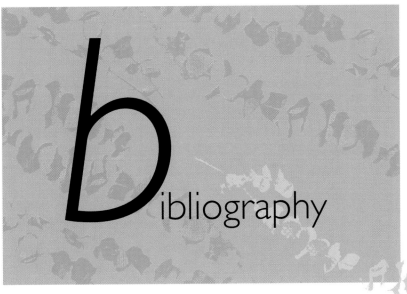

bibliography

Arey LB: The origin and form of Brenner tumors. *Am J Obstet Gynecol* 81:743, 1961.

Azoury RS, Woodruff JD: Primary ovarian sarcomas. *Obstet Gynecol* 37:920, 1971.

Blaustein A (ed.): *Pathology of the Female Genital Tract*, 2nd ed. New York, Springer-Verlag, 1982.

Fenoglio CM, Ferenczy A, Richart RM: Mucinous tumors of the ovary. Ultrastructural studies of mucinous cystadenomas with histogenetic considerations. *Cancer* 36:1709, 1975.

Ferenczy A, Fenoglio CM, Richart RM: Observations on benign mesothelioma of the genital tract. *Cancer* 30:244, 1972.

Fox H, Langley FA: *Tumors of the ovary.* London, William Heinemann, 1976.

Genadry R, Parmley TH, Woodruff JD: Secondary malignancies in benign cystic teratomas. *Gynecol Oncol* 8:246, 1979.

Genadry R, Parmley TH, Woodruff JD: The origin and behavior of parovarian tumors. *Am J Obstet Gynecol* 129:873, 1977.

Hart WR, Norris HJ: Borderline and malignant mucinous tumors of the ovary. Histologic criteria and clinical behavior. *Cancer* 31:1031, 1973.

Hernandez E, Rosenshein NB, Bhagavan BS, et al: Tumor heterogeneity and histopathology in epithelial ovarian cancer. *Obstet Gynecol* 63:330, 1984.

Hertig AT: Gestational hyperplasia of the endometrium. *Lab Invest* 13:1153, 1964.

Ireland K, Woodruff JD: Masculinizing ovarian tumors. *Obstet Gynecol Survey* 31:83, 1975.

Konishi I, Fujii S, Okamura H, et al: Development of interstitial cells and ovigerous cords in the human fetal ovary: An ultrastructural study. *J Anat* 148:121, 1986.

Kramer DW, Welch WR, Scully RE, Wojciechowski CA: Ovarian cancer and talc. *Cancer* 50:372, 1982.

Kurman RJ, Norris HJ: Embryonal carcinoma of the ovary. *Cancer* 38:2420, 1976.

Kurman RJ, Norris HJ: Endodermal sinus tumor of the ovary. *Cancer* 38:2403, 1976.

Kurman RJ, Craig JM: Endometrioid and clear cell carcinoma of the ovary. *Cancer* 29:1653, 1972.

Meigs JV: Fibroma of ovary with ascites and hydrothorax. *Am J Obstet Gynecol* 67:962, 1954.

Mostafa SAM, Bargeron CB, Flower RW, et al: Foreign body granulomas in normal ovaries. *Obstet Gynecol* 66:701, 1985.

Norris HJ, Taylor HB: Luteoma of pregnancy. *J Clin Pathol* 47:557, 1967.

Parmley TH, Woodruff JD: The ovarian mesothelioma. *Am J Obstet Gynecol* 120:234, 1974.

Richardson GS, Scully RE, Nikrui N, et al: Common epithelial cancer of the ovary (part I). *N Engl J Med* 312:415, 1985.

Richardson GS, Scully RE, Nikrui N, et al: Common epithelial cancer of the ovary (part II). *N Engl J Med* 312:474, 1985.

Roth LM, Sternberg WH: Proliferating Brenner tumors. *Cancer* 27:687, 1971.

Sampson JA: Development of the implantation theory for origin of the peritoneal endometriosis. *Am J Obstet Gynecol* 40:549, 1940.

Scully RE: Germ cell tumors of the ovary. *Prog Gynecol* 5:343, 1970.

Scully RE: Gonadoblastoma: A review of 74 cases. *Cancer* 25:1340, 1971.

Scully RE: Tumors of the ovary and maldeveloped gonads. In *Atlas of Tumor Pathology,* series 2, fascicle 16. Washington DC, Armed Forces Institute of Pathology, 1979.

Scully RE, Borrow JF: "Mesonephroma" of the ovary. Tumor of müllerian nature related to endometrioid carcinoma. *Cancer* 20:1405, 1967.

Stein IF, Leventhal ML: Amenorrhea as associated with bilateral polycystic ovaries. *Am J Obstet Gynecol* 29:181, 1935.

Takashina T, Kanda Y, Hayakawa O, et al: Yolk sac tumors of the ovary in the human yolk sac. *Am J Obstet Gynecol* 156:223, 1987.

Taylor HB, Norris HJ: Lipid cell tumors of the ovary. *Cancer* 20:1953, 1967.

Teilum G: *Special Tumors of Ovary and Testes.* Philadelphia, JB Lippincott, 1976.

Witschi E: Migration of the germ cells of human embryos from the yolk sac to the primitive gonadal folds. *Contrib Embryol* 32:67, 1948.

placenta

development and histology

The placenta develops from the blastocystic trophoblast and is the first fetal organ to differentiate. Before implantation occurs, the blastocystic trophoblast is a flattened mesothelial cell layer. As these surface cells make contact with the endometrium, they become cuboidal and are called cytotrophoblast. The cytotrophoblast produces an underlying layer of fibroblastic-type cells (the extraembryonic mesoderm) and an overlying layer, a syncytium of multinucleated cells (the syncytiotrophoblast), which further invade the endometrial tissue (Fig. 8.1). The combination of extra embryonic mesoderm, cytotrophoblast, and syncytiotrophoblast constitutes the chorionic membrane. As the blastocyst becomes completely buried, its entire surface is converted first to cytotrophoblast and then to syncytium. The syncytiotrophoblast develops multiple intracellular vacuoles that coalesce, producing an intercommunicating labyrinth that extends entirely around the blastocyst and is contained within the syncytium (Fig. 8.2; see Fig. 8.1). The syncytiotrophoblast invades maternal endometrial glands and capillaries so that they empty their contents into the labyrinth contained within the syncytium (Fig. 8.3). There, blood and gland secretions passively circulate around the embryo and then passively reenter the maternal vascular spaces.

Subsequently, the cytotrophoblast produces first buds and then columns of undifferentiated cells that penetrate the syncytium and reach the maternal tissues (Fig. 8.4). These columns are invaded from below by the underlying extraembryonic mesoderm and subsequently by fetal blood vessels (Fig. 8.5). The entire column is termed an anchoring villus. Where the cellular tips of the columns reach the maternal tissue, they begin to spread out, and, by merging with spreading tips from adjacent columns or anchoring villi,

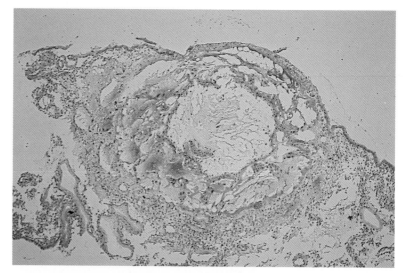

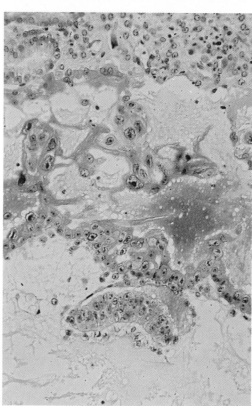

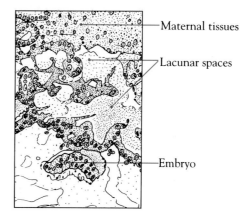

Maternal tissues

Lacunar spaces

Embryo

figure 8.1

About 12 days from fertilization, this blastocyst (top) is entirely buried within the endometrium. The bilaminar embryo is central and is associated with a small amniotic space. A labyrinth of lacunar spaces surrounds the entire structure. The bilaminar embryo (bottom) is suspended within the amniotic space. The whole is attached to the surrounding chorionic membrane, which consists of extraembryonic mesoderm, cytotrophoblast, and syncytiotrophoblast containing lacunae. Maternal tissue is above.

8.2

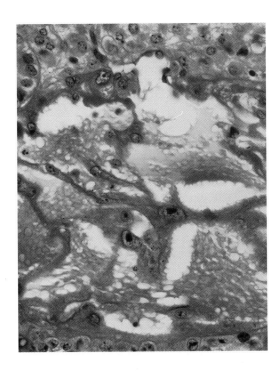

figure 8.2

The base of the chorionic membrane is below, while the labyrinthine portion is in the middle. Above is maternal tissue. A capillary is opening into the labyrinthine space.

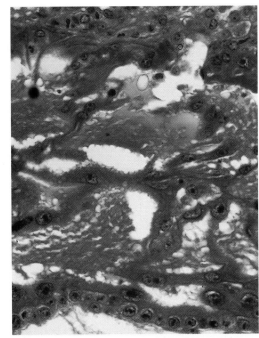

figure 8.3

This view (top) is similar to that of Figure 8.2. A gland is seen opening into the labyrinthine space above. Two capillaries (bottom) are directly invaded by the advancing trophoblast.

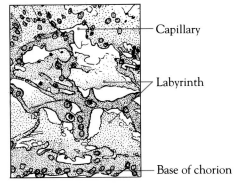

Capillary

Labyrinth

Base of chorion

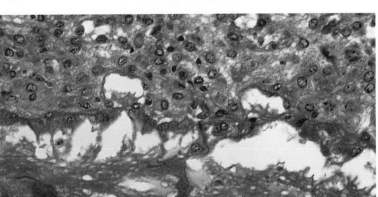

8.3

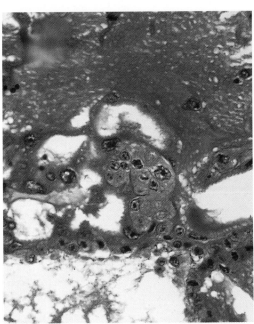

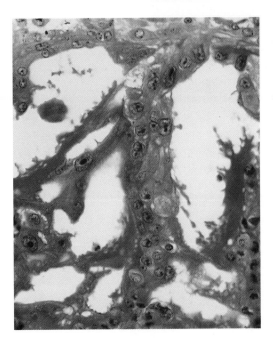

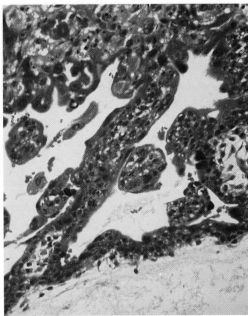

figure 8.4

Cytotrophoblastic proliferation (left) has produced a column of basal-type cells that protrude into the syncytial labyrinth. Cytotrophoblastic proliferation (right) has produced a column of cytotrophoblast that protrudes through the syncytial labyrinth from the base of the chorionic membrane to the maternal tissue above.

figure 8.5

The amount of extraembryonic mesoderm has grown, and some of it is protruding into the base of the cytotrophoblastic columns that extend across the labyrinthine space.

placenta

they form a complete shell around the blastocyst (Fig. 8.6). This has been called a *cytotrophoblastic shell*. In the sense that this shell is composed of nonsyncytial cells with discrete cell membranes, this nomenclature is accurate, but these cells are more differentiated than the basal cytotrophoblast. The cytotrophoblastic shell also contains a few multinucleated giant cells. Soon, a layer of fibrinoid known as *Nitabuch's layer* develops between the maternal tissue and the cytotrophoblastic shell (Fig. 8.7).

The syncytium now lines an interior space defined by the cytotrophoblastic shell and the basal cytotrophoblast that will become the intervillous space (Fig. 8.8). The columns, or anchoring villi, which extend from the fetal side (the chorionic plate) to the maternal side (the basal plate) will become the placental septa (Fig. 8.9). The cytotrophoblastic shell is penetrated by channels that connect maternal endometrial glands and blood vessels with the syncytial labyrinth (Fig. 8.10). Isolated trophoblastic cells invade the endometrium and the myometrium immediately beneath the implantation site and differentiate into large mononuclear or multinuclear intermediate trophoblastic cells (Fig. 8.11). This is termed syncytial endomyometritis. Occasionally, this process is exaggerated, and a mass of intermediate trophoblast produces a so-called placental site tumor (described below).

Trophoblastic cells also invade the walls of the spiral arterioles that supply the implantation site; there they differentiate into large intermediate trophoblastic cells (Fig. 8.12). In the process, they destroy the muscular walls of the spiral arterioles. With the subsequent degeneration of the trophoblastic cells themselves, the vascular walls become hyalinized and physiologically nonresponsive. This hyalinized structure persists after delivery and may produce enlarged, hyalinized vessels in the myometrium for months postpartum (Fig. 8.13).

Meanwhile, cotyledons have begun to develop within the intervillous space. The cotyledons develop from the fetal surface of the intervillous space, the chorionic plate. First as trophoblastic proliferations but soon supported by mesodermal cores containing fetal vasculature, they form sprouts that grow toward the basal plate (Fig. 8.14). They divide many times, with the initial divisions resulting in branches that are nearly as large as the original stem, so that the bulk of the cotyledon expands. Subsequent division reverses this process, and the terminal villi are much smaller. The cotyledon becomes a squat, bush-shaped collection of branches of the chorionic membrane, all containing fetal vasculature. As the cotyledons grow in relation to the maternal blood supply, they tend to become arranged so that spiral arterioles, piercing the basal plate, open into the center of the bush. This pattern of cotyledonary growth is such that the larger originating branches of the cotyledons are nearer the fetal surface of the placenta (Fig. 8.15). Nearer the maternal surface, terminal villi dominate (Fig. 8.16).

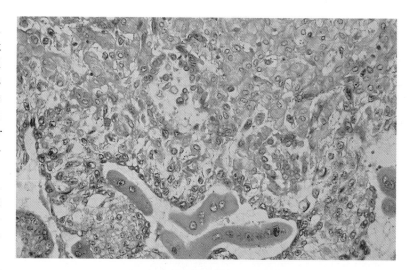

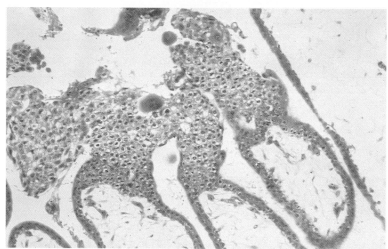

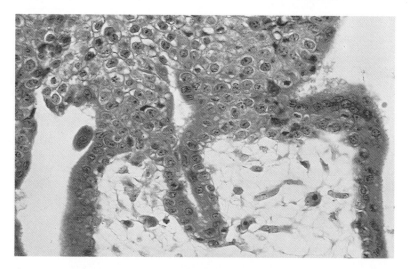

figure 8.6

Two anchoring villi (top) are attached to the maternal tissue on the left and right. The cytotrophoblast at their anchoring sites extends from each, to meet in the middle, forming a continuous layer that separates the maternal tissue above from the syncytiotrophoblast below. Three anchoring villi (center) are attached to a fragment of the cytotrophoblastic shell in these curettings. A large, multinucleated giant cell in the cytotrophoblastic shell represents intermediate trophoblast. Two anchoring villi below (bottom) are joined in the cytotrophoblastic shell above. The cells in the shell are more differentiated, possessing a moderate amount of light clear cytoplasm, than those basal cytotrophoblastic cells immediately adjacent to the extraembryonic mesodermal stroma.

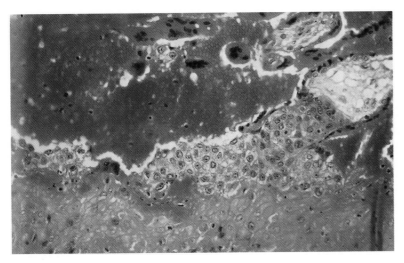

figure 8.7

An anchoring villus extends from the upper right. The cytotrophoblastic bud on its tip is attached to the decidua below. To the left, a dense eosinophilic material, Nitabuch's layer, is developing between the decidua and the cytotrophoblast.

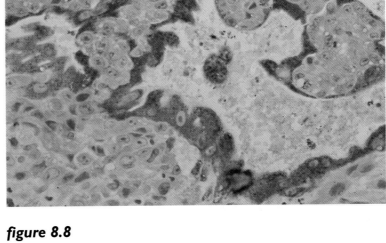

figure 8.8

This immunoperoxidase stain for the protein SP-1 clearly outlines the syncytiotrophoblast lining the intervillous space. The cytotrophoblast is unstained. (Courtesy of Dr. Frank Kuhajda.)

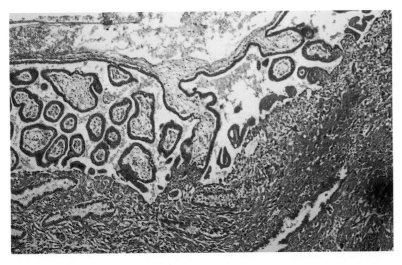

figure 8.9

In this photomicrograph, the chorionic membrane above is attached to the maternal tissue below by an anchoring villus. Both to the left and to the right of this anchoring villus, other villous structures are seen filling the now-defined intervillous space.

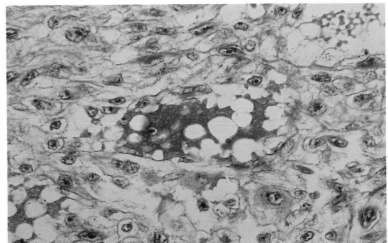

figure 8.10

A blood-filled channel lies in the midst of this sheet of cytotrophoblast.

8.5

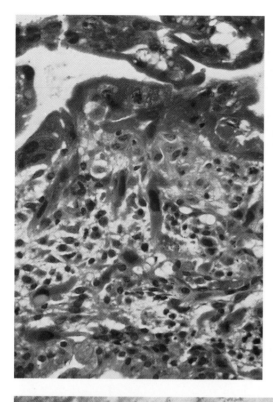

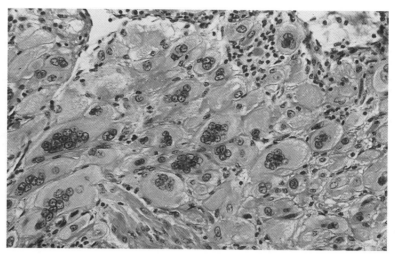

figure 8.11

Isolated large trophoblastic cells (left) have penetrated into the maternal tissue below this implantation site. Here they have differentiated into multinucleated giant cells, or so-called intermediate trophoblast. Deeper in the myometrium (right) a large collection of intermediate trophoblastic cells have resulted in the picture termed syncytial endomyometritis.

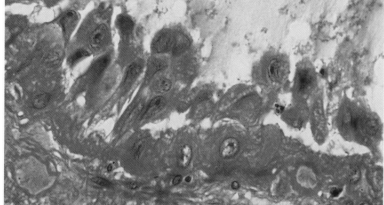

figure 8.13

This hyalinized spiral arteriole lies at the endomyometrial junction immediately beneath an old implantation site.

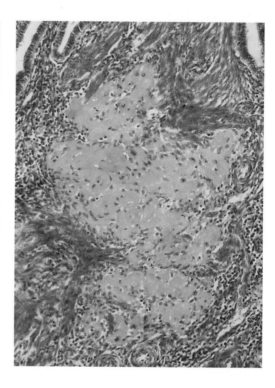

figure 8.12

Trophoblastic cells above fill the lumen of this vessel; furthermore, they have invaded its wall.

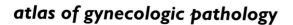

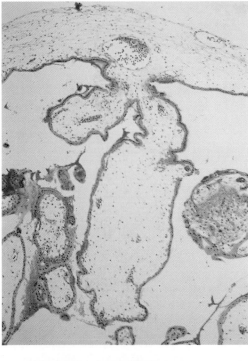

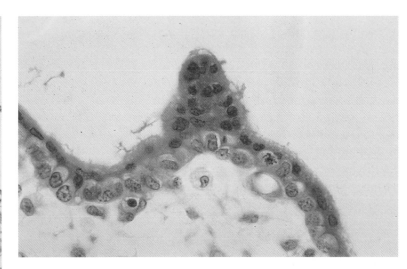

figure 8.14

This cotyledonary stem (left) is developing from the chorionic plate.
It has already divided into two large trunks. This focus of trophoblastic
proliferation (right) is the first sign of a developing cotyledonary stem.

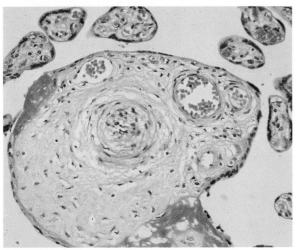

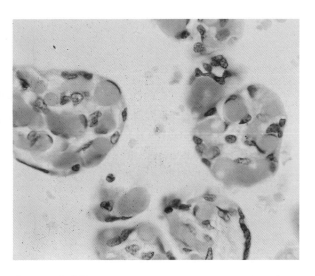

figure 8.15

This large vascular stalk is near the base of the
cotyledon, close to the fetal surface of the placenta.

figure 8.16

The terminal villi in this photomicrograph are on the
periphery of the cotyledon. They are composed
of multiple small capillaries with little associated
stroma and thin trophoblastic covering.

As the entire conceptus enlarges, the portion that reemerges above the endometrial surface is deprived of a blood supply and ceases to grow. Atrophy of cotyledons occurs, and this portion of the chorionic membrane becomes the decidua capsularis. Ghosts of the cotyledons are present at term (Fig. 8.17). The portion of the chorionic membrane that remains attached to the endometrium continues to grow. Multiple cotyledons growing between the original anchoring villi further excavate the maternal tissues and grossly merge, forming a placental lobe. This leaves a septum between the lobes (Fig. 8.18). It is composed of the original anchoring villus, extending from the chorionic plate, attached to a column of maternal tissue extending from the endometrium. The maternal tissue is embedded with so-called X cells, which are the remnants of the cytotrophoblastic shell (Fig. 8.19). For unknown reasons, septal cysts frequently develop and may be lined by X cells. These may become large and present on the surface of the chorionic plate (Fig. 8.20). Sonographically, the septa are not well defined in the second trimester, but they are at term (Fig. 8.21).

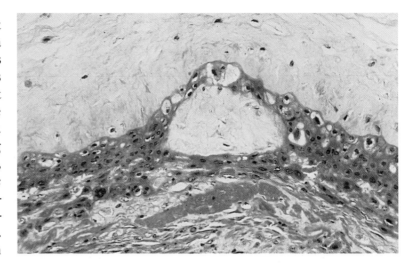

figure 8.17
This ghost of a chorionic villus lies in the chorionic membrane, where it has been pushed against the maternal decidua.

8.8 Implantation-related anomalies

The site and depth of the original implantation and the orientation of the blastocyst to the endometrial surface all have consequences for placental development. Maximal reproductive efficiency occurs when the blastocyst implants in the middle of the functional portion of the anterior or posterior wall. If it implants elsewhere, abortion may occur. Implantation at or near the internal os results in a placenta previa (Fig. 8.22). If implantation occurs at a site where the decidua is poorly developed, placenta accreta may result. Because trophoblastic invasion of the myometrium is routine, villi must be seen attached to muscle before the diagnosis of placenta accreta can be made (Fig. 8.23). It is traditional to use the term *increta* when villi invade to a significant depth in the myometrium, and *percreta* when they invade to the serosal surface.

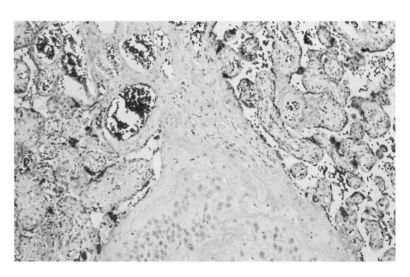

figure 8.18
This placental septum contains large vascular channels. It is joining the basal plate below. Two placental lobes lie on either side of it.

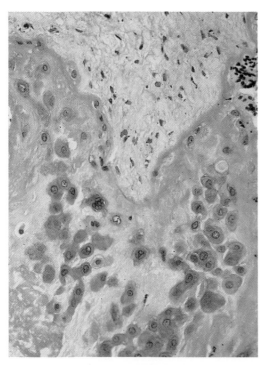

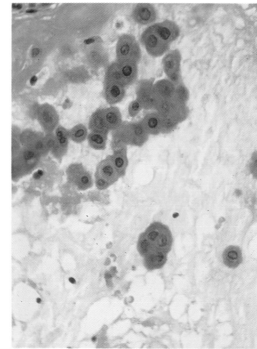

figure 8.19

Extraembryonic mesoderm (left) lies above and joins the maternal tissue below. This tissue is infiltrated by the remnants of the cytotrophoblastic shell, or the so-called X cells. X cells (right) are seen here lying in hyalinized maternal tissue.

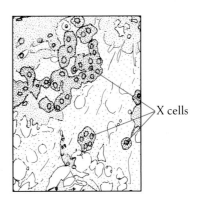

X cells

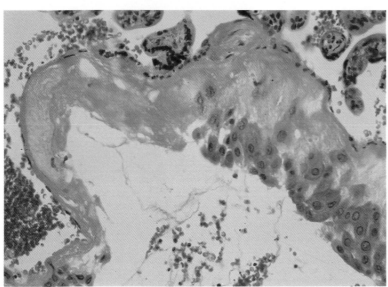

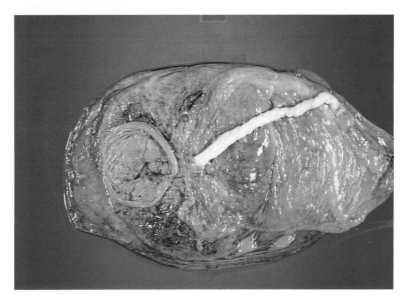

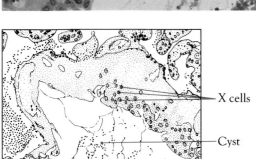

X cells

Cyst

figure 8.20

A cyst (left) within a septum below is lined by hyalinized maternal tissue and X cells. A large septal cyst (right) has produced a grossly visible structure on the chorionic surface.

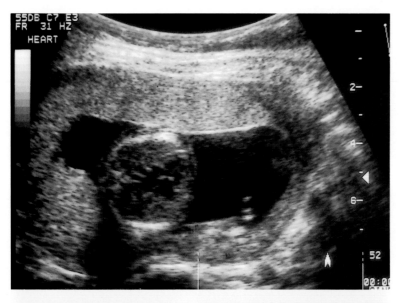

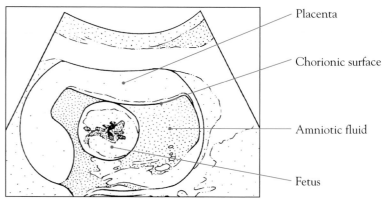

Placenta

Chorionic surface

Amniotic fluid

Fetus

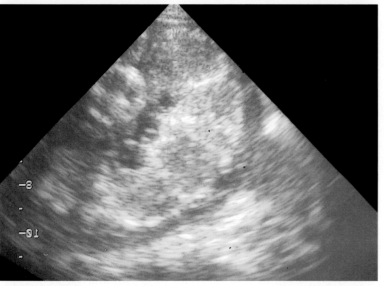

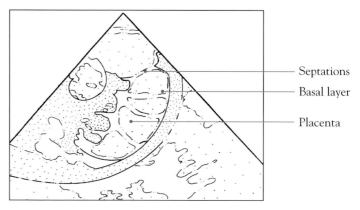

Septations

Basal layer

Placenta

8.10

figure 8.21

Transverse transabdominal ultrasound of an immature placenta (top) that is located predominantly along the anterior uterine wall. There is no evidence of calcifications within the placental substance. The chorionic surface is smooth. There is adequate amniotic fluid surrounding the fetus. Transverse transabdominal ultrasound of a mature placenta (bottom) that lines the left lateral uterine wall. Densities seen at the basal layer of the placenta represent calcifications. Sepatations are demonstrated to run perpendicular to the basal layer, separating the placenta into sections. These features are usually seen in the late third trimester of gestation.

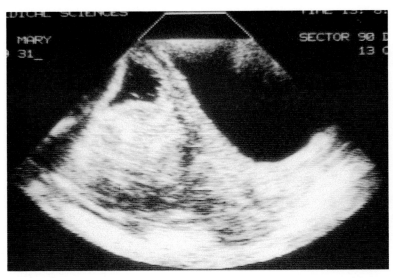

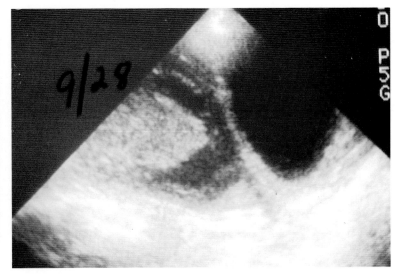

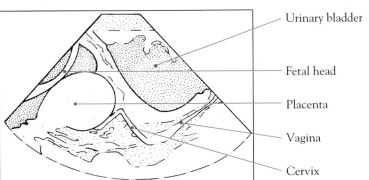

Urinary bladder

Fetal head

Placenta

Vagina

Cervix

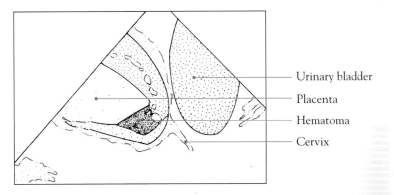

Urinary bladder

Placenta

Hematoma

Cervix

8.11

figure 8.22

Longitudinal transabdominal ultrasound of a placenta previa (left) taken along the axis of the vagina and cervix. The caudal termination of the placenta covers the cervical internal os completely. A pocket of amniotic fluid separates the placenta from the presenting fetal head.

Longitudinal transabdominal ultrasound of a placenta previa with hematoma (right) taken at the level of the cervical internal os. The placenta and the os are separated by a hypoechoic collection representing a hematoma.

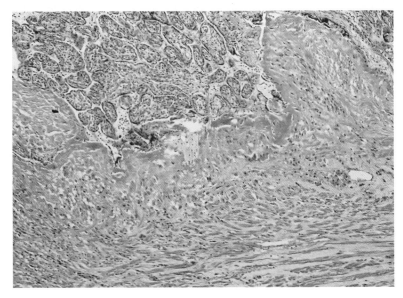

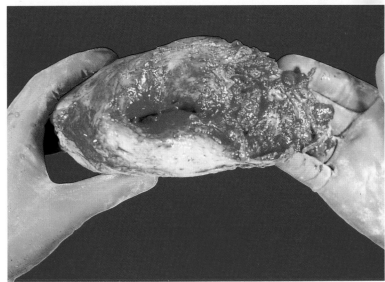

figure 8.23

In this case of placenta accreta (left), placental tissue is directly implanted upon myometrium without any intervening decidua. The

lower uterine segment (right) to the right has been totally destroyed in this case of a placenta previa, percreta.

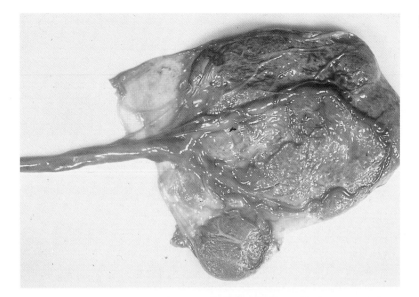

figure 8.24

In this specimen, a small succenturiate lobe lies below. It is connected to the main placental cake by multiple vascular channels.

8.12

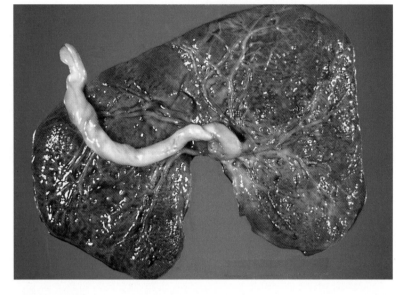

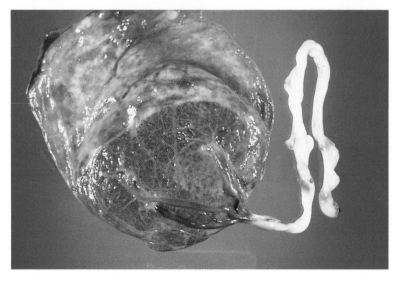

figure 8.25

This bilobed placenta (left) demonstrates the type of abnormal shape attributed to implantation in an unusual intrauterine site. Gross specimen of a bilobate placenta (right) showing the fetal side of the placen-

ta. The two placental masses are separated by membrane. The umbilical cord is inserted very close to the margin of one mass of chorionic villi.

figure 8.26

Redundant membrane produces an apparent hood over the upper rim of this placenta marginata.

Comparative studies suggest that too superficial an implantation may provide for simultaneous implantation on different walls of the cavity, with the production of accessory placental lobes (Fig. 8.24). Other studies suggest that complexly shaped placentas are from implantations in unusual sites, such as the cornual region or the sides of the cavity (Fig. 8.25).

Too deep an implantation has been related to placenta marginata or circumvallata. In the case of placenta marginata, the villous portion of the placenta extends beyond the edge of the fetal surface of the chorion (Fig. 8.26). In circumvallata, the chorionic and amnionic membranes are folded back upon the fetal surface and may contain villi or blood clot (Fig. 8.27). The two conditions are often associated.

The site on the sphere of the blastocyst at which the placental villi will develop is determined by which portion implants first and remains in contact with the endometrium and the maternal blood supply. If the embryo is located in this implantation pole, the umbilical cord develops at the same site as the placenta. However, if the embryo is rotated away from the implantation pole of the blastocyst, the umbilical cord will develop at a site remote from the placenta and will have to run in the membranes to the placental cake (Fig. 8.28). This velamentous insertion can result in vasa previa.

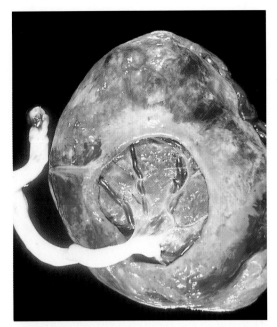

figure 8.27

A thick, well-developed, redundant membrane in this specimen produces the characteristic appearance of placenta circumvallata. (Courtesy of Dr. Kevin Winn.)

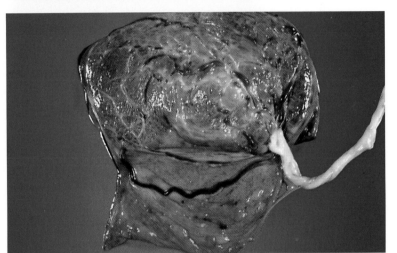

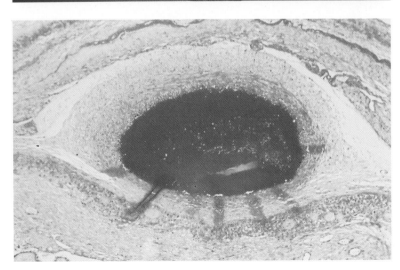

figure 8.28

This velamentous insertion (top) is associated with a large fetal vessel running in the membranes. A histologic cross section (bottom) of a fetal vessel in the membranes is seen.

If the embryo is located directly opposite the implantation, monozygotic twinning may occur. Dividing membranes may or may not define the type of twinning. If the membranes dividing two gestational sacs are composed of two opposed chorions and two surface amnions, then monozygotic or dizygotic twinning may have occurred, but if these dividing membranes consist only of two opposed amnions, only one chorion exists and the twins are monozygotic (Fig. 8.29). All of the placental anomalies related to implantation are highly associated with one another (Fig. 8.30).

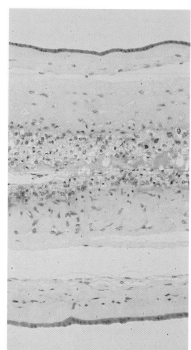

figure 8.29

Amnions (top) lie on both sides of this dividing membrane. In the center are two closely apposed chorions. Two amnions (bottom) are closely apposed without any intervening chorion.

Maturational Changes

During the course of gestation, the placenta undergoes development and maturation. Histologically, the apparent result is an increase in exchange area. This is dramatically illustrated in the changing morphology of the terminal villi.

CHANGES IN THE TERMINAL VILLI

During the first trimester, terminal villi are composed of a relatively large amount of stroma with a few capillaries (Fig. 8.31). Up to the tenth week of development, the capillaries contain nucleated fetal red blood cells. The villus itself is surrounded by two well-defined layers of trophoblast, an inner cytotrophoblast, and an outer layer of syncytium. An occasional syncytial sprout occurs.

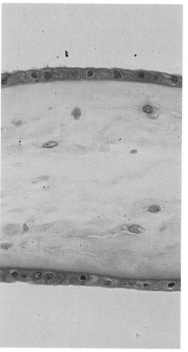

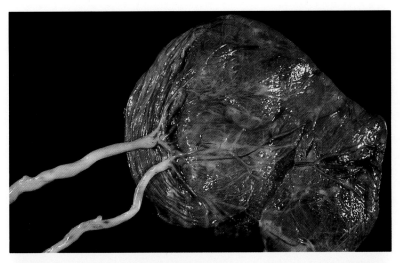

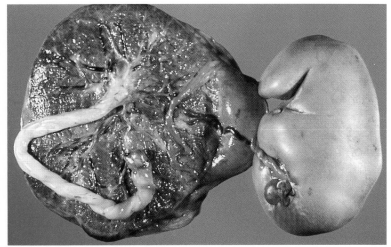

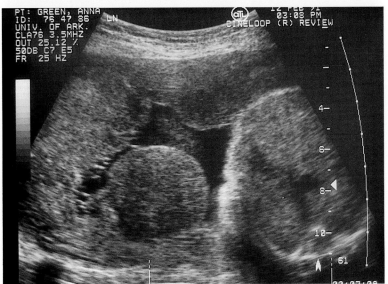

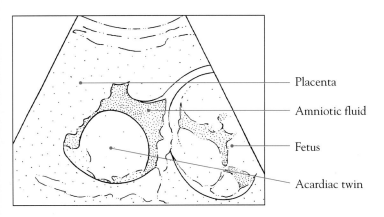

Placenta

Amniotic fluid

Fetus

Acardiac twin

figure 8.30

Two umbilical cords (top left) insert velamentously within the same amniotic sac, and the placental cake is bilobed. An acardiac monster (top right) is attached velamentously to this placenta, which also has a central cord that was associated with a normal twin. Transverse transabdominal ultrasound of an acardiac amorphous with the placenta (bottom) *implanted along the anterior and right uterine wall. There is a mass located at the edge of the placenta simulating a neoplasm. This mass turned out to be an acardiac twin with a separate umbilical cord. There is a normal amount of amniotic fluid.*

figure 8.31

This first-trimester villus possesses a large amount of stroma that contains capillaries with nucleated fetal red cells. The double-layered trophoblast is readily apparent, as are syncytial sprouts.

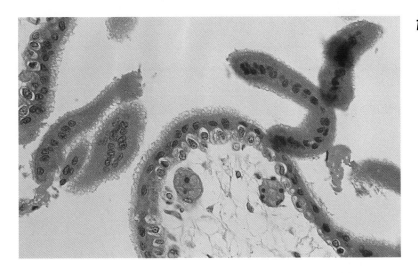

During the second trimester, the villi enlarge, primarily due to stromal proliferation (Fig. 8.32). While there is extensive proliferation of capillaries, the stromal growth is sufficiently great that the stroma remains the preponderant tissue within the villus. Both layers of trophoblast are maintained as well, although the cytotrophoblast may not be as clearly defined as in the first trimester.

During the third trimester, much of the stroma in the terminal villi is lost so that they become largely composed of capillaries (Fig. 8.33). In addition, the trophoblast is markedly thinned, with apparent loss of the cytotrophoblast. Vasculosyncytial membranes develop where only a thin layer of syncytial cell cytoplasm and a layer of endothelial cell cytoplasm separate the maternal and fetal compartments. In one way, however, the trophoblast becomes more prominent. The syncytial trophoblast contains more and more foci, in which numerous degenerating nuclei are collected in an amorphous mass, resulting in large, dark syncytial knots on the villous surface (Fig. 8.34). The number of syncytial knots increases as gestational age advances.

FIBRIN DEPOSITS

Other changes that occur in the placenta include the development of fibrin deposits. The term *fibrin* should be understood in this context as only descriptive. The homogeneous eosinophilic material seen in H & E sections may represent immune complexes (Fig. 8.35). It accumulates particularly under the chorionic plate and in the periphery of the placenta. If it totally covers a villus, infarction of that villus is the result. Initial deposits seem to begin where there is a defect in the trophoblast (Fig. 8.36). Subsequently, they extend beneath the trophoblast, and finally encompass the villus. When the process is extensive, coalescence of many villi may

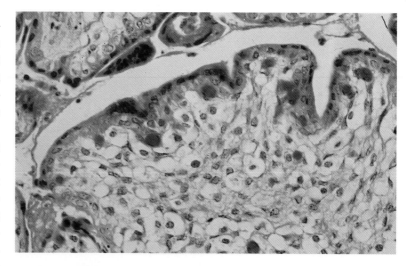

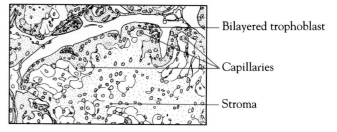

figure 8.32

During the second trimester, a large accumulation of mesodermal stroma has occurred and there are more capillaries, but they are still minor components of the total structure. The trophoblast is still bilayered, although less distinctly.

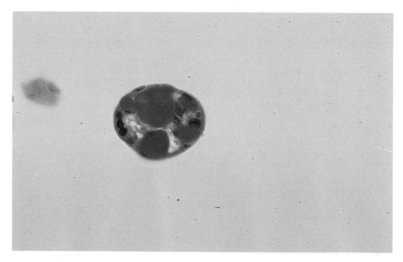

figure 8.33

Photomicrograph of a terminal villus consisting almost entirely of capillaries and a very thin trophoblastic layer. Other terminal villi are seen in Figure 8.16.

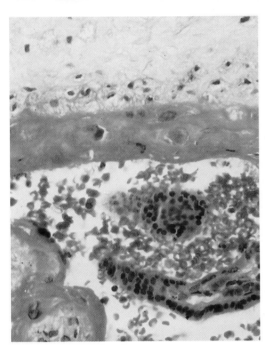

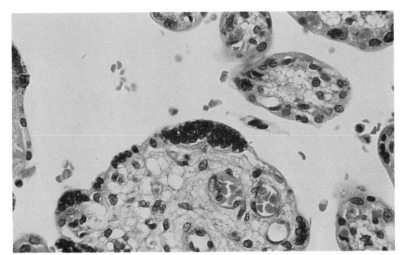

figure 8.34

A large collection of degenerating trophoblastic nuclei forms a syncytial knot.

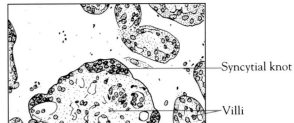

Syncytial knot

Villi

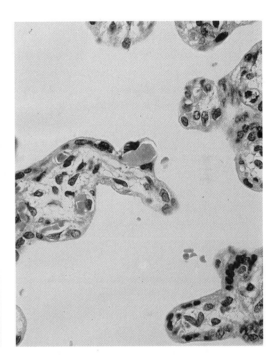

figure 8.35

A collection of homogenous eosinophilic material immediately beneath the chorionic plate of the placenta contains some necrotic trophoblastic cells.

figure 8.36

A small focus of homogenous eosinophilic material (left) appears to have formed on the surface of this terminal villus in a focal defect between two trophoblastic cells.

Here the fibrin (right) appears to be elevating the trophoblast and developing on the mesodermal surface.

occur, and large sheets of denuded villi and fibrin may result (Fig. 8.37). Focal calcification may occur anywhere in the placenta, but it is particularly likely in these sites (Fig. 8.38). Occasionally, the process of fibrin deposition is so dramatic that fetal compromise results. There are cases in which it recurs in subsequent pregnancies in this extensive form.

PLACENTAL INFARCTS

Placental infarcts are the result of compromise of a single maternal spiral arteriole and therefore are more frequent in the case of maternal vascular disease. The most common example of such disease is, of course, toxemia. These infarcts reveal the area over which the distribution of flow from a specific maternal vessel was physiologically important (Fig. 8.39). Histologically, they consist of a patch of necrotic villi surrounded by varying amounts of inflammation in the immediately adjacent healthy tissue. Abruptio placentae is also associated with maternal vascular disease. Grossly, this condition results in retroplacental blood clots, but unless it is of long standing, little histologic change in the underlying placenta occurs (Fig. 8.40). Although the classical clinical picture of abrutio placentae is one of the third trimester, there is ultrasound evidence that many early abortions are associated with a similar event (Fig. 8.41).

When the fetal vasculature is compromised, the result is infarction of only the central portion of the villus, as the external surface is maintained by intervillous space blood flow. A central zone of homogenization and scarring develops within an otherwise healthy-appearing villus (Fig. 8.42). The fetal vasculature also develops leaks as term is approached and passed, so that the frequency of fetomaternal hemorrhages increases with gestational age. Normally, when this occurs, clotting is initiated and a laminated intervillous thrombus develops (Fig. 8.43). If fetal clotting is defective, very large intervillous thrombi may result (Fig. 8.44). Meconium staining of the placenta and membranes has been associated with advanced gestational age, but may occur in any example of fetal compromise. If extensive, the placenta will appear grossly green and the macrophages immediately beneath the amniotic epithelium will contain ingested brown meconium (Fig. 8.45).

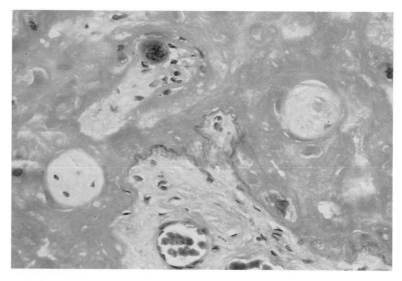

figure 8.37

Photomicrograph of a large sheet of fibrin, containing necrotic trophoblastic cells and infarcted villous stems.

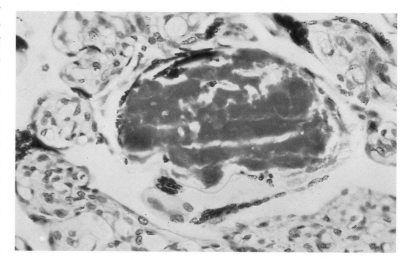

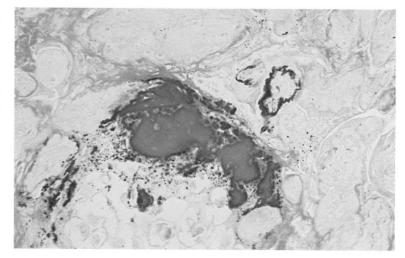

figure 8.38

Focal calcification (top) has developed within these terminal villi. A large focus of calcification (bottom) has developed within the fibrin and necrotic villi immediately beneath the chorionic plate.

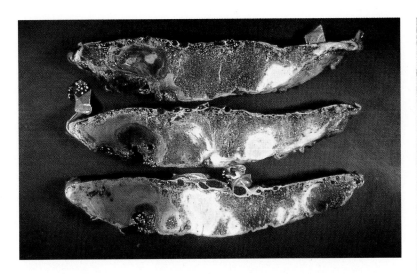

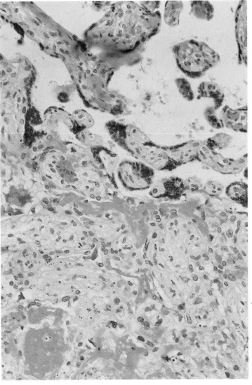

figure 8.39

Large white areas in this placental cake (left) are infarcts, histologically. (Courtesy of Dr. Kevin Winn.) Above, the terminal villi (right) are normal, while below they are agglutinated and necrotic. This was a portion of a large infarct.

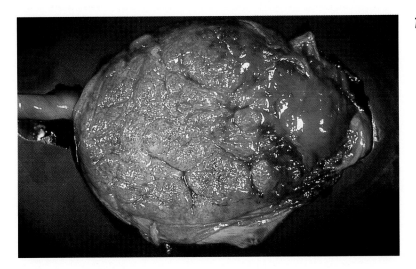

figure 8.40

Fresh and old retroplacental clots are adherent to the maternal surface of this newly delivered placenta. It was associated with a clinical abruption.

8.19

placenta

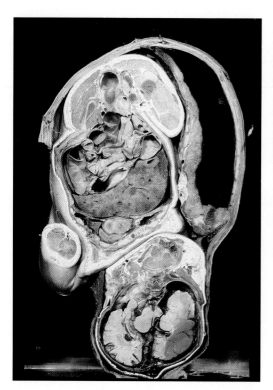

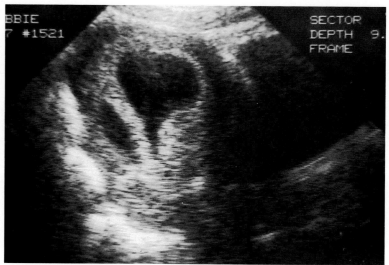

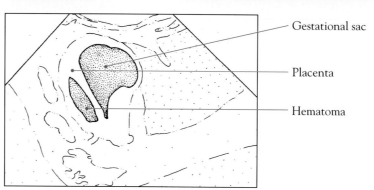

Gestational sac

Placenta

Hematoma

figure 8.41

This infant (left) died at term because of total placental separation (from Tuck and Fletcher, 1985). Longitudinal transabdominal ultrasound of an incomplete abortion (right) shows a gestational sac in the uterine cavity. The placenta has partially separated from the posterior uterine wall resulting in the formation of a subplacental hematoma. The fetal parts which were initially present are no longer visualized, suggesting an incomplete abortion.

figure 8.42

In this villus, the central portion is eosinophilic due to fetal vascular collapse and scarring.

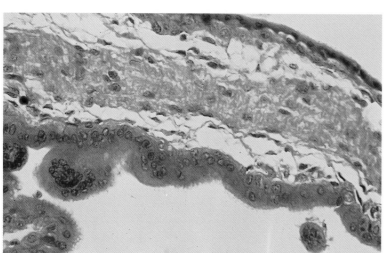

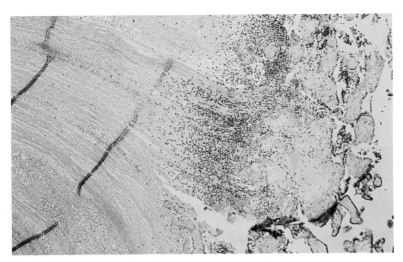

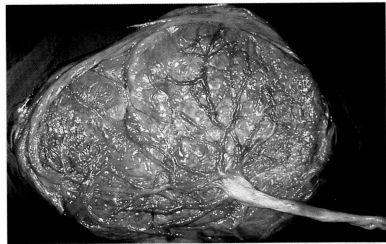

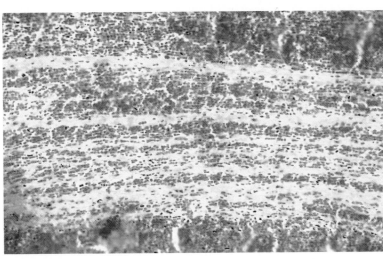

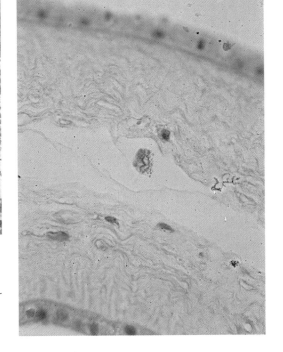

figure 8.43

The intervillous position (top) of this laminated thrombus is apparent. A higher power (bottom) reveals the sequential laminations of a similar thrombus.

figure 8.44

The large inter-villous throm-bus seen immediately beneath the chorionic plate was associated with a fetal bleeding disorder.

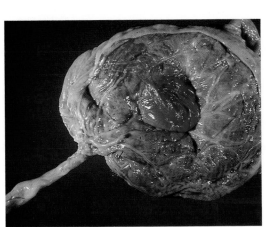

— Amniotic epithelium

— Macrophage with meconium

figure 8.45

The green discoloration of this placental surface (top) is produced by large amounts of meconium within the mesoderm beneath the amnion. (Courtesy of Dr. Kevin Winn.) In this unusual case (bottom), meconium existed in the amniotic sacs of a pair of monozygotic twins. A macro-phage within the dividing diamniotic membrane contains the orange-brown pigment associated with this condition.

placenta

Inflammatory Conditions

VILLITIS

Inflammation in the placenta takes several forms. Villitis is the term used for an inflammatory response in the villi. Specific fetal infections such as toxoplasmosis, rubella, or congenital syphilis may be responsible, but most cases of villitis are of unknown etiology. Villitis may consist of only slight villous edema and a scattered infiltrate (Fig. 8.46). More significant cases are characterized by infiltrates that tend to accumulate beneath the trophoblast, elevating it from the villous stroma (Fig. 8.47). In severe cases, trophoblastic epithelium is lost and necrosis of villi occurs (Fig. 8.48); agglutination of large masses of necrotic villi may be seen. Moreover, villitis may be associated with apparent vascular sclerosis (Fig. 8.49). Another type of vascular lesion is *hemorrhagic endovasculitis;* the term is applied when intact and fragmented red cells are extravasated into the walls of collapsed fetal vessels (Fig. 8.50). This condition is probably due to cessation of flow.

CHORIOAMNIONITIS

Chorioamnionitis is the most common inflammation seen in the placenta and its membranes. A histologic definition is the presence of an inflammatory infiltrate in the mesoderm, between the chorionic epithelium and the amniotic epithelium (Fig. 8.51). However, the case is more complex than this, as infection in the amniotic space elicits an inflammatory response in the cord, placenta, and membranes.

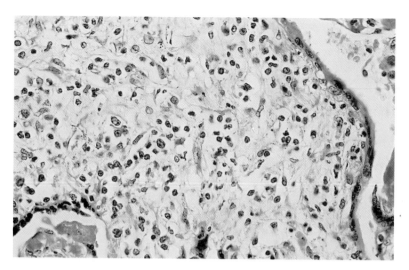

figure 8.46

The villus in this photomicrograph is swollen with edema and filled with an inflammatory infiltrate.

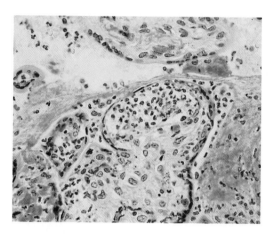

figure 8.47

The trophoblast is elevated off of this villus by an underlying collection of leukocytes.

8.22

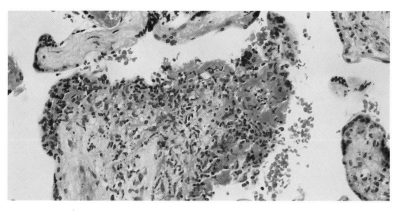

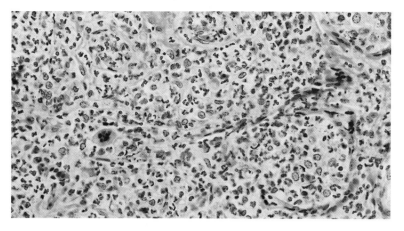

figure 8.48

The tip of this villus (left) is necrotic and covered with a purulent exudate. Multiple villi are agglutinated into one inflammatory mass. Scattered foci (right) of trophoblast persist.

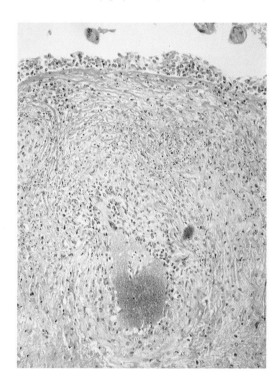

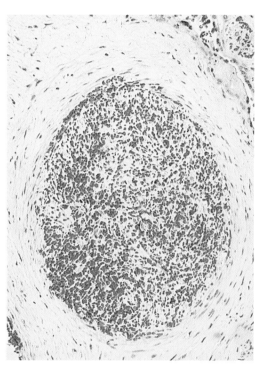

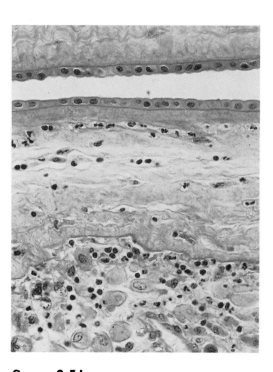

8.23

figure 8.51

An inflammatory infiltrate rises from the chorion below into the mesodermal layer between amnion and chorion.

figure 8.49

This sclerotic vessel is intensely inflamed throughout its thickened wall. The trophoblast has been lost from the villous surface.

figure 8.50

The wall of this collapsed vessel contains both intact and fragmented fetal red blood cells.

Both chronic and acute inflammatory infiltrates may be seen in the placental membranes. The chronic type is unusual and of unknown etiology (Fig. 8.52). Certainly, most clinical chorioamnionitis is associated with an acute response. In its earliest form, polymorphonuclear leukocytes accumulate in the chorion where they destroy the trophoblastic layer; they then migrate into the mesoderm immediately beneath the amnion (Fig. 8.53). In most cases, they progress to the level just below the dense stroma that supports the amniotic epithelium. Here the infiltrate stops for a time and is associated with bacteria. Basophilic deposits, which when appropriately stained reveal themselves to contain bacteria, are a feature of more advanced cases; in severe cases, focal microabscesses destroy the overlying amnion (Fig. 8.54). Destruction of the dense stroma beneath the amnion occurs, and the amniotic epithelium is lost, at first focally, but eventually over broad areas. Dense basophilia throughout the membranes indicates large numbers of bacteria (Fig. 8.55). If post-delivery bacterial growth has occurred, large colonies of bacteria may be seen in the sites at which they were originally located (Fig. 8.56). Such observations suggest that bacteria are commonly halted by the defense mechanisms in the layer immediately beneath the amnion.

In the body of the placenta, the maternal inflammatory response to a chorioamniotic infection is first seen in the margination of leukocytes along the chorionic plate in the intervillous space (Fig. 8.57). Subsequently, the leukocytes migrate in the chorionic plate toward the amniotic surface. In this tissue, they may be joined by a fetal inflammatory response emanating from the fetal vessels in the chorionic plate. In this case, the fetal inflammatory response emanates only from the side of the vessel that is closest to the amniotic space (Fig. 8.58). Again, post-delivery bacterial growth occa-

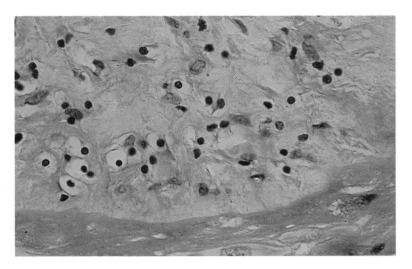

figure 8.52

This small focus of chronic inflammatory cells lies in the mesoderm, immediately above the chorion.

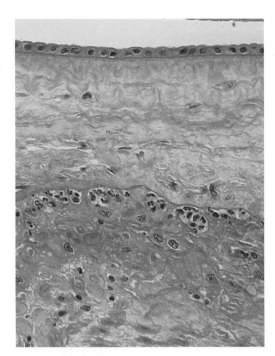

figure 8.53

An acute inflammatory reaction (top) occupies the chorion, but has not yet risen into the mesoderm above. An acute inflammatory infiltrate (bottom) occupies the mesoderm just below the dense layer that supports the amniotic epithelium.

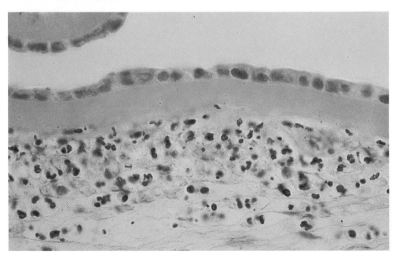

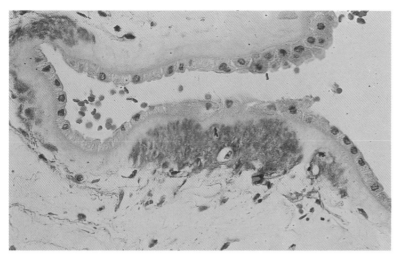

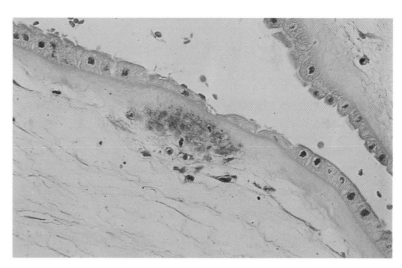

figure 8.54

The dense basophilia seen in this photomicrograph (left) represents bacteria. It is associated with an acute infiltrate, just beneath the sub-

amniotic dense zone. Here (right) the process has resulted in the focal loss of amniotic epithelium.

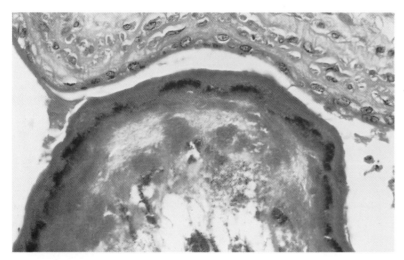

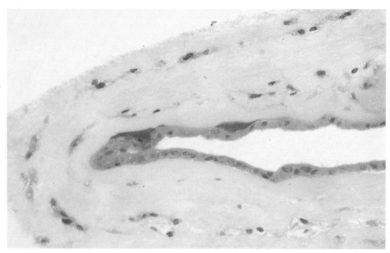

figure 8.55

The amniotic epithelium is totally lost from this membrane, which is heavily infested with bacteria.

figure 8.56

Dense basophilic deposits immediately beneath the amniotic epithelium represent large accumulations of group B streptococci.

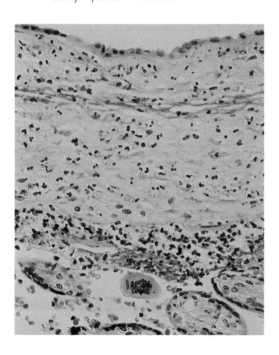

figure 8.57

An inflammatory infiltrate has collected in the intervillous space immediately beneath the chorionic plate. It rises in the chorion toward the amniotic sac. The trophoblast has been lost.

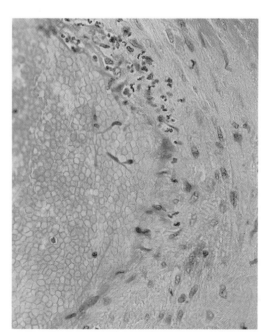

figure 8.58

In this photomicrograph, a fetal inflammatory infiltrate is migrating through the top (or amniotic) side of the chorionic plate vessel but not through the bottom side.

placenta

sionally manifests itself in the placenta as large basophilic deposits that, when stained, reveal themselves to be bacteria (Fig. 8.59).

FUNISITIS

The fetal inflammatory response in the umbilical cord is termed *funisitis*. It consists of inflammatory cells that first marginate along the inner surface of the umbilical vein or arteries and then migrate through their walls (Fig. 8.60). Initially, this process takes place only through the portion of the vascular wall closest to the amniotic surface. If the infection exists for several days without delivery of the infant, a circumvascular infiltrate will develop (Fig. 8.61).

Placental tumors

CHORIOANGIOMAS

Both benign and malignant tumors are seen in the placenta. The benign ones are chorioangiomas. They may be malformations rather than tumors, but in either case they consist of masses of fetal capillaries in the placental body (Fig. 8.62). Although usually nodular in form, they may be more diffuse, appearing to infiltrate and enlarge villi adjacent to the main mass (Fig. 8.63). Histologically, they also form a spectrum that extends from clear-cut dilated capillary spaces to a more dense cellular pattern, in which proliferating endothelial cells form a cellular mass without well-defined capillary spaces (Fig. 8.64). When large, chorioangiomas may result in arteriovenous shunts; in such cases, they result in fetal hydrops, polyhydramnios, and premature labor.

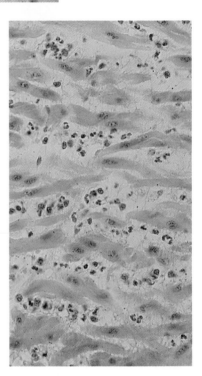

figure 8.59
Large basophilic deposits in the fetal blood vessels are due to bacterial growth subsequent to delivery; they suggest that fetal sepsis existed.

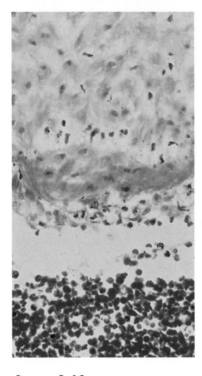

figure 8.60
Fetal inflammatory cells (left) are marginating along the luminal edge of this umbilical vessel and then moving into the vascular wall. The muscular wall of an umbilical vessel (right) is heavily infiltrated with leukocytes.

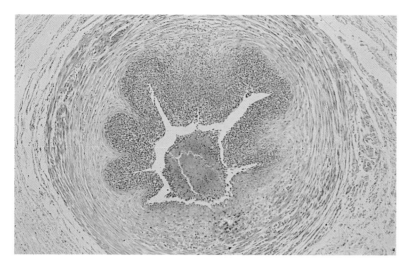

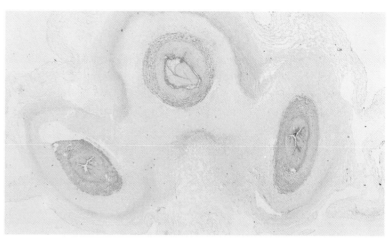

figure 8.61

Fetal inflammatory cells (left) are filtering through the portion of the vessel wall closest to the amniotic sac. A tripartite loop (right) formed by a continuous line of inflammatory cells in the umbilical cord, outlines the three vessels in this example of advanced funisitis.

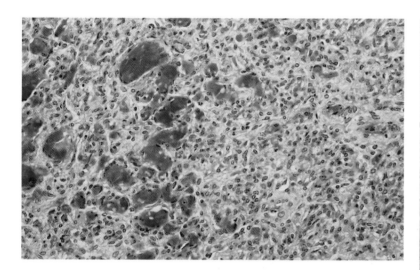

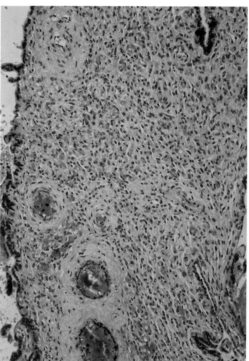

figure 8.63

This chorioangioma has invaded and expanded a villous stem.

figure 8.62

Dilated, blood-filled capillaries on the left contrast with a more cellular area on the right in this chorioangioma.

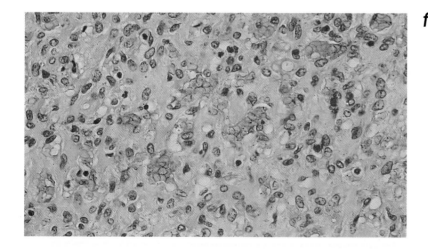

figure 8.64

Blood-containing capillaries are embedded in a more cellular matrix.

PLACENTAL SITE TUMORS

Of intermediate potential are placental site tumors. When the trophoblast infiltrates beyond the cytotrophoblastic shell into the endometrium or myometrium, the process occasionally is so dramatic that a mass is formed; this constitutes a benign placental site tumor (Fig. 8.65). It consists of sheets of large mononuclear or multinuclear intermediate trophoblastic cells that infiltrate the maternal tissue without significant destruction. In addition, syncytium is lacking, cell borders remain distinct, and there is homogeneity of appearance. Rarely, however, choriocarcinoma develops in placental site tumors; in this case, syncytium occurs and the cell population becomes dual in appearance, with syncytiotrophoblast present (Fig. 8.66).

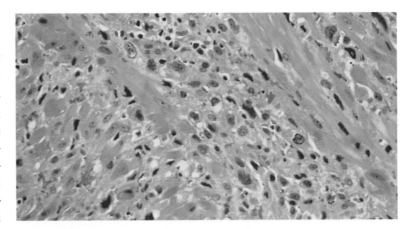

figure 8.65

A nodular mass within the uterus consists of muscle bundles that are separated but not destroyed by sheets of intermediate trophoblastic cells.

CHORIOCARCINOMA

Choriocarcinoma, a highly malignant trophoblastic tumor, may develop in normal placentas, where it may present as an asymptomatic nodule or as the site of a fetomaternal hemorrhage (Fig. 8.67). Most commonly, however, it develops from hydatidiform moles, which are the result of fertilization of an ovum by two sperm or by one sperm that splits. The maternal genome does not take part in the subsequent growth, so that only male genetic material is present.

Moles are characterized by hydropic villi and abnormal trophoblastic proliferation (Fig. 8.68). The hydrops is extreme and central. Cell-free, fluid-filled cisterns develop in the center of many villi (Fig. 8.69). The remaining stroma is pushed into a rim, just beneath the trophoblast. The trophoblast differs from normal trophoblastic proliferation in several ways: it occurs not only at the tips of anchoring villi, as in normal placentas, but on all surfaces of the villus; it may consist of large numbers of syncytial sprouts, producing a finely papillary appearance on the epithelial surface (Fig. 8.70); more often, however, it consists of cytotrophoblast, intermediate trophoblast, and syncytiotrophoblast intermingled without the organization that occurs in normal structures; the syncytium is of the primitive type with intracellular

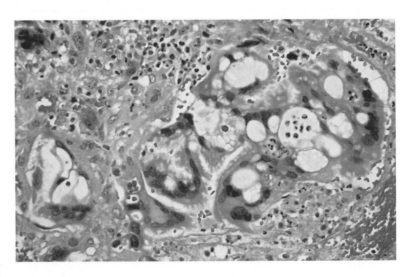

figure 8.66

At one site within the tumor seen in Figure 8.65, there is syncytiotrophoblastic differentiation. This may represent a site of developing choriocarcinoma.

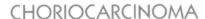

8.28

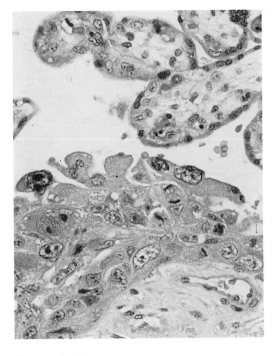

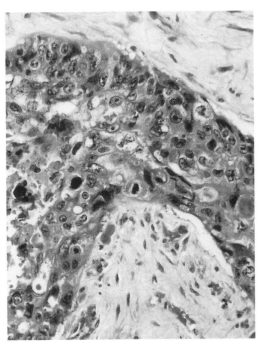

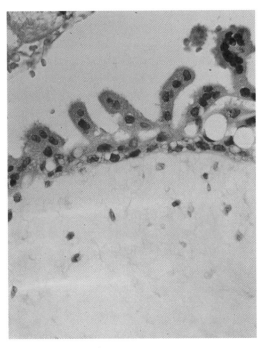

figure 8.67

Undifferentiated, highly atypical trophoblast (left) containing mitoses covers this villus. Agglutination of adjacent villi (right) has occurred as a result of malignant trophoblast between them.

figure 8.68

A fluid-filled cistern is apparent below. Stromal cells underlie the trophoblast, which shows multiple sprouts and vacuolated syncytium arising from the villous surface without organization.

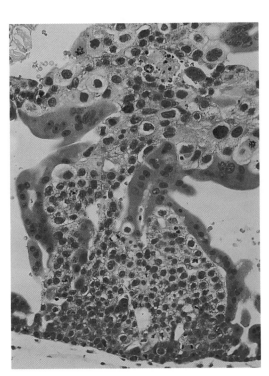

figure 8.69

A fluid-filled cistern is visible below, and the stromal cells are pushed against the trophoblast. The latter is proliferating as if it were on the anchoring tip of a villus, but it is on a free surface of the second-trimester villus.

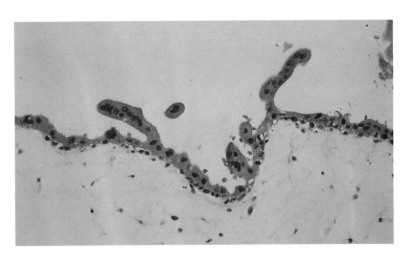

figure 8.70

Two large and two small syncytial sprouts occur in close proximity on the free surface of this villus.

spaces, and there is much cytologic atypia (Fig. 8.71); mitoses may be bizarre and at sites other than the basal cytotrophoblast. If moles are seen early as a result of elective termination of pregnancy, the hydrops may not be an important feature. If the entire uterus is seen and the case is advanced, the mole may have invaded the uterine wall (Fig. 8.72). Ovarian theca lutein cysts, commonly associated with hydatidiform moles, are thought to be the result of elevated levels of HCG, but the relationship is not always simple (Fig. 8.73).

So-called partial moles, which are due to triploidy, are an entirely separate entity from hydatidiform or true moles, and in this sense their name is misleading. While the villi are hydropic in partial moles, this feature is less dramatic than in hydatidiform moles, and central cisterns are much rarer (Fig. 8.74). Moreover, extreme hydrops is more focal in partial moles (Fig. 8.75). In addition, although the villi look enlarged, their surface is not distended in appearance, but is in fact scalloped, such that tangential sectioning of the clefts will result in apparent trophoblastic islands deep within the stroma (Fig. 8.76). Trophoblastic proliferation is minimal. As partial moles are associated with an embryo and a circulation, these villi may contain capillaries with blood cells. Although some partial moles have persisted, no clear-cut case of choriocarcinoma has been observed to arise from them.

Edema, occurring in the terminal villi of normal placentas associated with spontaneous abortion, may produce so-called hydropic degeneration that is usually much less dra-

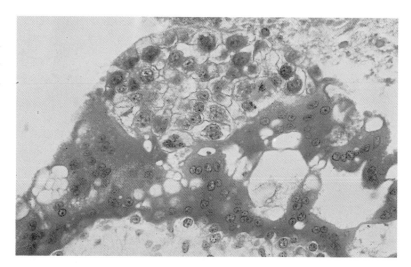

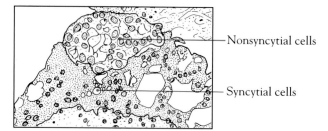

Nonsyncytial cells

Syncytial cells

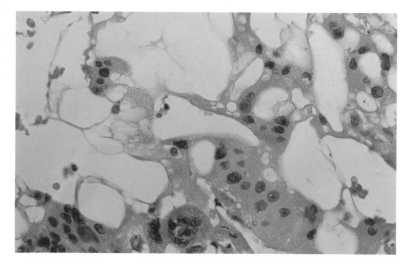

figure 8.71

Vacuolated syncytium (top) is immediately adjacent to the villus while a nonsyncytial cell population is above, the opposite of normal organization. Photomicrograph (bottom) of a mass of labyrinthine-type syncytium in an advanced mole is seen.

matic than that demonstrated by partial moles; trophoblastic proliferation in this case is normal (Fig. 8.77). Unusual cases of uncertain nature are seen, in which capillaries with nucleated fetal red blood cells imply an embryo, but the trophoblast is markedly abnormal (Fig. 8.78). The nature of these cases is unclear, but they should be viewed with suspicion.

When true choriocarcinoma develops from any of the types of trophoblastic abnormality described above, it has a similar histology consisting of mixtures of basal cytotrophoblastic and intermediate trophoblastic-type cells, with syncytial trophoblast producing a two-tissue picture (Fig. 8.79). The two will be intermixed without obvious organization. There will be syncytial immaturity in the form of lacunar spaces, and there is frequent cytologic atypia (Fig. 8.80). Although of unknown clinical significance, there is a spectrum of differentiation, with poorly differentiated examples displaying little or no syncytial development (Fig. 8.81). Invasive choriocarcinoma is highly destructive and is usually associated with dramatic amounts of tissue necrosis and hemorrhage; these are some of its characteristic features (Fig. 8.82).

Very rarely, metastatic tumors occur in the placenta. While historically melanoma has been the one most likely to do so, carcinoma of the lung also seems to be capable of doing so, and indeed the incidence of this disease is rising in young women (Fig. 8.83).

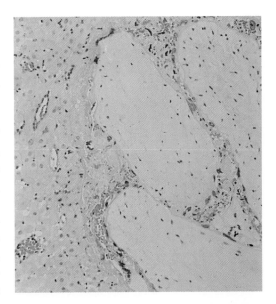

figure 8.72
This invasive mole shows three villi deep within the uterine tissue.

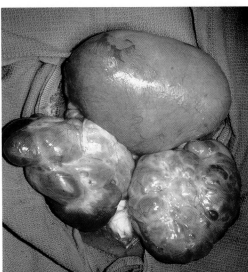

figure 8.73
In this example of a patient with a hydatidiform mole, the uterus is anterior. Both ovaries, enlarged with multiple theca lutein cysts, are seen posterior to the uterus.

8.31

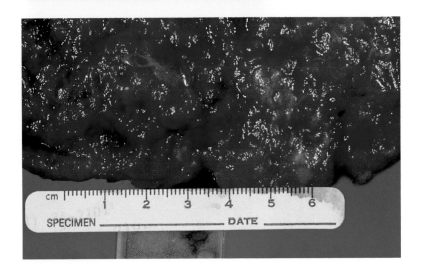

figure 8.74
The hydropic nature of this placenta is obvious, but the vesicles are less dramatic than those of a true mole.

placenta

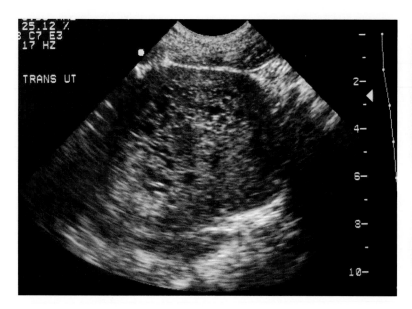

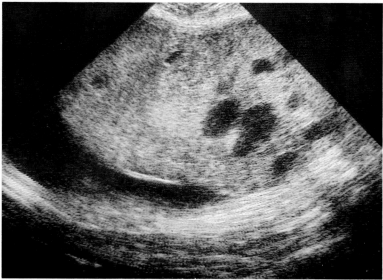

TRANS UT

Placenta

Partial mole

Amniotic fluid

8.32

Mole

figure 8.75

Transverse transabdominal ultrasound of a hydatidiform mole. The uterine cavity (left) shows alternating cystic and solid areas. They correspond to the proliferative trophoblastic tissue and cysts within the mole. Transverse abdominal ultrasound of a partial mole. An enlarged

placenta (right) is seen attached to the anterior uterine wall. Multiple cysts are demonstrated within the placenta representing hydropic degeneration.

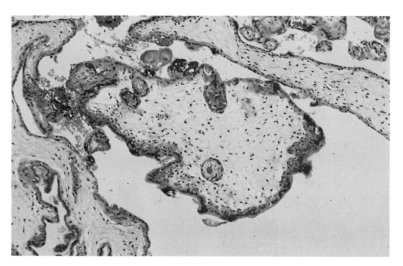

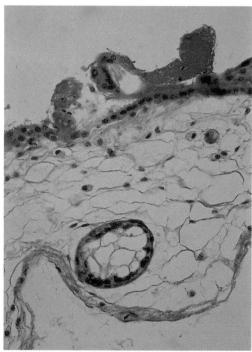

figure 8.76

This swollen villus (left) has a scalloped appearance. An apparent trophoblastic island (right) is seen in the mesoderm. In this unusual case, a central cistern is present below.

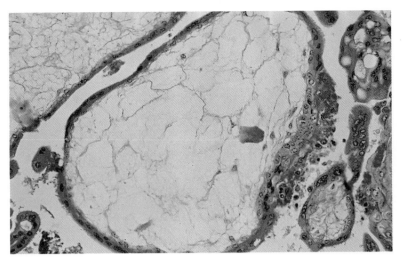

figure 8.77

This villus is swollen with generalized edema, but only normal trophoblastic proliferation is present.

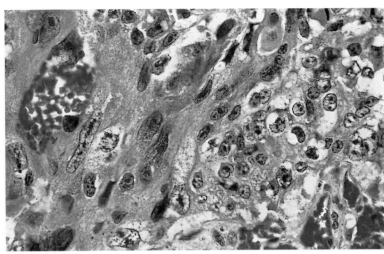

figure 8.79

To the left, a blood vessel is surrounded by a syncytiotrophoblast. On the right, the cell population more clearly consists of individual cytotrophoblastic-type cells.

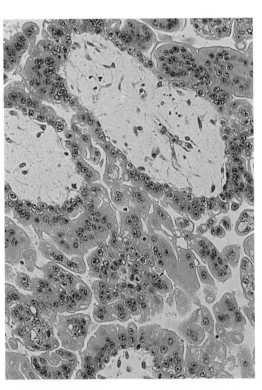

figure 8.78

This villus (top) contains a capillary with nucleated fetal red blood cells but markedly abnormal amounts of syncytial proliferation. In an adjacent field (bottom), there is marked development of labyrinthine syncytium.

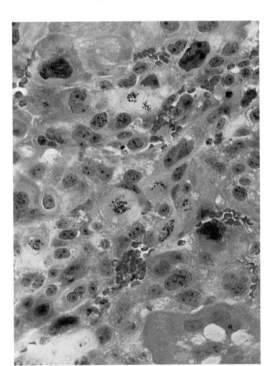

figure 8.80

In this photomicrograph, a vacuolated syncytial cell lies below, and several atypical mitotic figures are mixed with large mononucleated and multinucleated cells above.

8.33

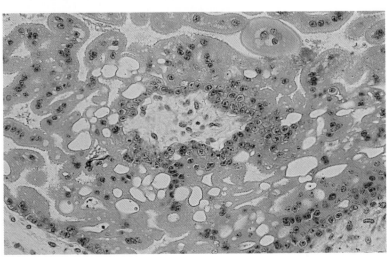

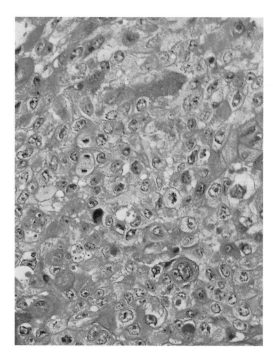

figure 8.81

Although a few cells are larger, with more syncytial-type features, most of the cell population in this photomicrograph is cytotrophoblastic in type.

8.34

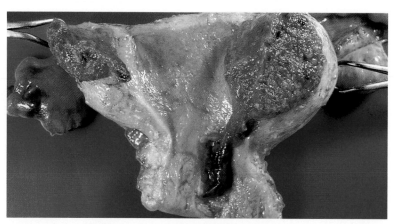

figure 8.82

A large mass of choriocarcinoma (top) is attached to the fundus and produces a prolapsing polyp. The typical invasive choriocarcinoma (center) seen here is characterized by a large amount of hemorrhage and very little tumor. Myometrium to the left (bottom) is being destroyed by a mixture of malignant cytotrophoblast and syncytiotrophoblast to the right.

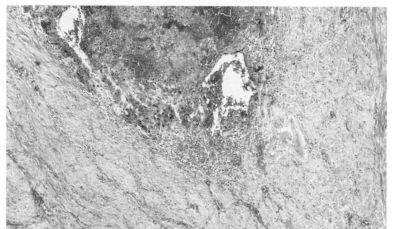

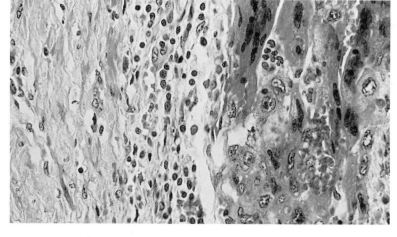

figure 8.83

The intervillous space is filled with malignant cells derived from an undifferentiated carcinoma in the maternal lung.

atlas of gynecologic pathology

bibliography

Batson JL, Winn K, Dubin NH, et al: Placental immaturity associated with anencephaly. *Obstet Gynecol* 65:846, 1985.

Benirschke K, Driscoll SG: The pathology of the human placenta, in *Handbuch der speziellen.* Pathologischen Anatomie Und Histologie 7. New York, Springer-Verlag, 1967.

Cernobilsky B, Brash A, Lancet M: Partial moles: A clinicopathologic study of 25 cases. *Obstet Gynecol* 59:75, 1982.

Dao AH, Rogers CW, Long SW: Chorioangioma of the placenta. Report of 2 cases with ultrasound study in one. *Obstet Gynecol* 57:46S, 1981.

Fox H: Pathology of the placenta. In Bennington JL (ed.): *Major Problems in Pathology,* vol. 7. Philadelphia, WB Saunders, 1978.

Goldstein DP, Berkowitz RS: *Gestational Trophoblastic Neoplasms.* Philadelphia, WB Saunders, 1982.

Hamilton JW, Boyd JD: Development of the human placenta. In Phillip EE, Barnes J, Newton M (eds.): *Scientific Foundations of Obstetrics and Gynecology.* Philadelphia, FA Davis, 1970.

Harris MJ, Poland BJ, Dill FJ: Triploidy in 40 human spontaneous abortuses: Assessment of phenotype and embryos. *Obstet Gynecol* 57:600, 1981.

Kurman RJ, Scully RE, Norris HJ: Trophoblastic pseudotumor of the uterus. An exaggerated form of syncytial endometritis simulating a malignant tumor. *Cancer* 38:1214, 1976.

Pattillo RA, Hussa RO (eds.): Human trophoblast neoplasms. In *Advances in Experimental Medicine and Biology.* New York, Plenum Press, 1984.

Scully RE, Young RH: Trophoblastic pseudotumor: A reappraisal. *Am J Surg Pathol* 5:75, 1981.

Strong SJ, Corney G: *The Placenta in Twin Pregnancy.* New York, Pergamon, 1967.

Surti U, Szulman AE, O'Brien S: Dispermic origin and clinical outcome of 3 complete hydatidiform moles with 46, XY karyotype. *Am J Obstet Gynecol* 144:84, 1982.

Torpin R: *The Human Placenta.* Springfield, Ill., Charles C Thomas, 1969.

Tuck JL, Fletcher CDM: *Royal College of Surgeons in England Slide Atlas of Pathology: Reproductive System.* London, Gower Medical Publishing Ltd, 1985.

Index

d

e

f

i.4

g

h

i

k

l

i.7

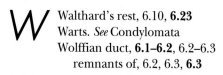
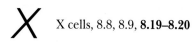
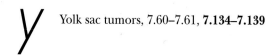